Textbook of

Echocardiography

VINCENT E. FRIEDEWALD, Jr., M.D.

Assistant Professor of Medicine, John A. Burns School of Medicine,
University of Hawaii; Director, Ultrasound Department,
The Honolulu Medical Group, Honolulu, Hawaii;
Formerly, Director, Robert S. Flinn Ultrasound Laboratory,
St. Joseph's Hospital and Medical Center, Phoenix, Arizona

1977

W. B. SAUNDERS COMPANY

PHILADELPHIA / LONDON / TORONTO

W. B. Saunders Company: West Washington Square
Philadelphia, PA   19105

1 St. Anne's Road
Eastbourne, East Sussex BN21 3UN, England

833 Oxford Street
Toronto, Ontario M8Z 5T9, Canada

Library of Congress Cataloging in Publication Data

Friedewald, Vincent E

Textbook of echocardiography.

Includes index.

1. Ultrasonic cardiography.   I. Title. [DNLM:
   1. Echocardiography. WG141 F899t]

RC683.5.U5F74   616.1′2′0754   76–4247

ISBN 0–7216–3919–4

Textbook of Echocardiography   ISBN   0-7216-3919-4

Last digit is the print number: 9   8   7   6   5   4   3   2   1

To my wife Julie
and
our children, Natalie and Vincent

Foreword

During the last several years physicians have sought noninvasive techniques that would assist them in the understanding of cardiac problems. Echocardiography is such a technique. Each physician has his or her own learning curve and during that period it is essential to correlate echocardiographic findings with other clinical findings. From this growing experience one soon learns when certain findings are pathognomonic of specific conditions and when the findings are merely corroborative. There are now a large number of echocardiographic machines and a number of individuals interested in echocardiography. Many scientific papers and books have been generated describing the use of this new technique and describing the echocardiographic findings in various conditions. Doctor Friedewald delineates the echocardiographic characteristics of the cardiac structures in health and disease in a simple, straightforward fashion.

New challenges will face all physicians and echocardiographers in the future. As time passes and the characteristics of the majority of cardiac conditions are delineated, it will be necessary to view the entire field in another way. The new challenge will be to carefully define the indications for echocardiography. If cardiac catheterization is to be done on a patient, is it also necessary to do an echocardiogram? If medical care decisions are not based on the echocardiogram but are based on the findings of some other technique, is the echocardiogram necessary? Who should pay for an echocardiogram when the information gained is known in advance to be merely corroborative? It is already clear that the echocardiogram is useful in the diagnosis of pericardial effusion, mitral valve disease, and certain cardiomyopathies. Perhaps new findings that will be considered to be pathognomonic of cardiac diseases will be forthcoming. The point is, as time passes and the learning curves are over, will it be possible for us to justify the recording of an echocardiogram "as a matter of interest"?

In summary, echocardiography has been a great advance. We have been in the midst of an exciting learning period. We are now entering the period in which each of us must utilize the technique wisely. The abuse of the technique could produce the difficulty that we have encountered in the abuse of electrocardiography.

Doctor Friedewald's book is excellent. It teaches us all a great deal. I am sure that he will face the challenge I mentioned without difficulty and that subsequent editions of his book will continue to be outstanding.

J. WILLIS HURST, M.D.

Professor and Chairman
Department of Medicine
Emory University School
of Medicine

Preface

In the few years since its introduction into clinical medicine, diagnostic ultrasound has become established as one of the most effective means of assessing cardiac anatomy and function.

The growth of echocardiography has been all the more remarkable in view of two imposing factors: first, that the recording methods require exceptional technical skill, and second, that interpretation is deceptively complex. The *Textbook of Echocardiography* is intended to enhance the interpretative skills of the physician working with the single-beam M-mode echocardiographic examination.

Echocardiography is most useful when considered in the context of all available information about the patient and his disease. Therefore, historical, physical, electrocardiographic, hemodynamic, and other relevant features of each major disease have been interwoven into the text to demonstrate that the echocardiogram is only one part of the overall evaluation of each patient.

Organization of the book has been into three parts. Part I consists of three chapters that deal with certain fundamentals of echocardiography and include discourses that are admittedly philosophical and assuredly are not dogma. Part II comprises nine chapters, each devoted to the normal and abnormal features of a major cardiac structure. Part III contains three chapters which deal with subjects that merit special attention because of their unique importance in the application of echocardiography.

Exclusion of discussions relating to cardiac ultrasound techniques other than the standard time-motion mode echocardiography is not a denial of the importance of these other modalities. Certainly, Doppler techniques, real-time multiple-transducer and sector scanning and ultrasonotomography all have become established methods for the diagnosis of cardiovascular disease. Furthermore, these and other yet-to-be-developed approaches, as well as the addition of computer assistance, promise many exciting refinements in diagnostic ultrasound.

Finally, it is important to recognize that information relating to M-mode echocardiography itself is expanding at a pace that, for most physicians, is much too rapid for digestion. Therefore, many of the concepts presented here will undoubtedly be extended, or in some cases even cast aside, by current and future scientific investigations. Such changes, however, should be embraced, not feared or ignored, because they are stimulated by the desire for truth that lies at the foundation of our profession.

VINCENT E. FRIEDEWALD

Acknowledgments

A few years ago my father assured me that as a physician I would encounter abundant opportunities to write. The *Textbook of Echocardiography* is an effect of his wisdom as well as the love and support of both my mother and father.

My wife Julie has participated in so many essential roles in the development of this book that only literary tradition precludes her recognition as a coauthor. Her work with the manuscript in the capacity of both critic (as an echocardiography technologist herself) and secretary has been invaluable. Furthermore, her unwavering enthusiasm has been a vital source of inspiration throughout the endeavor, causing me to wonder how anyone alone could ever write a book.

The generosity of Dr. and Mrs. Robert S. Flinn, through the Flinn Foundation, made possible the laboratories in which we obtained almost all the illustrated clinical material. I am also grateful to the good people of St. Joseph's Hospital and Medical Center in Phoenix, Arizona, especially the Sisters of Mercy and the administration, for their support of this project.

Within the text I have emphasized the indispensability of the skilled technologist to the correct echocardiographic examination. I am particularly thankful for the assistance of several talented and dedicated persons whose work pervades this book. Among them, I am most indebted to our laboratory supervisor, Ms. Betty Phillips. Ms. Jacklyn Ellis, Ms. Carol Hughes, and Mr. Mike Smith have also made valuable contributions.

It has been my good fortune to enjoy the superb editorial assistance of Ms. Susan Hannan. Her dedication to this book during all phases of its development was of inestimable value.

The numerous and tedious secretarial tasks, including typing the many drafts, were the excellent work of my personal secretary, Ms. Linda Decker. Mr. Isaac Carbajal, Mr. Larry Repp, Mr. Ron Brandon, and the remainder of the staff of the Department of Medical Communications of St. Joseph's Hospital produced the illustrations. I also owe special thanks to Ms. Karen Keeton, who is the artist responsible for the sagittal drawings of the heart. Mr. David Sansbury gave his time to review the passages related to the basic principles of ultrasound. The staff of Ultrasound Diagnostic Services of Phoenix also made many important contributions to the book.

I am most appreciative to Mr. John Hanley, the Medical Editor of W. B. Saunders Company, for his confidence in this book from its inception. The members of the Saunders staff, particularly Ms. Donna Musser for her editorial assistance, Ms. Lorraine Battista for the book design, Mr. Ray Kersey for the art work, and Mr. Herb Powell for his efforts in production, deserve my special thanks.

I am also indebted to Dr. J. Willis Hurst, who so generously accepted the task of writing the Foreword.

No amount of space or words could ever satisfy the recognition that so many peers and former teachers deserve for their indirect but nonetheless essential roles in the *Textbook of Echocardiography*. Among them I am proud to acknowledge Dr. Henry McIntosh and Dr. Ted Wright, who taught me those first fundamental lessons of cardiology.

Finally, it is important to recognize that a textbook is really only a compendium of facts and ideas that have been given to us previously by others. My hope is that they will regard this book as a fitting tribute to their work, which has provided us one of the truly valuable methods for diagnosing heart disease.

Contents

Part I

Fundamentals of Echocardiography

1
The Ultrasound Principle

The term "ultrasound" refers to sound waves with frequencies above the range of human hearing. Echocardiography involves the science of transmitting ultrasound waves and of receiving and recording those waves that have been reflected by cardiac structures. It also includes the art of analyzing and interpreting the patterns recorded.

The remaining chapters in this text deal with the clinical applications of echocardiography, with only secondary reference to the physics of ultrasound where this is pertinent to the discussion. Although an intimate knowledge of the physics of sound is best left to engineers and physicists, an understanding of certain of its principles is important to the technologist and the physician.

WAVES

Nature transmits energy from one point to another by wave motion.[1] Transmission is carried out by oscillations of particles, usually molecules, within the transmitting medium. In the case of sound waves, the particle oscillation is *longitudinal* in direction, i.e., the oscillations are along the direction of the wave (as opposed to *transverse* waves, which oscillate perpendicular to the wave direction, as in electromagnetic radiation).

When a particle involved in longitudinal wave transmission moves toward an adjacent particle, *compression* occurs as the interval between them narrows.

With the transfer of energy the second particle then moves in the same direction, and as the two particles diverge, *rarefaction* occurs. Thus, by compression and rarefaction of a series of particles within a medium, energy is transmitted through that medium although there is no *net* motion of the particles. The point that this transmission has reached within the medium at any time is the *wavefront.*

When two or more waves are propagated through a medium, the distance between successive wavefronts is the *wavelength* (λ). The frequency (v) of wave transmission is the number of wavefronts passing any point in one second. The *velocity* (V) of wave motion is the distance a wave travels in one second and is expressed by the formula

$$V = v\lambda$$

For example, if the wavelength is 1 mm and the frequency is 100,000 transmissions per second, then the velocity is $1 \times 100,000 = 100,000$ mm or 1,000 meters per second.

The velocity of wave transmission is a function of the density and the elastic properties of the medium through which the wave travels. Velocity increases with increasing elasticity and decreases with increasing density. In the case of the soft tissues of the body, the velocity of sound averages about 1,540 meters (M) per sec. Sound travels much more slowly in air, at 331.4 M per sec, and much faster through bone, at 3380.0 M per sec.

The frequency of waves is determined by the source from which they are generated. The more rapidly the material initiating a wave oscillates, the higher the frequency. The human ear can hear sound waves in the frequency range of 20 to 20,000 cycles per second (cps). Sound frequencies greater than the audible range for humans are termed *ultrasonic*. Medical diagnostic ultrasound utilizes sound waves in the range of 1 million to 10 million cps. One million cps is more conveniently expressed as 1 megahertz (MHz).

SOUND REFLECTION

A sound wave traveling in a homogeneous medium has constant velocity and direction. When it passes into a medium with different density and elasticity, however, the velocity changes, and a portion of the sound energy is reflected (Fig. 1–1). The reflected sound is an *echo*. The point at which the sound encounters the medium change is termed the *acoustic interface*. If the acoustic interface is perpendicular to the direction of the sound waves, then the echoes are reflected back toward the source of transmission. As the difference in the transmission properties of the adjacent media (the *acoustic impedances*) increases, a greater portion of the sound energy is reflected. In echocardiography, for example, after the ultrasound beam traverses the chamber of the right ventricle, it intercepts the edge of the interventricular septum. Because the blood within the right ventricle and the tissue comprising the interventricular septum possess sufficiently different acoustical impedances, a heavy echo is reflected from the right ventricular edge of the septum.

Sound waves can be reflected more than once before returning to the transducer. This delays the reflected wave and gives the appearance of a struc-

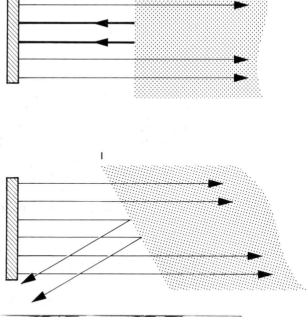

FIGURE 1-1. Some of the sound waves traveling from one medium to another with a different acoustic impedance are reflected at the boundary between the two media, termed the acoustic interface (I). *A,* When the acoustic interface is perpendicular to the direction of transmission, the reflection is back toward the sound source (S). *B,* When the acoustic interface is not perpendicular to the direction of sound transmission, then the sound waves are reflected at an angle.

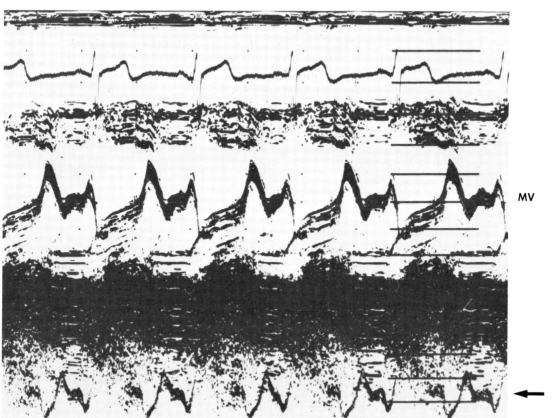

FIGURE 1-2. "Ring around" effect. The mirror image of the anterior mitral valve leaflet (arrow) behind the posterior cardiac wall occurs because some of the returning echoes from the mitral valve (MV) reflect off two other structures such as the chest wall and septum, before returning to the receiver.

ture, most often the mitral valve, behind the heart (Fig. 1–2). This is termed the "ring around" effect.

INTENSITY

The *intensity* is the energy per unit area possessed by a sound wave, and the *amplitude* is the energy density. As the sound wave is propagated through a medium, it loses energy to the medium. Such energy loss is termed *attenuation*. The deeper into a medium the sound wave has penetrated, the greater its attenuation. Furthermore, reflected sound waves are also more attenuated the further the acoustical interface is from the sound source. In addition to the distance traveled, the frequency of the wave also affects attenuation. The higher the frequency, the greater the attenuation and consequently, the shorter the distance the wave can travel. The medium also affects the energy loss, as the greater its density, the greater the sound attenuation for the distance traveled.

THE SOUND BEAM

Sound waves are propagated in a direction initially parallel to the oscillations of the sound source. Close to the source, the width of the sound beam and the width of the oscillating source are equal; this is termed the near field, or Fresnel region (Fig. 1–3). With the distance from the sound source, however, the beam width progressively widens; this is the far field, or Fraunhofer region. The intensity rapidly decreases in the far field as the beam spreading occurs. The distance (d) from the sound source to the point of beam di-

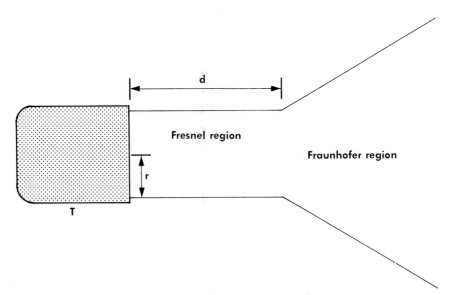

FIGURE 1–3. The sound beam. In the near field, or Fresnel region, the beam width remains equal to the diameter of the transducer (T). The length of the near field (d) is determined by the radius (r) of the transducer and by the wavelength. In the far field, or Fraunhofer region, beam divergence occurs.

vergence is determined directly by the square of the radius (r) of the oscillating source and inversely by its wavelength (λ), according to the formula

$$d = r^2/\lambda$$

For example, a 2.25 MHz transducer width with a one-quarter-inch radius and 0.06-mm wavelength has a near-field distance of only 15 mm before beam divergence of the far field begins.[2]

Because of the beam width, the ultrasound view of the cardiac structures may encompass a rather broad area. This sometimes results in the confusing presentation on the echocardiogram of two adjacent structures that appear to occupy the same position. A structure anywhere within the beam target area is displayed as though it actually lies within the center axis.

THE SOUND SOURCE

Sound waves are initiated by a mechanical disturbance within the transmitting medium. A vivid example of this is lightning, which causes a temporary dispersion of molecules of the air surrounding an electrical discharge, followed by a succession of compressions and rarefactions of air outward. These air disturbances are audible to the human ear as thunder.

The key element in artificial ultrasound wave generation is a piezoelectric material, such as crystalline quartz or lead-zirconate-titanate (Fig. 1–4). The piezoelectric quality is the property of a polarized crystalline substance to change its shape when an electrical charge is applied to it. When a piezoelectric material is excited by an electrical charge of alternating polarity, the resulting mechanical deformations are oscillatory, setting up sound waves that can be coupled with the biological medium. In the case of medical ultrasound, the biological media are the skin and underlying tissues. (Coupling is done with a transmission gel between the face of the transducer and the skin surface and is necessary to ensure overall, direct contact with the body, without interposed air.)

For the purposes of diagnostic ultrasound, the piezoelectric crystal is

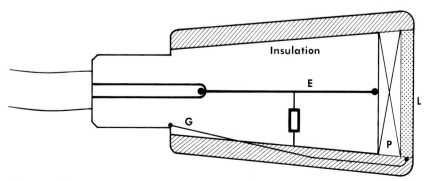

FIGURE 1–4.   The ultrasound transducer. The piezoelectric crystal (P) is positioned immediately behind the lens (L). The crystal oscillates when voltage is applied to it through an electrode (E) from the machine cable. Sound waves generated back into the transducer are quickly absorbed by insulating material within the transducer housing (G = ground lead).

mounted in such a way that the sound waves are transmitted in only one direction, with all other waves being absorbed in the transducer housing. The characteristic frequency of the piezoelectric substance depends both on its composition and on its thickness. The frequency is inversely proportional to the thickness of the crystal.

The piezoelectric crystal is separated from the skin surface by a lens. The lens may be flat, or it may be convex, in which case it will alter the beam shape, i.e., to focus the beam at a distance approximately equal to the diameter of the curved lens. Beyond the focus point the beam diverges. The use of focused transducers is discussed in Chapter 2.

Echocardiography does not employ a continuous voltage to the piezoelectric crystal. Instead, short bursts are delivered to the transducer, a technique termed *pulse-echo* ultrasound. The optimal pulse repetition frequency is twice the transducer frequency. (Continuously excited "Doppler" ultrasound is used for velocity measurements, whereas distance determinations are made with pulsed ultrasound.)

THE RECEIVER

The piezoelectric crystal, which oscillates in response to an electrical excitation, also has the quality of producing electrical signals when deformed by mechanical energy. Reflected sound waves impinge on the transducer, causing it to generate electrical information. The electrical signal is processed by circuitry that displays the converted ultrasound signal on the cathode-ray tube. This display may be in the A-mode, the B-mode or the M-mode (Fig. 1–5).[3]

A-mode (Amplitude): In the A-mode, the sound waves are displayed as spikes whose amplitudes are determined by the relative intensities of the corresponding echoes. Their position is dictated by the depth of the reflection from

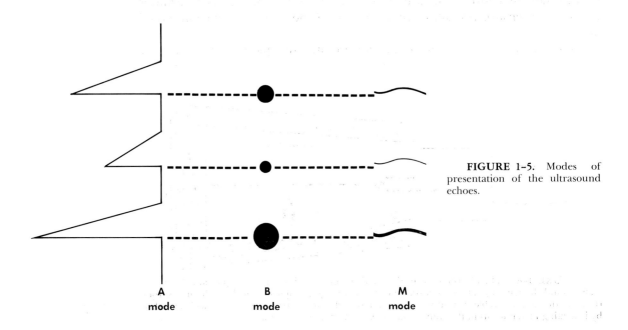

FIGURE 1–5. Modes of presentation of the ultrasound echoes.

A
mode

B
mode

M
mode

the reflected target. The early studies of cardiac ultrasound dealt exclusively with the A-mode presentation.

B-mode (Brightness): The B-mode is simply the A-mode signals turned "on end." Cardiac echoes then appear only as a line of moving dots, the size of which corresponds to the echo intensity. This mode has been used in cross-sectional studies of the heart by some investigators and is the conventional basis for displaying abdominal scans.

M-(T-M) Mode (Motion): The M-mode appearance is created by "sweeping" the B-mode display, usually at the rate of 50 mm per sec. Because the heart is a dynamic structure, the analysis of its component structures as they move in time provides an essential dimension in cardiac ultrasonic evaluation. For this reason the time-motion mode (M-mode) has been devised and is now the standard means of cardiac ultrasound display and recording.

References

1. Smith AW, and Cooper JN: Elements of Physics. New York, McGraw-Hill Book Company, 1964, pp. 193–232.
2. Goldberg SJ, Allen HD, and Sahn DJ: Pediatric and Adolescent Echocardiography. Chicago, Year Book Medical Publishers, 1975.
3. Wells PNT: Physical Principles of Ultrasonic Diagnosis. New York, Academic Press, 1969.

2
The Examination

The quality of the echocardiographic examination is more dependent on the expertise of the technologist than on any other single factor. Until formal guidelines for training are established and generally accepted, the methods for the development of the necessary technical skill are dependent principally on the capabilities of the individual learning to perform the test.

Whereas both written and didactic instruction are valuable, experience remains the essential element in developing technical competence. Six months of experience in a high-volume echocardiography laboratory with intensive physician involvement is probably a minimum training period for most persons before they are able to perform consistently excellent tests.

Prior experience in related medical areas, with basic knowledge of cardiac anatomy and physiology, is helpful in the understanding of the techniques of echocardiography, but this background should not be held as an inflexible prerequisite to training. Enthusiasm and dedication go a long way in compensating for a basic science deficit that can be overcome during the practical training experience.

THE PATIENT

It is not necessary to instruct the patient beyond a simple explanation of what is entailed in the test and the assurance that there is no discomfort or known hazard involved. This type of preliminary discussion at the time the test is scheduled allays unnecessary fears so the patient will be more at ease when he arrives at the laboratory.

It has not been established whether an acknowledgment of informed consent should be obtained from the patient. Some laboratories require that the patient sign a statement acknowledging that he understands that the potential hazards of ultrasound are under investigation but that no dangers have yet been demonstrated. A definitive answer to the question of informed consent should be forthcoming, and until then all persons involved in ultrasound testing should be current on this issue, as well as the related issue of possible hazards associated with ultrasound.

The success of the test requires that both the technologist and the patient be comfortable throughout the examination. Patient comfort often results in somnolence, and it is sometimes necessary to awaken the patient when his cooperation in breathing and special positioning is required.

Most patients find the test interesting and are inquisitive about the machine and what the technologist sees. This interest should not be discouraged, but the technologist must exercise great discretion to avoid suggesting that the test is either normal or abnormal. This is especially difficult when observers are present for learning purposes. Nevertheless, respect for the patient's feelings and the physician's exclusive prerogative for personally discussing the findings cannot be abridged for any reason.

THE TECHNOLOGIST

It is imperative that the technologist understand the reason for the test in every case. Whereas a routine examination in which an attempt is made to study all major cardiac structures is standard, special attention to certain aspects of the examination is often necessary to resolve the questions that led to the test. For example, a ventricular aneurysm may be missed unless slow scanning of the ventricular walls is accomplished, a technique that many laboratories do not incorporate in the routine examination. Furthermore, special procedures sometimes are indicated, as in the use of amyl nitrite inhalation in the detection of mitral valve prolapse.

TRANSDUCER SELECTION

The most important considerations in choosing a transducer for each examination are the depth of penetration and the resolution necessary for the desired information.

The depth of penetration is a function of the transducer frequency. Lower frequency allows greater beam depth penetration. However, the resolution of the recorded structures diminishes with decreasing frequency. In most adults the optimal frequency for adequate depth penetration with satisfactory resolution is 2.25 MHz. In patients with large chests, in whom the heart is located at a greater distance from the anterior chest wall, a lower frequency transducer is necessary, but unfortunately the quality of resolution is affected. In general, it is best to begin the adult examination with the 2.25-MHz transducer. In other words, starting the test with the highest frequency transducer and then changing to a lower frequency if necessary is the best approach.

In the pediatric examination, a much smaller depth of penetration will encompass the entire anteroposterior cardiac dimension. Therefore, a high-frequency transducer should be employed. This allows the better resolution required for the smaller structures encountered, a particularly important factor in newborns and in infants. Conventional transducers with frequencies of 3.5 MHz and 5.0 MHz are commercially available for this purpose.

The width of the transducer is another important factor to be considered. As discussed in Chapter 1, the larger the transducer width, the greater the near-field depth. Thus, while the logical choice would be to use very large transducers, the width of the intercostal space imposes a practical limitation. Furthermore as the beam width increases, the precision in recording various structures diminishes. For these reasons the standard transducer diameter does not exceed 6 mm for adult use, and is 3 mm for pediatric examinations.

A transducer may also be focused or nonfocused. Focusing becomes especially important in the employment of very narrow-width transducers which, without focusing, have a very small near field. The focused transducer requires more technical skill for its proper use, however, as the region of high resolution occurs at a limited range of depth (i.e., the focal zone).

With so many variations in the number of transducer combinations of size, frequency, and focusing characteristics, it is possible for a laboratory to become "transducer-poor." A bewildering array of shapes and sizes not only is unnecessary for the average clinical laboratory but also inhibits rather than promotes good performance. The technologist is well advised to learn how to use two or three transducers very well, realizing that the skill in using one transducer is more critical to quality than the number of transducers available.

INSTRUMENTATION

Instrument controls vary among the different echocardiograph machines, and detailed descriptions of their uses are provided by the manufacturers. Whatever the equipment design, the near gain and reject controls are particularly important because their misuse is especially prone to lead to erroneous interpretation.

The near gain is necessary because the sound waves lose their intensity (attenuate) as they travel deeper into the body tissue. Consequently, if all echoes are displayed and recorded without selective modification of their intensity according to depth, then those from structures near the chest wall will be very intense relative to those from more distant structures of similar density. The near gain control allows attentuation of the echoes close to the transducer to any depth desired by use of the *delay*. The range over which the gain of the far echoes is increased is varied by the *slope*. The greatest artifactual error induced by incorrect use of this control is the elimination of a portion of the echoes from the right ventricular side of the interventricular septum, or even the entire septum itself (Fig. 2–1). This results in a septal width recording smaller than the true thickness, a critical dimension in the diagnosis of asymmetric septal hypertrophy. In the same way, the echoes from the pulmonic valve, which lies very close to the chest wall, may be missed. The best way to avoid this error is to place the delay at the chest wall during at least some of the recordings of the septum and mitral valve in every examination (Fig. 2–2), and when attempting to locate the pulmonic valve as well.

The reject control is employed to eliminate all signals that fail to reach a

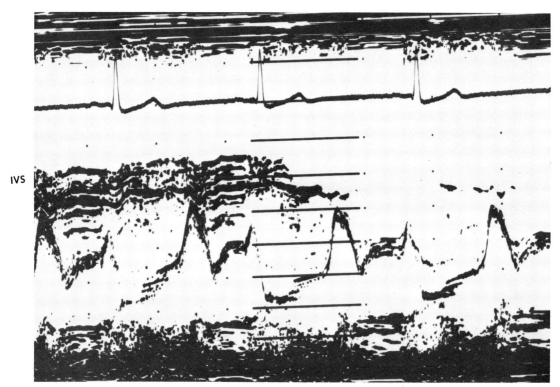

IVS

FIGURE 2–1. The near gain control (not visible) is properly positioned anterior to the interventricular septum (IVS) during the first two beats; as a result, the full width of the septum is evident. After the second beat, however, the delay has been moved to a position slightly deeper than the septum, causing total eradication of septal echoes.

given level of intensity. The result is to produce a much less cluttered recording, which is particularly helpful in eliminating unimportant intracavity echoes (presumably from blood). Overzealous use of reject, however, can eliminate relatively weak echoes such as those reflected from the endocardium. Furthermore, abnormally thick structures such as a fibrosed, stenotic mitral valve, can appear as very thin echoes (Fig. 2–3).

THE RECORDER

Echocardiography recently left the "Polaroid era" and entered the "strip chart era." Once a status-symbol, the strip-chart recorder has truly had a valuable impact on the applications of cardiac ultrasound. Before the final death knell for Polaroid is sounded, however, it must be said that despite its four-heart-beat limitation, many accurate diagnoses have been made in many laboratories with this recording technique. Furthermore, the Polaroid camera provides a reliable substitute for a malfunctioning strip-chart recorder. Therefore, the technologist should maintain proficiency in the use of the Polaroid or other type of camera for those instances in which the recorder is not available.

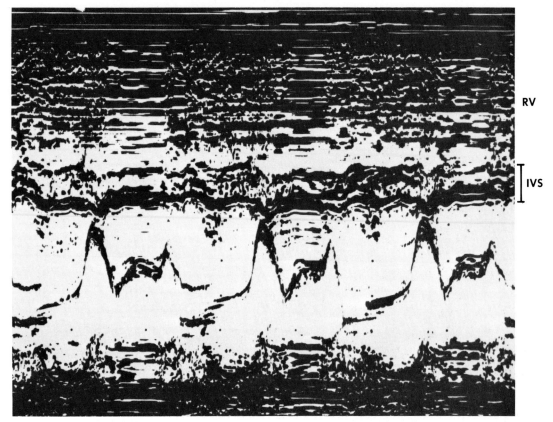

FIGURE 2–2.   The delay of the near gain control has been positioned at the anterior chest wall. This ensures that the true width of the interventricular septum (IVS) is seen. The internal dimension of the right ventricle (RV), however, cannot be measured on this recording, as the intracavitary right ventricular echoes have obscured the anterior myocardium.

STRUCTURE IDENTIFICATION AND RECORDING

The technologist may prefer to use either the A-mode or M-mode display during the course of the examination. While this is mainly a function of habit, we have found that the best technique is to use the A-mode primarily, and to refer to a separate, simultaneous M-mode display for fine control adjustments prior to each recording. (Although it is possible to employ a single oscilloscope and to switch from A-mode to M-mode, the use of two oscilloscopes greatly facilitates the examination.)

Art knows no absolutes, and the art of recording the heart with ultrasound is not an exception. From individual to individual, the cardiac anatomy does not have a fixed relation to the chest wall, so recommendations for transducer position can be made only in general terms. Once a landmark has been identified in any patient, the location of all other structures is accomplished through a knowledge of the positions of those structures relative to that landmark.

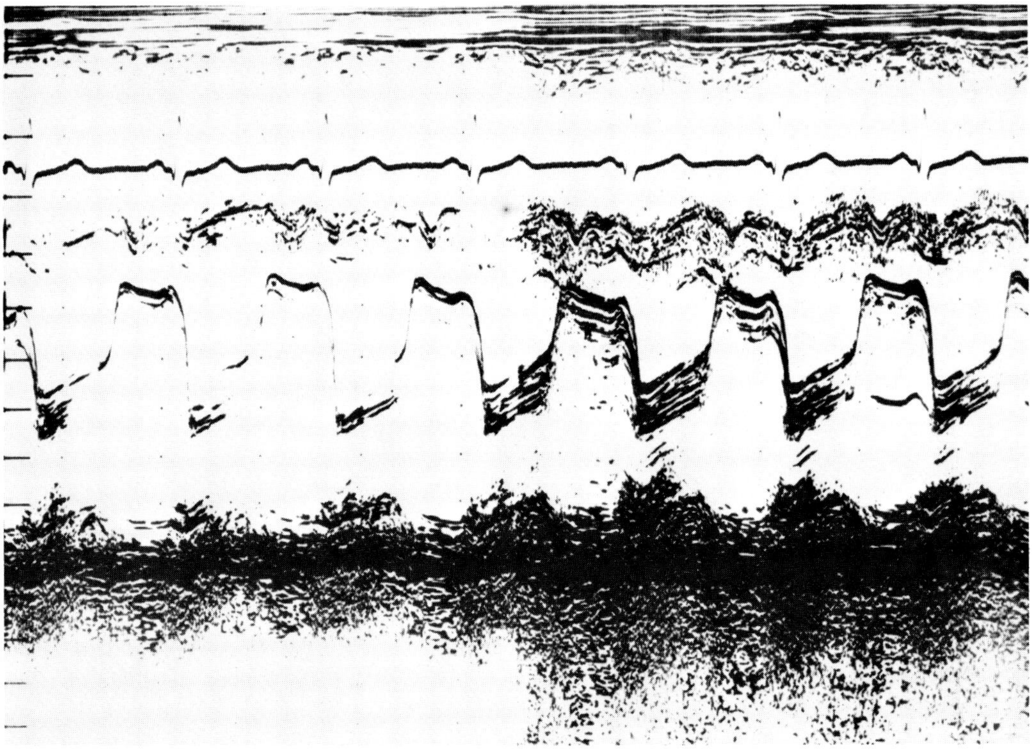

FIGURE 2-3. During the first half of this recording, the echoes have been over-rejected, causing the mitral valve (MV) to appear normal in thickness and the septal width to be indistinct. When the reject is decreased, the true thickness of the stenotic mitral valve becomes apparent, and the full septum (IVS) comes into view.

For reasons discussed in Chapter 4, the best reference structure is the anterior leaflet of the mitral valve, which almost invariably can be readily identified as a rapidly moving and intense echo 6 to 8 cm from the anterior chest wall in adults. Slightly anterior, superior, and medial of the anterior mitral leaflet are the heavy, parallel echoes from the root of the aorta, which also serve as an important reference point. The technologist should be well versed in the three-dimensional relationships of all other cardiac structures to the anterior mitral leaflet and the aortic root.

One of the most difficult, albeit most important, techniques is the sweep or sector scan (Fig. 2-4). In this way, the anatomical relationships among cardiac structures that lie on different planes can be documented. For example, the identity of the mitral valve is verified by its contiguous relationship to the posterior wall of the root of the aorta. In some instances, the scan is facilitated by recording at a slow paper speed.

Whereas most of the examination can be accomplished with the patient in the supine position, many structures, especially the interventricular septum, the mitral valve, and the posterior left ventricular wall, are better defined with the patient positioned on his left side (Fig. 2-5).

Also, it is not mandatory that the transducer be kept near the left sternal border. It is often surprising how far over the anterior chest wall the heart can be penetrated without intercepting overlying lung. The "cardiac window" is

Text continued on page 18

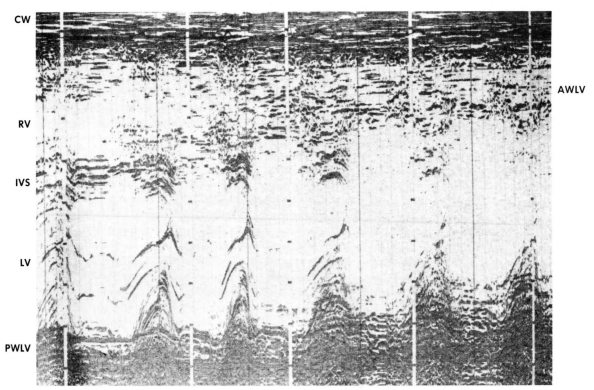

FIGURE 2-4. Sector scan from the left (LV) and right ventricles (RV) laterally to the anterolateral wall of the left ventricle (AWLV). Note that the septum (IVS) is contiguous with the anterior left ventricular wall (AWLV) (PWLV = posterior wall of left ventricle; CW = chest wall).

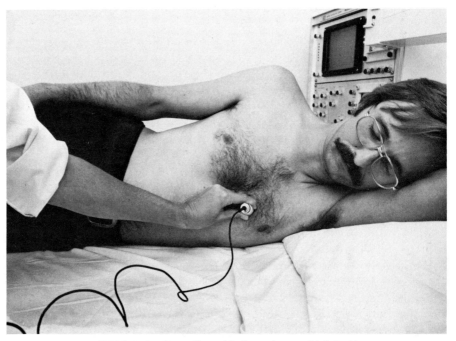

FIGURE 2-5. Recording with the patient on his left side.

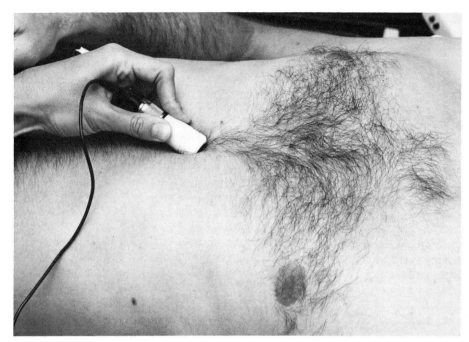

FIGURE 2-6. The subxiphoid transducer postion.

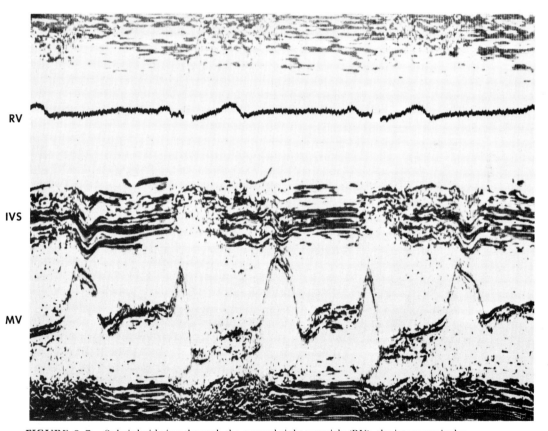

FIGURE 2-7. Subxiphoid view through the normal right ventricle (RV), the interventricular septum (IVS), and the mitral valve (MV). Note that the right ventricle appears slightly larger than it would appear from the standard precordial position.

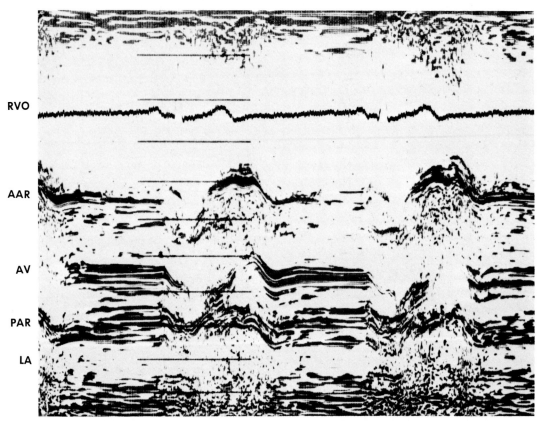

FIGURE 2–8. Subxiphoid view through the normal right ventricular outflow tract (RVO), the aortic root, the aortic valve (AV), and the left atrium (LA). The right ventricular outflow tract is slightly larger in this view than it appears from the precordial approach, and the left atrial dimension is markedly reduced (AAR = anterior wall of aortic root; PAR = posterior wall of aortic root).

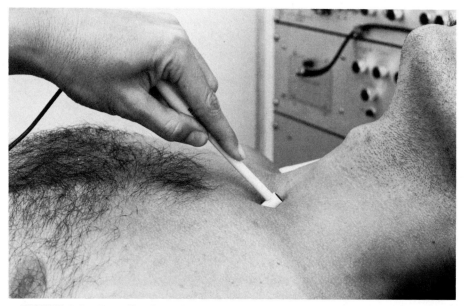

FIGURE 2–9. Recording from the suprasternal notch, utilizing a special transducer for this position.

much larger in many patients than might be anticipated. Nevertheless, in patients with extensive overlying lung tissue (usually those with chronic obstructive lung disease), anterior penetration may be impossible. In such cases the subxiphoid approach is the best alternative, and except for the left atrial dimension, a complete examination can often be accomplished from this position (Figs. 2–6 through 2–8).[1] An alternative approach that can be utilized for study of the great vessels involves positioning the transducer in the suprasternal notch and angling it acutely inferiorly (Fig. 2–9).[2] The principal difficulty with both the subxiphoid and the suprasternal positions is that they are used only in exceptional circumstances, and consequently most technologists have little experience with them, which seriously reduces their reliability.

It is important to note that the normal values established from the precordial approach should not be applied to the findings made from the suprasternal and subxiphoid approaches until such extrapolation has been validated, as in the study by Chang and Feigenbaum.[1]

_____ *References*

1. Chang S, and Feigenbaum H: Subxiphoid echocardiography. J Clin Ultrasound *1*:14–20, 1973.
2. Goldberg BB: Suprasternal ultrasonography. JAMA *215*:245–250, 1971.

3
The Interpretation

The general tendency among physicians who have not become thoroughly acquainted with echocardiography is to underestimate both its difficulties and the enormous extent of its applications. This tendency derives for the most part from an all-too-frequent casual approach to echocardiography. Generally, unless a physician develops an interest that is sufficiently serious to lead him to spend a period of devoted study in a high-volume echocardiography laboratory before attempting his own interpretations, he will meet with frustration and incorrect and inadequate diagnoses. Very often this leads to abandonment of the technique altogether. This is not to imply that total self-education is impossible, but it is the most difficult approach to the complexities of echocardiography.

QUALIFICATIONS

Currently echocardiography is most commonly performed under the auspices of a cardiologist or a radiologist, and there is widespread concern over where the responsibility for supervision and interpretation lies. It is certain that there is insufficient justification for the establishment of echocardiography within the domain of a single specialty or subspecialty to the exclusion of all others. It is equally certain, however, that such responsibility should be assumed only by a physician-interpreter whose knowledge of ultrasound diagnostic techniques is equivalent to his understanding of his primary specialty.

The *Report of the Inter-Society Commission for Heart Disease Resources*[1] outlines the physician requirements for echocardiogram interpretation:

1. *A thorough background in cardiac anatomy, physiology, hemodynamics, and pathology and the ability to conceptualize three-dimensional spatial relationships in func-*

tioning cardiac structures. The cardiologist, even without formal exposure to ultrasound during his subspecialty training, is best suited to gain proficiency in cardiac ultrasound because of his essential basic knowledge of cardiology. Nevertheless, the noncardiologist can attain this necessary background; deficiencies in fundamental cardiology among those physicians engaged in echocardiography are more often a result of failure to recognize its importance than an inability to gain this knowledge. It must be pointed out also that simply being a cardiologist does not qualify an individual for echocardiographic interpretation.

2. *The ability to recognize and interpret variations of normal and pathologic patterns on the echocardiographic tracing.* No test in medicine presents the physician with as many "variations of normal." These variations are both real (anatomical) and artifactual (machine–technologist induced), and to discern them from disease is often the greatest challenge facing the interpreter.

3. *A thorough understanding of the physical and technical principles of ultrasound instrumentation and its proper and safe use.* In addition to understanding the fundamental physics of ultrasound, every physician engaged in echocardiographic interpretation should know how to perform a complete, high-quality examination. Certainly it is impossible to appreciate the limitations of the technique

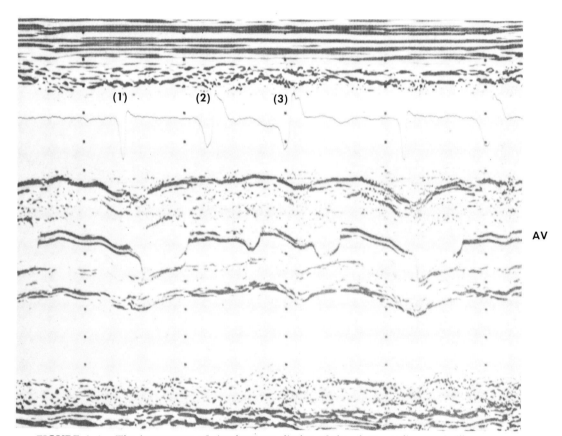

FIGURE 3-1. The importance of simultaneous display of the electrocardiogram is illustrated in this recording of the aortic valve (AV). The first beat (1) is associated with normal aortic leaflet separation during ventricular systole. The second (2) and third (3) beats are premature contractions with abbreviated valve opening. Without the concurrent ECG display, this aortic valve motion would be confusing to the interpreter.

until the physician himself has gained this experience. Only when he has achieved technical proficiency is he capable of exercising proper judgment in his interpretations, and only then is he qualified to judge for himself the suitability of the tests performed in his laboratory.

4. *A working knowledge of the electrocardiogram and phonocardiogram to facilitate their correlation with the echocardiographic tracing.* Every echocardiogram should

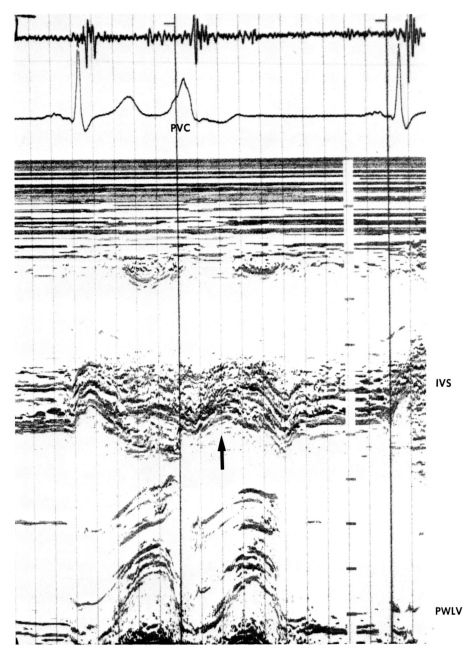

FIGURE 3-2.   Paradoxical septal motion after premature ventricular contraction (PVC). The first contraction, after a normal ECG complex, exhibits normal posterior systolic motion of the interventricular septum (IVS). The second complex (PVC), which is prolonged and premature and probably originates in the right ventricle, causes the septum to move abnormally anterior during ventricular ejection (arrow). (PWLV = posterior wall of left ventricle)

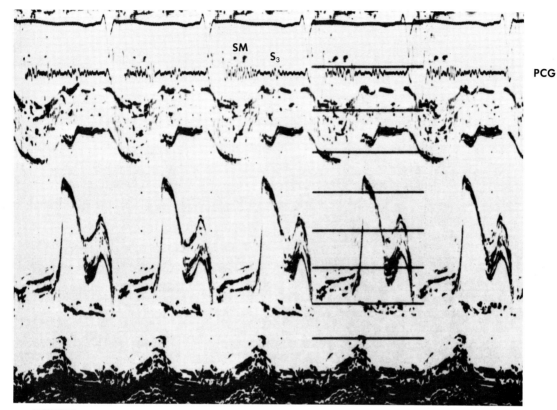

PCG

FIGURE 3-3. The phonocardiogram (PCG) in a patient with mitral regurgitation. In addition to the systolic murmur (SM) of mitral regurgitation, a third heart sound (S_3) is recorded at the time of initial mitral valve opening during the period of rapid ventricular filling.

include simultaneous recording of an electrocardiographic lead. The simultaneous electrocardiogram elucidates alterations in valve and wall motion caused by arrhythmias and permits timing of cardiac anatomical events in terms of the electrical activity of the heart (Figs. 3–1 and 3–2). Furthermore, the QRS complex of the electrocardiogram serves as the best fixed reference point within each cardiac cycle. For example, the initial inscription of the QRS complex is the beginning of ventricular electrical systole for each cardiac cycle. This point is used in the calculation of ejection time indices (see Chapters 5 and 8). It is also useful in timing the relative motion of individual cardiac structures that cannot be recorded simultaneously, as in demonstrating the delay in tricuspid valve closure relative to mitral valve closure in Ebstein's anomaly (see Chapter 10).

The phonocardiogram is not essential in most instances, but it is very useful when the timing of intracardiac events relative to auscultatory phenomena is desirable. Important information regarding the genesis of heart sounds has been brought to light by phonoechocardiographic correlation (Figs. 3–3 to 3–6).[2-4] Finally, the timing of prosthetic mitral valve opening relative to the aortic component of the second heart sound carries diagnostic importance (see Chapter 15).

5. *A knowledge and understanding of each patient's clinical problem.* The echo-

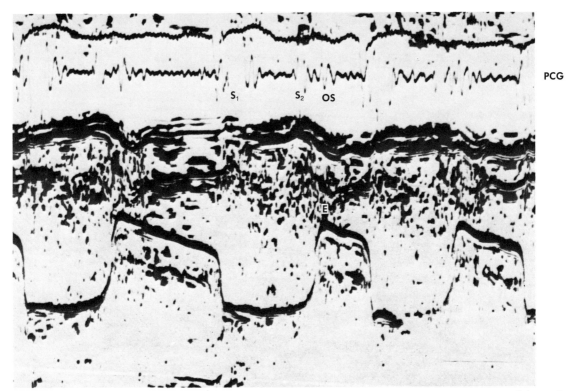

FIGURE 3-4. Mitral stenosis. The relationship between the opening snap (OS) and the peak mitral valve opening (E point) is demonstrated by the simultaneous phonocardiogram (PCG). (S₁ = first heart sound, S₂ = second heart sound)

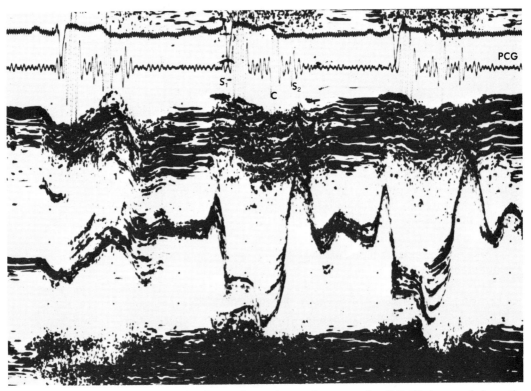

FIGURE 3-5. Mitral valve prolapse. A prominent systolic click (C) is recorded on the phonocardiogram (PCG) immediately following the point of maximal prolapse. A systolic murmur is also present. (S₁ = first heart sound; S₂ = second heart sound)

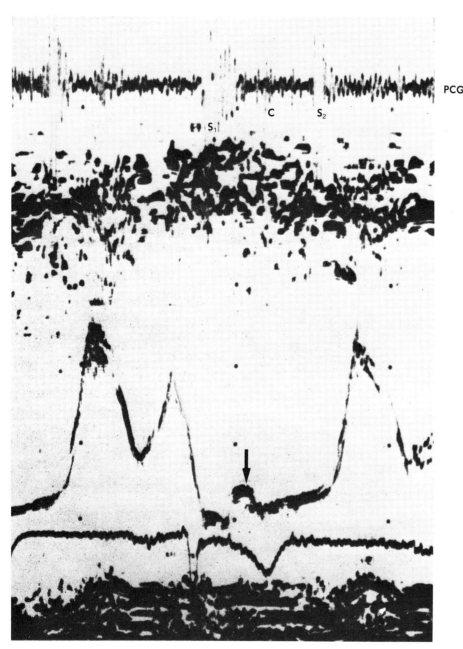

FIGURE 3–6. A short anterior-posterior motion (arrow) of the mitral valve in early systole occurs at the time of a systolic click (C) recorded on the phonocardiogram (PCG) (S₁ = first heart sound; S₂ = second heart sound).

cardiogram is of minimal value without such additional patient information as pertinent medical history, physical (especially auscultatory) findings, and a 12-lead electrocardiogram. In other words, the routine clinical use of the echocardiogram is not as part of an exercise to determine test superiority but rather as a single test that attains its ultimate value when used in the context of all available information about each patient.

INTERPRETATION

Ideally, the interpreting physician can be present at the time the examination is performed. When this is not possible, he should at least be available to assist the technologist in circumventing any problems that might arise. Observation of the cardiac motion in "real time," on the A-mode in particular, often provides a valuable dimension to the physician's interpretation. Also, listening to the patient's heart should not be regarded as "cheating" but as the mark of a good physician seeking the widest possible range of information.

When it is possible, echocardiograms should be read and interpreted in the presence of the technologist who performed the examination. Interchange between physician and technologist on a daily basis is a means of improving the quality of the examinations by increasing the technologist's understanding of the data the physician needs for intelligent interpretation and by informing the physician of the practical problems encountered by the technologist.

Chamber and great vessel dimensions, wall thicknesses, and valve motion can be measured by the technologist before the physician begins his reading. This serves to allow the technologist to look closely and critically at his own work. Furthermore, it permits the physician to devote his time to the actual interpretation of the test. Frequent spot-checking of the technologist's measurements should be made by the responsible physician, however.

As the cardiac ultrasound literature continues to expand, the number of proposed measurements increases proportionately. All of these cannot be measured, but a complete routine echocardiographic examination should include certain measurements, with others added as necessary. While the routine measurements vary among laboratories, those of fundamental importance are listed in the sample report form included here as Figure 3–7. The echocardiographic report form should include all routine measurements and those of special pertinence to the case at hand. Descriptions of recorded structures should also be included.

Because marked variations in cardiac motion may be recorded with changes in ultrasound beam direction, great care must be taken in the selection of appropriate recordings for measurement of each structure. This is dealt with in detail throughout Parts II and III of this text.

Use of the terms "anterior" and "posterior" direction of movement must be clarified, as they really refer to movements that are "toward" and "away from" the transducer. Therefore, a structure moving away from a transducer angled toward the patient's left may actually be exhibiting a more lateral than true posterior motion; nonetheless, the term "posterior" is acceptable as long as this is understood. It should also be noted that the term "diameter" is not used in chamber and great vessel measurements. "Dimension" is the preferred term because cardiac chambers are neither circles nor spheres, nor can it be assumed that the ultrasound beam traverses their centers.

Absolute measurements of dimensions often are of greater value when compared with a standard measurement determined in each subject. In other words, each patient serves as his own control. This may be accomplished in two ways. First, a dimension may be corrected for (i.e., divided by) the body surface area. The rationale for this approach is that cardiac structural size has a direct relationship to body size. In general this is true, and this assumption adds to the accuracy of such measurements as the right ventricular internal dimension and the left atrial dimension. This is not valid, however, for certain other parameters, including myocardial thickness.

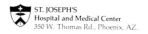

ST. JOSEPH'S
Hospital and Medical Center
350 W. Thomas Rd., Phoenix, AZ.

THE ROBERT S. FLINN ULTRASOUND LABORATORY

ADULT CARDIAC ULTRASOUND REPORT

NAME:_____   HOSPITAL NO._____   HT:_____

DIAGNOSIS:_____   ECHO NO._____   WT:_____

REASON FOR TEST:_____   AGE:_____

REFERRING PHYSICIAN:_____   BSA:_____ M^2

	Measured	(Normal)
MITRAL VALVE EF Slope		(> 70 mm/sec)
Description		
TRICUSPID VALVE EF Slope		(> 60 mm/sec)
Description		
AORTIC ROOT AND AORTIC VALVE End-Systolic Dimension		(28-35 mm)
Systolic Leaflet Separation		(17-21 mm)
Description		
PULMONIC VALVE EF Slope		(> 20 mm/sec)
A Wave Amplitude:		(2-7 mm)
Description		
LEFT VENTRICLE Septal Thickness		(< 1.2 cm)
Septal Motion		
End-Diastolic Dimension		(< 5.0 cm)
Posterior Wall Thickness		(< 1.1 cm)
Septal: Posterior Wall Thickness (Ratio)		(< 1.5:1)
LEFT ATRIUM Internal Dimension		(< 4.0cm)
Corrected for Body Surface Area		(< 2.0 cm/M2)
RIGHT VENTRICLE Internal Dimension		(< 3.0 cm)

SPECIAL MEASUREMENTS AND COMMENTS:

IMPRESSION:

_____
Physician

FIGURE 3-7. Sample echocardiographic report form.

The second means is to compare the size of one cardiac structure with another. This has been of particular value in assessing the width of the interventricular septum relative to the posterior left ventricular wall thickness in patients with asymmetric septal hypertrophy. Other ratios include left atrium–aortic root, left atrium–right ventricular outflow tract, and left ventricle–right ventricle.

The echocardiographic time-motion mode allows a detailed study of the movements of the cardiac valves and walls that is not duplicated by any other test. Measurement of the closure rate of the anterior mitral valve leaflet following the early left ventricular filling phase is an example that has achieved universal acceptance as an excellent indicator of the flow rate from the left atrium to the left ventricle. This measurement is now routine in echocardiography. Similarly, the rate of pulmonic valve excursion during diastole reflects the pressure within the pulmonary artery. Also, it is probable that the characteristic motions of the interventricular septum and of the posterior left ventricular wall are indicators of myocardial function.

The timing of intracardiac events is detected with unequaled precision by the echocardiogram. For example, left ventricular ejection time indices, most often determined by external carotid pulse tracings, are easily measured by ultrasound with careful recording of the aortic valve. An extension of this technique, which is not possible by other noninvasive methods, is assessment of right ventricular ejection time indices by pulmonic valve recording. The timing of mitral valve opening and closure is yet another means by which left ventricular function can be evaluated.

Interpretation should not be restricted to a single cardiac structure, regardless of the reason for the test. The motion, appearance, and pertinent measurements of all the cardiac structures that can be recorded should be made routinely. The only exception to this policy is examination of the acutely ill patient, for whom an abbreviated examination may be necessary. Even in these cases, a complete examination should be performed when the patient's condition has stabilized.

Proficiency in test interpretation by an individual physician can be maintained only by frequent reading, probably of no fewer than two tests per day. Therefore, despite the interest demonstrated by many physicians, it is not feasible in the average laboratory to have several doctors available as interpreters when only four or five echocardiographic examinations are performed each day. Furthermore, disproportionate numbers of physician–interpreters and technologists interferes with the technologist–physician interchange that is so important in maintaining satisfactory quality.

Finally, as simply another aspect of the practice of medicine, echocardiographic results should be correlated with catheterization data and surgical tissue findings whenever possible. Only when this is accomplished in a high percentage of cases are self-evaluation and self-education possible. Skilled echocardiography cannot be practiced in a vacuum.

References

1. Gramiak F, Fortuin N, King DC, Popp RL, and Feigenbaum H: Report of the Inter-Society Commission for Heart Disease Resources: Optimal resources for ultrasonic examination of the heart. Circulation *51*:A–1–7, 1975.
2. Waider W, and Craige E: First heart sound and ejection sounds: Echocardiographic and phonocardiographic correlation with valvular events. Am J Cardiol *35*:346–356, 1975.
3. Towne WD, Saudye A, Loeb HS, and Gunnar RM: Pseudoatrial gallop with atrioventricular block. Am J Med *57*:299–302, 1974.
4. Burggraf GW, and Craige E: The first heart sound in complete heart block. Circulation *50*:17–24, 1974.

Part II

Cardiac Structure

4

The Mitral Valve

The vast amount of literature describing echocardiographic studies of the mitral valve attests to the relative technical ease in recording this structure. Out of this has come an added appreciation for the complex nature of mitral valve structure and function and increased awareness of the critical position it holds within the left side of the heart. Therefore, the motion of the mitral valve is a reflection not only of the function of the valve itself but also of the hemodynamics of the left atrium and left ventricle.

NORMAL ANATOMY

The mitral valve is a complex apparatus[1] made up of the following basic components: (1) two valve leaflets, (2) the annulus, (3) the chordae tendineae, and (4) the papillary muscles. The performance of the valve is dependent not only on the functional integrity of these components, but also on the left ventricular walls, to which the papillary muscles and the mitral annulus are attached, and the posterior left atrial wall, which is continuous with the posterior mitral leaflet.[2]

The Leaflets

The two mitral leaflets have been designated the anterior and posterior mitral leaflets. Furthermore, the portion defined as the posterior leaflet has indentations that have been termed "accessory leaflets." While they are thus described as independent structures, in reality the mitral valve cusps form a continuous veil covering the mitral orifice. Although we recognize that the designation of the mitral leaflets as "anterior" and "posterior" is a semantic oversimplification, this distinction is conveniently suited to a current discussion of the state of the art of echocardiography, and the terms will be used in this text.

The anterior leaflet, which reflects the most distinctive echo in the cardiac ultrasound examination, is located in an anterior and medial relation to the mitral orifice. In its open position, this leaflet borders the left ventricular outflow tract, with its ventricular surface facing the upper portion of the interventricular septum. Its base is principally connected to the posterior aortic root and to the noncoronary and left coronary aortic cusps.[2] The posterior leaflet opens toward the posterior wall of the left ventricle. Its base is continuous with the left atrial endocardium and also forms part of the mitral annulus. The shape of the two leaflets differs in that the anterior leaflet has a smaller base but

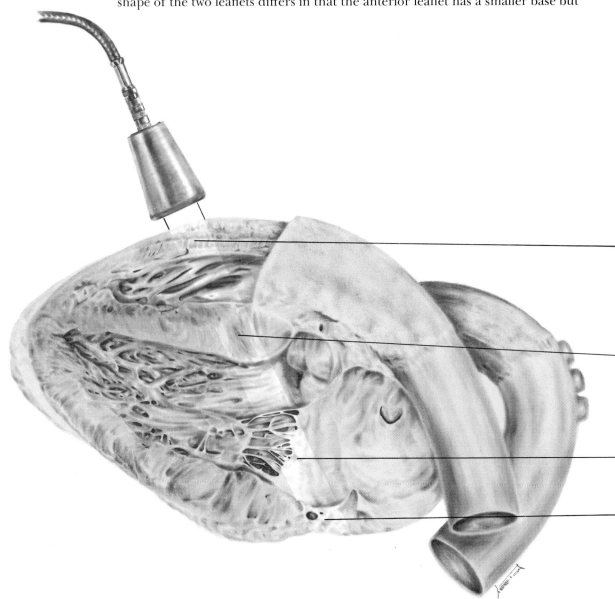

FIGURE 4-1. Ultrasonic beam through the heart, viewed from the left lateral projection. See opposite page for key.

is considerably longer from base to apex, and therefore has a broader range of motion from closure to full opening than the posterior leaflet.

The Chordae Tendineae

The chordae tendineae are strands of fibrous tissue of varying lengths and thicknesses that extend from the anterolateral and posteromedial papillary muscles to both valve leaflets.[3] While the chordae to the anterior leaflet join its ventricular surface at or near its free edge, those to the posterior leaflet attach both at the cusp's margin and at its base.

Possessed of remarkable strength, the chordae tendineae function to assist in maintaining mitral leaflet closure during ventricular systole when the pressure differential between the left ventricle and left atrium is high.

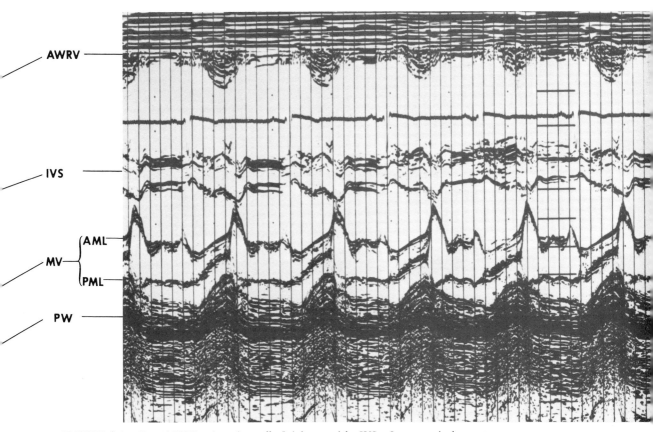

FIGURE 4–1.   Key: AWRV = Anterior wall of right ventricle. IVS = Interventricular septum. MV = Mitral valve. AML = Anterior leaflet of mitral valve. PML = Posterior leaflet of mitral valve. PW = Posterior wall.

The Papillary Muscles

The anterolateral papillary muscle extends from both the septum and the left ventricular free wall and lies in a plane parallel to the main axis of the left ventricle. The posteromedial papillary muscle arises solely from the ventricular free wall and also parallels the left ventricular main axis.

The papillary muscles are especially vulnerable to vascular compromise in that they are end-organs in the coronary arterial system.[4] The blood supply to the anterolateral papillary muscle is provided by both the left anterior descending and the circumflex coronary arteries. The dominant coronary artery, which in 90 percent of cases is the right coronary artery, is the principal source of blood supply to the posteromedial papillary muscle. In the remaining 10 percent of cases, the circumflex coronary artery is dominant and is the main artery to the posteromedial papillary muscle.

Both muscles have several finger-like protrusions to which approximately 12 chordae tendineae are attached. In all, each papillary muscle supports approximately 60 chordae.

Because the papillary muscles are extensions of the muscular walls of the left ventricle, the integrity of the mitral valve is in part dependent on left ventricular myocardial function. For example, hypokinesia of the wall at a site of papillary muscle attachment may result in papillary muscle dysfunction and secondary mitral regurgitation.

The Mitral Annulus

The mitral annulus is part of the fibrous skeleton from which muscle bundles are suspended to form the cardiac chamber walls. The annulus surrounds the mitral orifice and is contiguous with the membranous septum, the aortic ring, and the tricuspid annulus.

ECHOCARDIOGRAPHIC FEATURES OF THE NORMAL MITRAL VALVE

The echocardiographic examination begins with recording the mitral valve (Fig. 4–1). The characteristic double-peaked diastolic configuration of the anterior mitral valve leaflet on the M-mode serves as an essential reference point for the entire examination. Failure to record the valve usually foretells difficulty in adequate recording of other cardiac structures, and even when other structures are recorded, often leaves their identification in doubt. The skilled technologist frequently returns to the mitral valve throughout each test for reorientation.

Identification of the Structure

The anterior mitral valve leaflet is ideally situated for ultrasonic recording because its broad surface during ventricular diastole is perpendicular to the ul-

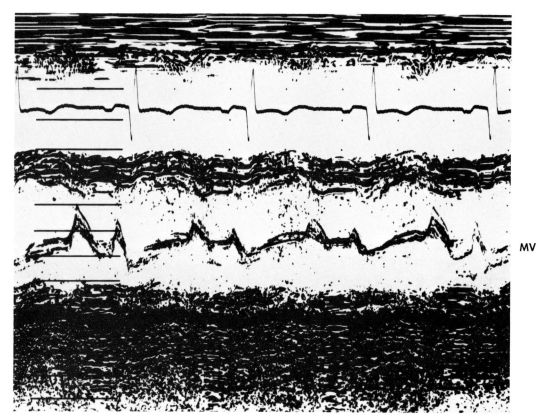

MV

FIGURE 4–2. Effect of transducer angulation on the mitral valve (MV) appearance. After the first beat, the transducer has been angled slightly superiorly and medially toward the leaflet base. Compared to the first beat, the second and third beats show reduced DE amplitude, a poorly defined E point, reduced EF slope, and reduced AC slope.

trasound beam, and its plane of motion parallels the beam. Furthermore, because it is a long leaflet, its apex possesses great amplitude of excursion in its opening and closing motions. While these features allow the anterior mitral leaflet to be identified quite easily, emphasis must be placed on the fact that most measurements and descriptions of mitral motion are valid only when recordings are made at or near the tip of this leaflet. Errors in transducer angulation become progressively magnified as the recorded area approaches the leaflet base (Fig. 4–2).[5] The posterior leaflet of the mitral valve provides a smaller target for the echo beam, and its motion is much less extensive (Fig. 4–3). In addition, diastolic opening carries the posterior leaflet into a position adjacent to the posterior heart wall where it may become lost in an array of other echoes. For this reason, the posterior leaflet is often more distinct in left ventricular failure as the posterior left ventricular wall is displaced from the tip of the posterior leaflet in its open position.

Once the mitral leaflets have been tentatively identified, the mitral–aortic sweep technique should be employed by angling the transducer superiorly and medially. The anterior leaflet will then appear continuous with the posterior wall of the aortic root (Fig. 4–4). This maneuver validates the identity of the mitral valve (whose motion pattern resembles that of the tricuspid valve) and facilitates location of the aortic root.

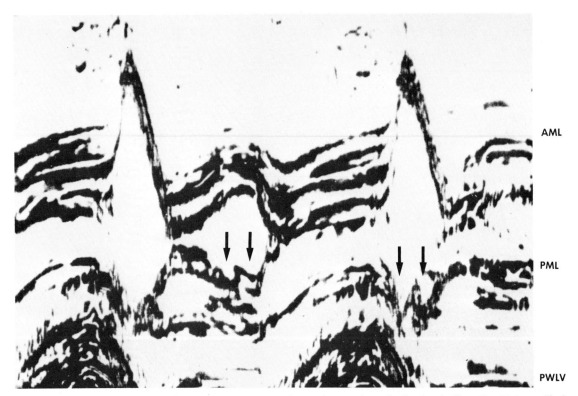

AML

PML

PWLV

FIGURE 4-3. The normal anterior and posterior mitral valve leaflets. In this magnified view, the posterior leaflet (PML) lies close to the posterior left ventricular wall (PWLV) and has considerably less amplitude of motion than the anterior leaflet (AML). Note also the double opening motion of the posterior leaflet during the A wave and the E wave (arrows), which is frequently observed in normal subjects. The multiple echoes recorded from the area of the anterior leaflet during diastole are reflections from the chordae and different parts of the leaflet and do not signify valve thickening.

Mitral Valve Motion

Many different measurements of mitral valve motion have been proposed to be of value in assessing valve and left heart function. Criteria for selecting the appropriate recording for such measurements are established. (1) The anterior mitral leaflet echo should be clearly discernible throughout the cardiac cycle. (2) The mitral valve recording should be performed with the beam angled toward the apex of the anterior leaflet. This beam direction is confirmed on the echocardiogram by the greatest amplitude of opening (DE distance) and the maximum early-diastolic closure rate (EF slope). (3) The posterior mitral leaflet should be visible during at least some portion of the cardiac cycle.

Pattern recognition in the interpretation of mitral valve motion is tempting but hazardous. Knowledge of transducer angulation and the simultaneous cardiac rhythm is essential before the interpretation of any recording is attempted. Furthermore, the mitral valve motion is intelligible only when viewed in the context of the electrical and pressure events of the left side of the heart throughout the cardiac cycle (Fig. 4-5).

The mitral valve is closed during ventricular systole, and at that time the entire mitral apparatus moves slowly in an anterior direction. During this time,

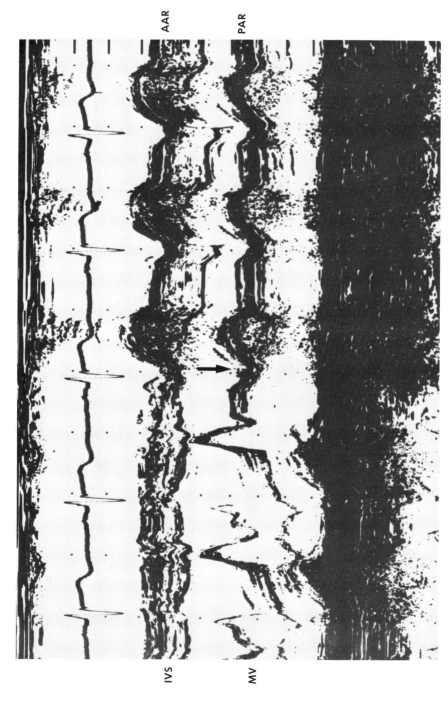

FIGURE 4-4. Scan from mitral valve (MV) to the aortic root. As the transducer is angled superiorly and medially from the mitral valve recording, the anterior leaflet is continuous with the posterior aortic root wall (PAR) (arrow), and the septum (IVS) is continuous with the anterior aortic root wall (AAR).

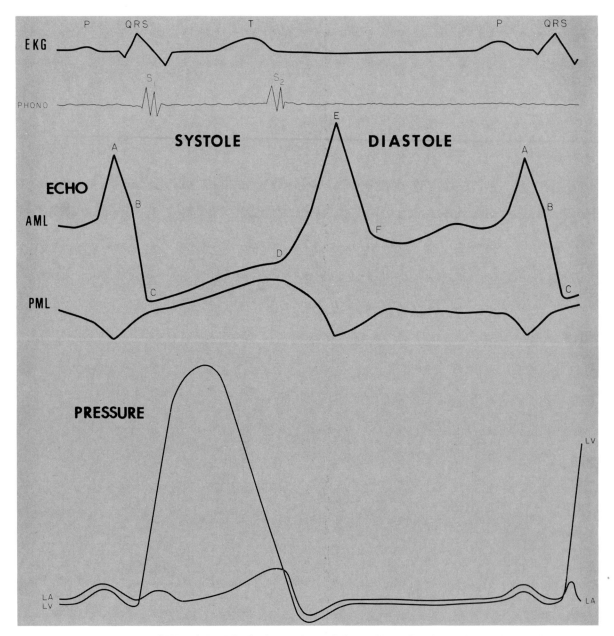

FIGURE 4–5. Mitral valve motion and the cardiac cycle. The motion of the anterior (AML) and posterior (PML) leaflets of the mitral valve is depicted relative to the pressure changes within the left atrium (LA) and left ventricle (LV).

left atrial filling is taking place. When ventricular systole ends, the aortic valve closes, and the pressure within the left ventricle falls below that in the left atrium; then the mitral valve opens. The time from aortic valve closure to mitral opening is the period of isovolumetric relaxation of the left ventricle. Immediately prior to mitral opening, the valve has a low-amplitude anterior excursion that begins at the time of crossover of the left ventricular and left atrial pressures; this is the D point. Actual leaflet separation is sometimes observed to occur after the D point and has been termed the D' point.[6,7] The two valve leaflets rapidly open to their maximal separation, the E point. This initial opening of the valve occurs during the rapid filling phase of the left ventricle; most of the blood entering the ventricle in the course of each cardiac cycle enters during this period of diastole. Both leaflets then return to a position of partial opening, corresponding to the F point, and remain basically in this position until late diastole. If diastole is sufficiently long, a low-amplitude, mid-diastolic opening is sometimes seen before the mitral A wave. Following the electrocardiographic P wave, the left atrium contracts and the valve again opens widely, usually with an excursion of two thirds to three fourths that of the E wave. The point of maximal opening occurring with atrial contraction is termed the A point. Valve closure begins immediately after atrial contraction,[8] and the cycle is completed when the valve completely shuts, shortly after the beginning of the electrocardiographic QRS complex as the left ventricular pressure exceeds that within the left atrium. The point of closure is the C point, which has been found to precede the peak intensity of the first heart sound by up to 50 msec.[9, 10] (Note: The B point occurs at the beginning of ventricular contraction and is not always distinctive on the AC slope of the echocardiogram. It can be visualized only when valve closure actually begins prior to the onset of ventricular contraction. Furthermore, Pohost et al.[6] and Rubenstein et al.[7] have identified the C_0 point, defined as the termination of the rapid posterior motion of the anterior leaflet, as the time of true leaflet

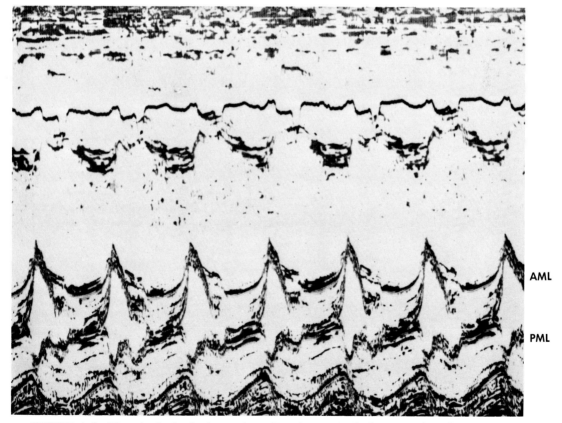

FIGURE 4-6. The mitral valve in sinus tachycardia. The anterior leaflet (AML) has a large single opening with only a small separate A wave as the early diastolic and atrial filling waves merge. The posterior leaflet (PML) E and A waves, however, remain distinct.

closure. The C point, which is the most posterior position of the anterior cusp, follows shortly thereafter.)

The position of the mitral leaflets in the normal heart (i.e., the degree of opening) at any time in diastole is dependent primarily on (1) the motion of the mitral annulus,[11] (2) the flow rate of blood across the valve at that instant, and (3) the relative pressures within the left atrium and the left ventricle. When the blood flow across the valve is plotted against time, it is apparent that the curve bears a strong resemblance to the normal motion of the anterior mitral leaflet.[12] During a tachycardia the "M" configuration of flow and the echocardiographic anterior mitral valve motion is lost, as the early diastolic and atrial filling phases merge (Fig. 4–6).

The time of left atrial contraction must also be considered in the analysis of mitral motion (Fig. 4–7). For example, in first-degree heart block (prolonged PR interval), atrial contraction occurs earlier, causing the two phases of ventricular filling to merge, and the distinct echocardiographic A point is lost. When the PR interval exceeds 0.18 sec in the presence of normal intra-atrial and intraventricular pressures, the mitral valve may close before the beginning of the QRS complex.[8]

Variations in the motion of the normal mitral valve also occur as a result of arrhythmias.[13, 14] The most important of these rhythm disturbances are prema-

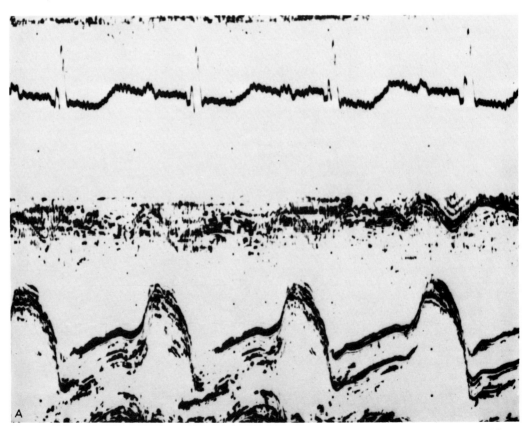

FIGURE 4–7. The effect of first-degree heart block on mitral valve motion. *A*, Mild PR prolongation (0.22 second). The E and A waves merge with a single diastolic opening. The time of valve closure is normal at the onset of the QRS complex.

ture contractions, atrial fibrillation and flutter, ventricular pacing, and atrioventricular dissociation.

With premature atrial contractions, the EA interval shortens during the diastolic opening preceding the premature beat (Fig. 4–8). During the longer diastolic period after the premature beat, the EA interval is correspondingly longer. In the case of premature ventricular beats, closure of the mitral valve occurs early (Fig. 4–9), usually without a preceding A wave. With marked prematurity of ventricular contraction, the mitral valve may be prevented from opening at all.

In atrial fibrillation, the early mitral opening (E wave) may appear normal, but in most cases, because synchronous atrial contraction does not occur, a distinct A wave is not present (Fig. 4–9). On these recordings, the mitral valve leaflets usually exhibit small-amplitude opening and closing movements for the duration of diastole. Occasionally, single high-amplitude openings resembling the normal A wave are seen late in diastole (Fig. 4–10). With atrial flutter, the mitral valve typically exhibits regular, low-amplitude diastolic excursions corresponding with the atrial flutter waves following the mitral E wave (see Fig. 3–2).

Mitral valve motion in the presence of ventricular pacing most often exhib-

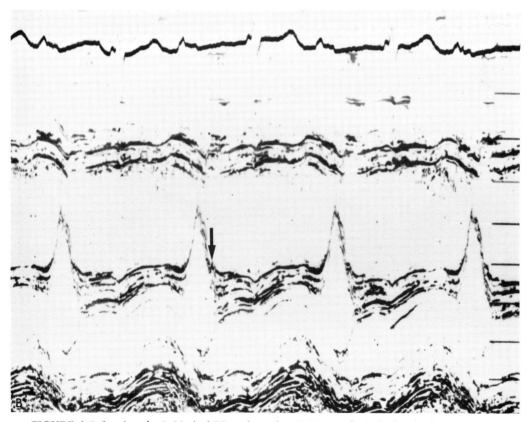

FIGURE 4-7 *Continued.* *B,* Marked PR prolongation (0.40 second). A single mitral opening is recorded with premature closure (arrow) well in advance of the electrocardiographic QRS complex.

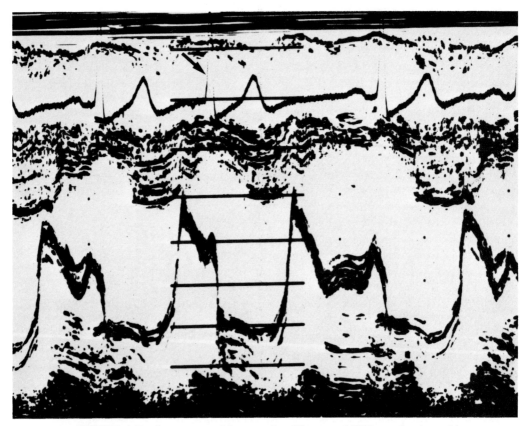

FIGURE 4-8. Premature atrial contraction. The second QRS complex (arrow) is premature, causing early ventricular systole and shortening in the duration of mitral valve opening during the previous diastole. The next diastolic period is slightly prolonged due to the compensatory pause. A mild late-systolic mitral prolapse is also present.

its an initial E wave, followed by partial or total valve closure for the remainder of diastole (Fig. 4–11). When atrial fibrillation is also present, slight opening and closing movements may be apparent during diastole. The mitral valve motion in a junctional rhythm is similar to the motion associated with ventricular pacing (Fig. 4–12).

The Chordae Tendineae

The chordae tendineae are most frequently recorded near their attachments to the mitral leaflets (Fig. 4–13), but they may be seen at any point within the ventricle along their extension from papillary muscles to mitral leaflets (Fig. 4–14). Their motion parallels that of the left ventricular posterior wall but with less systolic excursion than the endocardium (see Figs. 8–3 and 8–4). With careful angulation of the ultrasound beam toward the cardiac apex, it is possible to record the chordae where they join the papillary muscles.

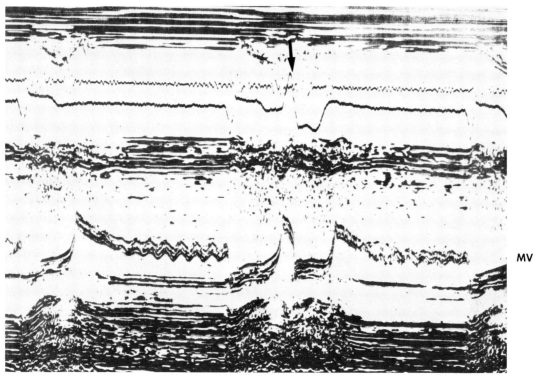

MV

FIGURE 4–9. Atrial fibrillation and premature ventricular contraction. Small diastolic undulations are seen during diastolic opening of the mitral valve (MV). There is no distinct A wave. A premature ventricular contraction (arrow) causes early closure after the second beat.

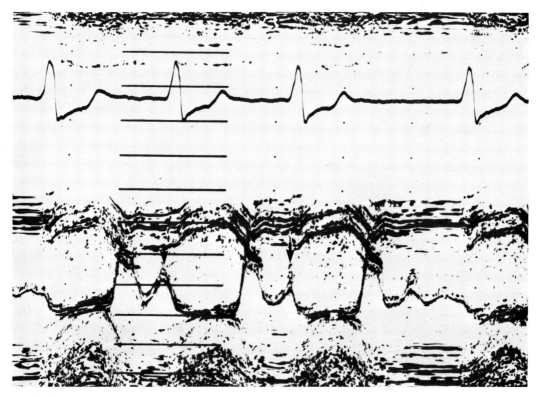

FIGURE 4–10. Atrial fibrillation. In this example, a distinct late-diastolic opening resembling an A wave is present, during some beats (arrows).

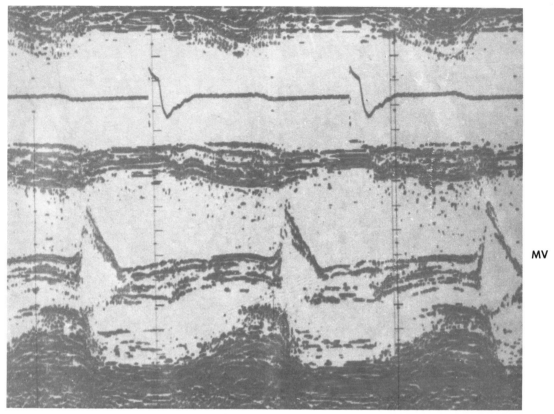

MV

FIGURE 4-11. Ventricular paced rhythm. The mitral valve has a single diastolic opening without an A wave. Mitral valve closure occurs before the QRS complex in this example but sometimes remains partially open throughout diastole.

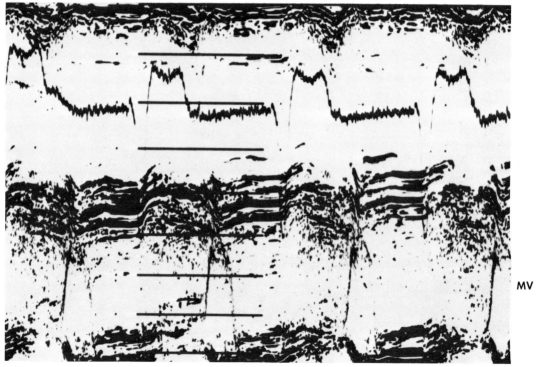

MV

FIGURE 4-12. Junctional rhythm. The mitral valve (MV) has a single diastolic opening (E wave) without an A wave. Very slight opening persists for the duration of diastole.

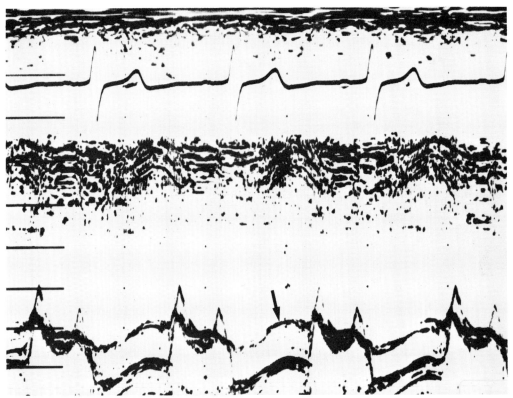

FIGURE 4-13. Chordae tendineae. A chordal echo (arrow) is seen near its point of attachment to the anterior mitral leaflet.

The Papillary Muscles

Both the anteromedial and the posterolateral papillary muscles may be recorded, and they can cause great confusion if they are not properly identified. The posteromedial papillary muscle can be visualized just below the left ventricular minor axis view as the echo beam is directed further inferiorly. It appears as a thickening in the posterior wall, with accentuated anterior excursion. The chordae may be seen at their point of attachment to this structure.

The anterolateral papillary muscle is seen less frequently but is sometimes recorded near the septum and may give the impression of greatly exaggerated septal motion during systole. Failure to identify this structure can lead to erroneously large measurement of the systolic thickness of the interventricular septum and a false reduction in the end-systolic intraventricular dimension.

The Mitral Annulus

The mitral annulus is recorded immediately behind and slightly superior to the optimal recording of the anterior and posterior mitral leaflets. Portions

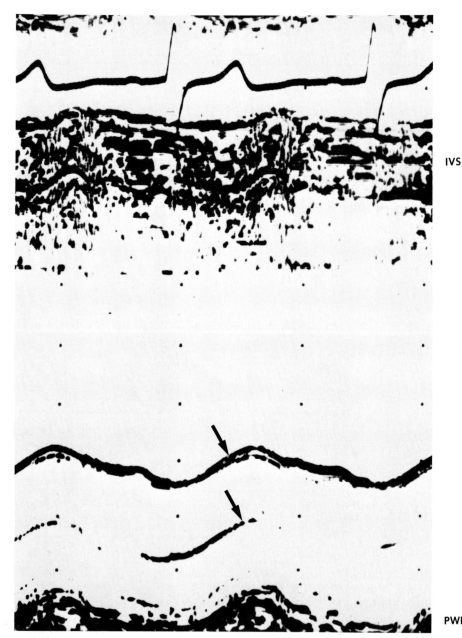

IVS

PWLV

FIGURE 4-14.   Chordae tendineae. Two chordal echoes (arrows) are observed within the left ventricle. Their motion parallels that of the posterior left ventricular wall (PWLV) (IVS = interventricular septum).

of the annulus may also be recorded as a discontinuous echo parallel and adjacent to the posterior wall within the left atrium.

Like all components of the cardiac skeleton, the annulus moves anteriorly in systole, posteriorly in diastole, and further posteriorly in late diastole, after the electrocardiographic P wave.[15-17] The annulus also moves downward toward the cardiac apex during ventricular systole and superiorly toward the left atrium in diastole.

Differentiation of the annulus from the true posterior left ventricular wall may be difficult. It may, however, be distinguished by variations in echo intensity, position, and motion. The echo reflected from the annulus appears much heavier than that from the endocardium and is located superior to the posterior mitral leaflet echo. Also, during atrial contraction, the annulus demonstrates a greater degree of posterior motion than the posterior left ventricular wall. While these characteristics will aid in the accurate identification of the mitral annulus, it often is not discernible unless it is abnormally thick (see Figs. 13–6 and 4–33).

MITRAL STENOSIS

Mitral stenosis most frequently is the end result of recurrent inflammation of the mitral valve secondary to rheumatic fever. A much less common form of mitral stenosis is the congenital variety, which in most cases leads to early death and is rarely seen in patients over the age of three.[18]

Rheumatic Mitral Stenosis

Recurrent rheumatic inflammation may cause three changes affecting the function of the mitral apparatus: commissural fusion, loss of valve pliability, and fusion and shortening of the chordae tendineae.[19] While fibrosis universally occurs in association with these changes, calcium deposition may or may not develop.

The normally functioning mitral valve permits blood to flow from the left atrium to the left ventricle in the absence of a pressure gradient of more than a few millimeters of mercury across the valve in diastole. However, as the valve and chordae undergo the changes of rheumatic valvulitis, the orifice begins to narrow. This process ordinarily does not result in symptoms until several years following the acute rheumatic episode.[20]

As the valve orifice narrows, the first hemodynamic alteration is a rise in the pressure within the left atrium.[21] This results in pulmonary hypertension and consequent dyspnea, the most common symptom of mitral stenosis. With further mitral narrowing, the left atrial pressure continues to rise, and the pulmonary hypertension becomes sufficiently severe to cause elevation of the right ventricular pressure. By this time, the mitral orifice has usually narrowed from its normal 4 to 6 cm^2 to approximately 0.5 to 1.0 cm^2. The full spectrum of signs and symptoms of mitral stenosis is usually apparent when this stage has been reached.

Echocardiographic Features

Specific changes in the components of the mitral valve, the ventricular walls, the papillary muscles, and the chordae tendineae are suggestive of mitral stenosis. Several investigations have been directed toward the identification of such changes on the echocardiogram.[5,11,22–29]

Early Diastolic Leaflet Closure (EF Slope). Although a reduction in the rate of early diastolic closure is a highly characteristic and sensitive index of mitral stenosis, (Figs. 4–15 to 4–17), it is not pathognomonic. As discussed elsewhere (see Chapters 6, 8, 11, and 14), reduced left ventricular compliance, left atrial myxoma, and pulmonary hypertension also decrease the EF slope. Furthermore, improper transducer angulation may result in a false reduction of this parameter. In spite of these possible causes of diminished EF slope, it is an invaluable echocardiographic indicator in the diagnosis and quantification of the severity of mitral stenosis. When the EF slope appears normal (greater than 80 mm per sec), a diagnosis of mitral stenosis can be excluded. The determination of a normal EF slope is therefore particularly helpful in ruling out mitral stenosis in patients with questionable diastolic murmurs or those with pulmonary hypertension of uncertain etiology.

While most investigators have shown a good general correlation between EF slope and the severity of stenosis as defined by other parameters,[30, 31] others[32] have found this to be unreliable in individual cases. Some variability in the slope independent of the severity of stenosis is not surprising, however, in view of the multiplicity of factors that affect the diastolic closure rate. For example, valve pliability itself will affect the slope. A highly calcified valve will exhibit a lesser slope than a valve with the same orifice size but no calcification.[31] Other factors include the degree of commissural fusion, left ventricular compliance, pulmonary hypertension, involvement of the chordae tendineae, and associated aortic valve disease.

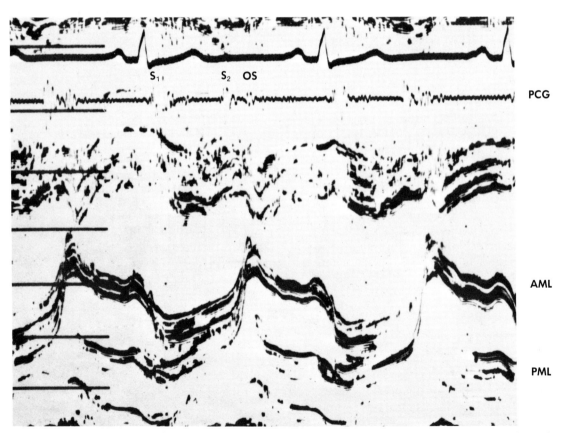

FIGURE 4–15.   Mild mitral stenosis. The valve leaflets are slightly thickened, with only modest (50 mm per sec) EF slope reduction. The valve appears pliable and shows a distinct A wave. The E point closely coincides with an opening snap (OS) recorded on the phonocardiogram (PCG). The posterior leaflet (PML) moves anteriorly during diastole in parallel with the anterior leaflet (AML).

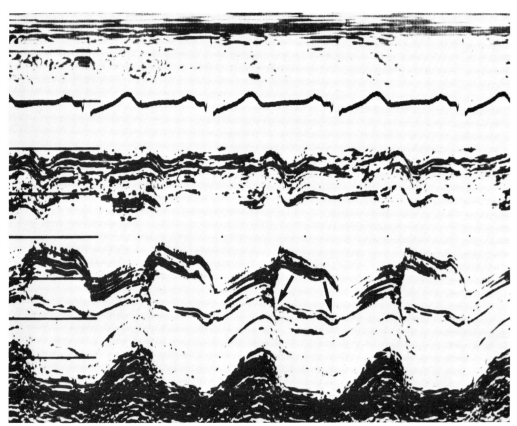

FIGURE 4-16. Moderate mitral stenosis. The cusps are slightly thickened and the EF slope is 24 mm per sec. Notice that the posterior leaflet appears to be pliable as its E wave and A wave move posteriorly (arrows).

Alterations in cardiac rate and rhythm may also have a significant effect on the diastolic closure rate in patients with mitral stenosis (Fig. 4–18). This is especially true in cases of atrial fibrillation with a rapid ventricular response. In these instances the closure rate should be measured during the longer diastolic periods, as measurement during rapid rates will result in a closure rate disproportionately slowed for the degree of stenosis.

It must also be reiterated that any conclusions based on the degree of EF slope presuppose optimal transducer angulation. Technique therefore remains highly critical in echocardiographic evaluation for mitral stenosis, because even small changes in beam direction factitiously reduce an already diminished EF slope. Multiple recordings must be examined, and the maximal slope selected for measurement. It is important to note that the posterior leaflet may not be useful as a parameter for selection of the optimal recording because its parallel motion may cause it to appear as part of the thickened anterior leaflet.

The primary reasons for the slowed EF slope in the presence of mitral stenosis continue to be debated, but several possibilities are well recognized. There is no doubt that in some cases loss of valve pliability is a factor. Also, it is apparent that stenosis causes a reduction in flow rate that results in persistence of flow across the valve orifice throughout diastole. This increased flow during mid- and late-diastole causes the valve leaflets to maintain a prolonged "open" and anterior position and slows the posterior–superior movement of the entire mitral apparatus during diastole because the rate of ventricular filling (and atrial emptying) slows.

The ventricular filling rate may also be reduced as a result of pulmonary hypertension or lowered left ventricular compliance. Subvalvular vortex forma-tion, subvalvular fusion, and increased traction of the leaflets by diseased chor-dae tendineae may also effect a reduction in EF slope.

While any or all of these factors may play a role, the reduced rate of ven-tricular filling and the associated loss of leaflet pliability are probably the most important mechanisms of decreased EF slope in the majority of patients with mitral stenosis.

Reliance on the valve thickness parameter in the assessment of mitral stenosis is unwise because the degree of thickening is a poor index of the sever-ity of the stenosis. This is true because orifice size is affected by the amount of commissural fusion rather than by the degree of leaflet thickening.[1] Further-more, if aortic regurgitation is also present, some leaflet thickening may occur as a result of that alone.

The presence of calcium in the valve, however, has more clinical impor-tance than leaflet thickening per se. Gross calcification with mitral stenosis

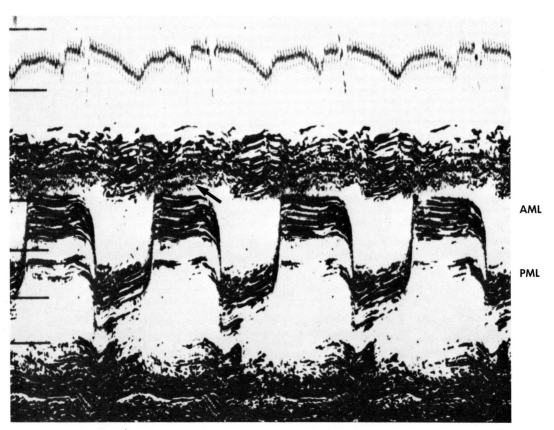

FIGURE 4–17.   Severe mitral stenosis. There is no measurable mitral early diastolic closure, and despite the fact that sinus rhythm is present, there is no discernible A wave. The anterior leaf-let (AML) is markedly thickened, and the posterior leaflet (PML) moves anteriorly during diastole. A fine fluttering motion of the interventricular septum (arrow) is due to concomitant aortic regurgitation.

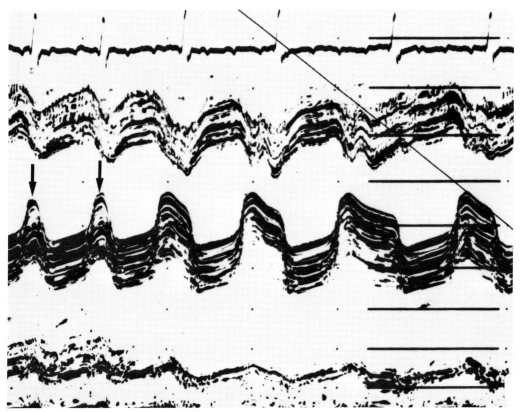

FIGURE 4-18. Mitral stenosis and atrial fibrillation. The rate of early diastolic closure cannot be measured during short diastolic periods (beats 1 and 2, arrows). Only when the rate slows is this measurement valid (beats 3 through 6).

occurs in less than 5 percent of afflicted patients under the age of 45.[1] Calcification portends a poor operative result if mitral commissurotomy is considered (see Chapter 15). With echocardiography, calcification is discernible on gray scale recordings as a heavier echo than that reflected by fibrous tissue. Often, a thickened annulus also is associated with leaflet calcification.

Diastolic Valve Opening. Friedman found that the E point and the phonocardiographic recording of the mitral valve opening snap occurred within 5 msec in patients with pure mitral stenosis and within 10 msec in those with mixed and bivalvular lesions (see Fig. 4–15).[33] The E point also has been noted to be rounded in patients with mitral stenosis.[11, 33]

The time from the closure of the aortic valve until opening of the mitral valve, termed the "A_2–OS interval" (A_2 = aortic component of the second heart sound; OS = opening snap of the mitral valve), has long been recognized as an important auscultatory and phonocardiographic parameter in the assessment of mitral stenosis. This interval is determined primarily by (1) the rate of fall of left ventricular pressure as the ventricle relaxes, (2) the aortic pressure at the time of aortic valve closure, and (3) the left atrial pressure at the time of mitral valve opening.[34] The mitral valve will open earlier as (1) and (3) increase and (2) decreases. With increasing severity of mitral stenosis, the left atrial pressure rises, and as a consequence the A_2–OS interval shortens. On auscultation the clinician recognizes this as the opening snap occurs more closely after the aortic component of the second heart sound.

Edler has correlated valve orifice size with the time interval from the aortic closure sound (A_2) to the E point on the echocardiogram in patients in sinus rhythm with and without valvular calcification.[31] He found that as orifice size narrowed, the A_2–E interval is shortened. (In the case of atrial fibrillation, the A_2–E interval varies in the same patient with the varying length of each preceding R–R interval.) If the timing of the mitral opening is normal or delayed in mitral stenosis, it is possible that the left ventricular end-systolic pressure is elevated, in which case concomitant aortic valve disease or ventricular myocardial dysfunction are to be suspected.

A loss of valve pliability and chordal shortening sometimes results in a reduction in valve excursion and diminished DE amplitude.[27, 30] It is important to note, however, that any other cause of reduced flow across the mitral valve or increased left ventricular end-systolic pressure may also reduce mitral opening amplitude.

Parallel Anterior and Posterior Leaflet Motion.   Duchak et al. have pointed out the great value in recording the posterior leaflet in patients with mitral stenosis.[22] The normal posteriorly directed diastolic opening motions of the posterior leaflet are usually reversed in patients with significant mitral stenosis; thus the leaflet appears to move in parallel with the anterior leaflet (see Figs. 4–15 and 4–17). The reversed posterior leaflet motion, however, is not seen in cases in which the reduction in EF slope is caused by such other factors as reduced left ventricular compliance (see Fig. 8–12).

The reversed posterior leaflet motion probably results when the motion of independent components of the valve lessens as stenosis increases and the motion of the entire mitral apparatus, which is anterior during diastole, governs the direction of leaflet motion. Indeed, in the most severe cases of mitral stenosis, the valve becomes a totally fixed structure in which all parts move in concert.

Levisman et al. have shown that in approximately 10 percent of patients with mitral stenosis, the posterior leaflet maintains its normal diastolic posterior motion (opposite to that of the anterior leaflet) (see Fig. 4–16).[35] They did not find that the degree of stenosis is a factor in whether posterior leaflet direction is normal or reversed. Flaherty et al. have also described a single case of mitral stenosis in which the normal motion of a thickened posterior leaflet was present.[36]

The A Wave.   The A wave is lost in mitral stenosis both when atrial fibrillation occurs and when the stenosis is severe. Preservation of a prominent A wave in sinus rhythm is sometimes a useful echocardiographic feature in differentiating mitral stenosis from other causes of reduced rate of early-diastolic closure. A reduced EF slope associated with an A point more anterior than the E point is against the diagnosis of pure mitral stenosis. This is an especially useful sign in patients with poor early-diastolic mitral opening due to aortic regurgitation (see Fig. 5–23).

The Mitral Annulus.   The mitral annulus sometimes is thickened and calcified in rheumatic valvulitis[37] and may appear abnormally thickened on the echocardiogram.

In mitral stenosis, the posterior excursion of the annulus during diastole becomes reduced as ventricular filling is decreased. Furthermore, the loss of atrial contraction in atrial fibrillation, the most common arrhythmia in advanced mitral stenosis, results in the absence of the characteristic late-diastolic posterior motion of the annulus.

The Chordae Tendineae. While the chordae tendineae frequently become calcified and thickened in rheumatic mitral valve disease,[37] this condition has not been associated with noticeable chordal changes on the echocardiogram. Chordal retraction is associated with reduced early-diastolic mitral opening of less than 13 mm, but chordal function is normal when the opening amplitude exceeds 25 mm.[30]

The Left Atrium. The characteristic increase in the internal dimension of the left atrium is evident on the echocardiogram of the patient with mitral stenosis (Fig. 4–19). Among 27 patients with mitral stenosis, it was reported that the LA–AO ratio was 1.93 (S.D. ± 0.48) compared to a mean among normals of 0.90 (S.D. ± 0.13).[38]

Mural thrombi that may result in arterial embolism frequently occur within the left atrium in association with mitral stenosis.[39] For this reason, systemic embolism is an indication for echocardiographic evaluation for "silent" mitral stenosis, as well as for left atrial myxoma (see Chapter 6). Echocardiography is not, however, a reliable technique for detection of a thrombus itself.

The Left Ventricle. Chronic rheumatic changes affecting the left ventricular performance may occur in pure mitral stenosis.[40–43] Marked enlargement of the left ventricle, however, is not a feature of mitral stenosis. Therefore, when the ventricle appears dilated, this finding should invoke the possibility of simultaneous mitral regurgitation or rheumatic aortic valve in-

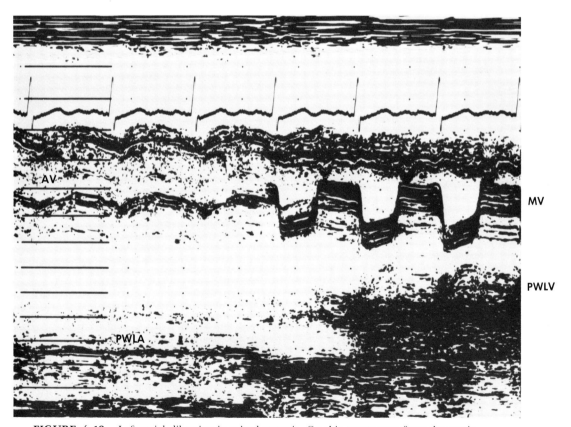

FIGURE 4–19. Left atrial dilatation in mitral stenosis. On this sector scan from the aortic root to the highly stenotic mitral valve (MV), the left atrial wall (PWLA) is displaced posteriorly relative to the position of the posterior left ventricular wall (PWLV). The left atrial dimension measures 6 cm. The aortic valve (AV) appears to be pliable.

volvement. Other concomitant diseases such as congestive cardiomyopathy and coronary atherosclerosis should also be considered.

Posterior left ventricular wall contractions, which appear on the echocardiogram immediately inferior to the mitral valve echoes, may become reduced if the rheumatic process involves that area of the myocardium visualized on the recording.[41] Also, the interventricular septum may exhibit an exaggeration of the post-systolic notch which immediately follows the mitral E point.

The Aortic Root and Aortic Valve. Many patients with mitral stenosis also have chronic rheumatic involvement of the aortic valve. In the case of concomitant aortic insufficiency (AI), the rigid mitral leaflets may fail to exhibit the echo oscillations typical of AI. Aortic insufficiency in the presence of severe mitral stenosis may be unsuspected on clinical grounds as well because of reduced cardiac output that results from the mitral involvement.[44] For the same reasons, aortic stenosis also may go undetected clinically,[45] but it should be suspected if the aortic valve leaflets appear on the echocardiogram to be thickened by calcification and fibrosis (Fig. 4–20).

When the cardiac output is diminished by severe mitral stenosis, the duration of aortic valve opening (left ventricular ejection) is reduced and the aortic root may be narrowed.

The Tricuspid Valve. In patients with mitral stenosis, the tricuspid valve is frequently easily visualized, probably as a result of pulmonary hypertension (Fig. 4–21). Rheumatic involvement of the tricuspid valve itself is another con-

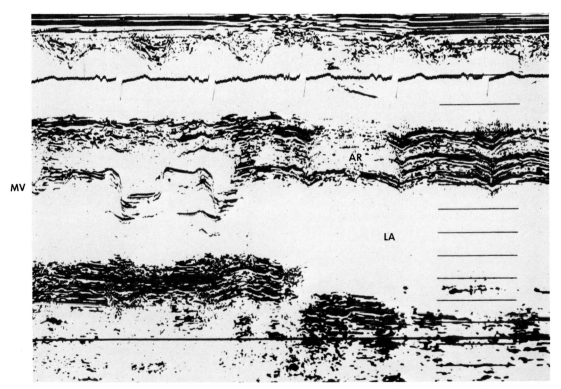

FIGURE 4-20. Concomitant rheumatic aortic stenosis and mitral stenosis. Discrete aortic valve leaflet motion is not discernible as the aortic root (AR) is filled with echoes due to scarring of the valve. The mitral valve (MV) is markedly thickened with a flattened EF slope. The left atrium (LA) is dilated.

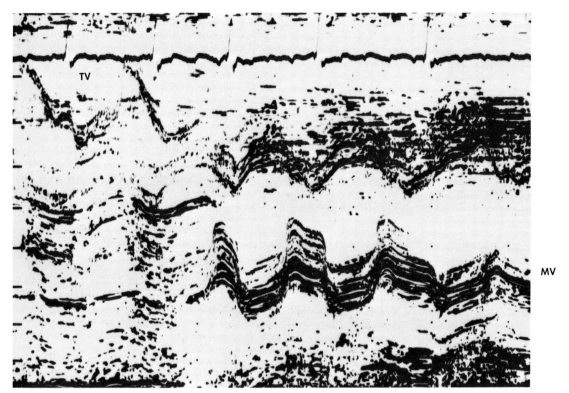

FIGURE 4-21. Moderate mitral stenosis. The tricuspid valve (TV) is often easily visualized anterior and medial of the stenotic mitral valve (MV).

sideration, although this occurs in only 10 percent of patients with rheumatic disease.[19] Because tricuspid stenosis is often clinically unsuspected in the presence of mitral stenosis, echocardiographic assessment of the tricuspid valve should always be attempted (see Chapter 10).[46] The echocardiogram is also useful in differentiating the murmur of tricuspid regurgitation secondary to mitral stenosis from significant mitral regurgitaiton.[47]

The Pulmonic Valve. The mean pulmonary artery pressure is usually elevated above 40 mm Hg in patients with moderate mitral stenosis.[19] This is reflected by a diminished or absent A wave and a reduced or flat EF slope of the pulmonic valve motion.[48-50] These changes are discussed in greater detail in Chapter 11.

Congenital Mitral Stenosis

Isolated congenital mitral stenosis is rare and usually occurs in association with such cardiac anomalies as endocardial fibrosis, aortic stenosis, patent ductus arteriosus, and coarctation of the aorta.[51] Lundström found that among seven infants ranging in age from 3 days to 7 months, with congenital mitral stenosis, all had an EF slope of less than 40 mm per sec.[52] In two of these cases, the EF slope exceeded 30 mm per sec, and the mitral stenosis was slight. In the remaining five infants with EF slopes of less than 25 mm per sec, the stenosis was severe. The amplitude of opening was reduced in two cases, and it was at the lower limit of normal in the remainder. In none of these patients was the mitral valve calcified. The marked reduction in the opening amplitude may also be associated with combined hypoplasia of the left ventricle.

MITRAL REGURGITAITON

Competence of the mitral valve may be lost if any one of the components of this complex apparatus fails to function properly. Thus mitral regurgitation may occur in varying degrees of severity as a result of one or more diverse causes.

Mild mitral regurgitation results primarily in an increased volume within the left atrium and an increase in the flow across the mitral valve in diastole equal to the retrograde systolic flow through the incompetent mitral valve. In an experimental study in dogs, Braunwald found that until the regurgitant flow was approximately double that of the total systemic (forward) blood flow, only a mild change in the systemic circulation was observed.[53] This correlates well with the clinical observation in humans in whom even severe chronic mitral regurgitation can occur without serious circulatory compromise. The ability of the left ventricle to function well despite the increased volume imposed by mitral regurgitation may be explained by the fact that the myocardial tension is lessened in this state, thus allowing the left ventricle to expend its energy in circumferential fiber shortening rather than in tension development. The myocardial oxygen demand is not significantly changed with increased fiber shortening alone.

In chronic mitral regurgitation, the left atrium accommodates the regurgitant flow by its increased volume. Therefore, the patient with chronic mitral insufficiency may develop a greatly dilated left atrium, with normal intra-atrial pressures and very little effect on the pulmonary circulation. Other patients do not adapt as well to mitral regurgitation. In such cases the atrium fails to dilate enough to accommodate the regurgitant flow. This results in increasing left atrial pressure, hypertrophy of the left atrial myocardium, pulmonary hypertension, and ultimately, right ventricular hypertrophy and failure.

Acute mitral regurgitation, as in rupture of the chordae tendineae, also causes an immediate marked increase in the left intra-atrial pressure because the atrium does not have time to accommodate by dilatation. Pronounced pulmonary hypertension accompanies the acute form of mitral regurgitation.

Rheumatic Mitral Regurgitation

Edwards has pointed out that three structural changes in chronic rheumatic disease may result in incompetence of the mitral valve.[2] These are (1) commissural calcification, which keeps the valve orifice open during ventricular systole, (2) actual shortening of the posterior mitral leaflet, and (3) relative shortening of the posterior leaflet secondary to left atrial dilatation. This is due to the "pulling" effect on the posterior leaflet by the dilating left atrium, the posterior wall of which is continuous with the posterior mitral leaflet. In addition, chordal shortening contributes to the insufficiency when the leaflets are retracted.

Echocardiographic Features

Valve Leaflets. Unfortunately the pre-eminent structural change that results in mitral regurgitation, i.e., failure of the leaflet edges to coapt during ventricular systole, is at present impossible to diagnose with certainty from the standard echocardiogram.[5] Systolic leaflet separation would be a reliable sign only if it could be determined that both leaflet edges were being recorded.

Steinfeld and associates have reported that systolic prolapse of the mitral leaflets, with a mid- or late-systolic murmur or click, may occur in chronic rheumatic mitral insufficiency.[54] These findings were observed in 34 of their 184 patients studied.

Characteristically, the leaflets are thickened in mitral regurgitation of rheumatic origin (Fig. 4–22),[55] but they are also thickened in myxomatous degeneration, which may also result in mitral insufficiency.

Increased flow across the incompetent valve may result in an increased opening (DE) rate[55] and amplitude of excursion. Segal et al.[56] found the opening amplitude to be increased to an average of 34 mm in patients with severe mitral insufficiency, but others have failed to confirm this finding.[55, 57] In cases of pure mitral regurgitation with preservation of valve pliability, the early diastolic closure rate (EF slope) usually remains normal or increased.[5, 23, 30, 56, 57] Because valve pliability is often diminished, however, the EF slope actually may be reduced.[30]

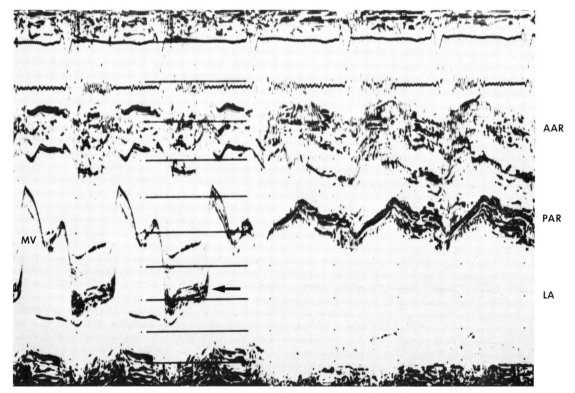

FIGURE 4–22. Mitral regurgitation secondary to infective endocarditis. The mitral valve (MV) systolic closure position (arrow) is displaced over 20 mm behind the posterior wall of the aortic root (PAR). The left atrium (LA) is dilated (AAR = anterior wall of aortic root).

It must be emphasized that the increased amplitude and EF slope sometimes present in mitral insufficiency are secondary effects characteristic of any circulatory state of increased flow across the mitral valve, including other causes of mitral incompetence and the high cardiac output states. Even in the presence of normal flow, patients with "large" mitral valves such as in Marfan's disease, may exhibit the same features of increased amplitude and EF slope.

Johnson et al. have shown that in patients with mitral insufficiency, closure of the anterior leaflet is greater than 8 mm from (behind) the posterior aortic wall, regardless of cause (Fig. 4–22).[58] This is demonstrable on the mitral-aortic root sweep. They did not, however, find a correlation between the severity of mitral insufficiency and the amount of mitral posterior displacement. Among patients in whom the closure was less than 8 mm from the posterior aortic root, 95 percent had no angiographic evidence of mitral insufficiency.

The Aortic Valve.   In the absence of rheumatic involvement of the aortic valve, significant mitral insufficiency sometimes shortens the duration of opening of the aortic valve during left ventricular systole. As blood flows from the left ventricle into the left atrium during left ventricular ejection, the left ventricle is unable to sustain its pressure for the usual duration, which results in early aortic valve closure. This correlates with two clinical characteristics of mitral regurgitation: increased splitting of the second heart sound as aortic closure occurs earlier, and a sudden fall-off in the peripheral pulse contour.[53]

The Left Atrium.   Massive dilatation of the left atrium is common in severe chronic mitral regurgitation. Increased left atrial size should always raise the possibility of mitral insufficiency, even when the echocardiographic features of the mitral valve appear normal. A normal or minimally dilated left atrium, however, does not exclude even severe mitral regurgitation, particularly in its acute form. In their study of 48 patients with mitral regurgitation of various causes, Burgess et al.[55] found the left atrial dimension, corrected for body surface area, to range from 1.4 to 4.7 cm per M^2 (mean 2.7 cm per M^2). Among normals, the range is 1.2 to 2.0 cm per M^2 (mean 1.6).

The Left Ventricle.   The increased volume of blood pumped by the left ventricle causes dilatation of the chamber, which is reflected by an increased end-diastolic dimension. In the study by Burgess et al.,[55] severe mitral regurgitation was associated with increases in left ventricular end-diastolic dimension, ranging from 5.6 to 9.3 cm, and with exaggerated motion of the interventricular septum (see Fig. 4–23). The increased septal motion contributes to a normal cardiac output. Decreased septal systolic motion in the presence of significant mitral regurgitation may signify myocardial dysfunction. The posterior wall systolic motion may also be exaggerated.

Combined Mitral Stenosis and Mitral Regurgitation

Rheumatic involvement of the mitral apparatus frequently results in a diastolic gradient across the rigid valve as well as systolic incompetence due to failure of leaflet coaptation caused by the scarring and retraction of the leaflets and chordae. Detection of significant mitral regurgitation in the patient with mitral stenosis is important in that such patients are candidates for valve replacement rather than mitral commissurotomy.

While the mitral valve motion is highly variable in combined mitral stenosis

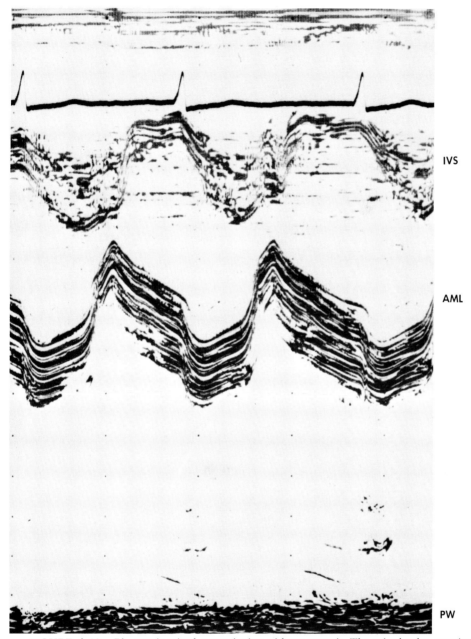

IVS

AML

PW

FIGURE 4-23. Rheumatic mitral regurgitation without stenosis. The mitral valve anterior leaflet (AML) is thickened and is displaced from the posterior wall (PW) as a result of chamber dilatation. The rate of early diastolic closure is reduced due to decreased valve pliability. The systolic motion of the interventricular septum (IVS) is increased as a result of the increased left ventricular volume load.

and insufficiency,[30] insufficiency should be suspected in the patient with stenosis who has the following echocardiographic findings:

1. Normal or increased opening mitral valve amplitude
2. Normal or only slightly diminished EF slope
3. Markedly dilated left atrium
4. Dilated left ventricle
5. Systolic prolapse of either or both leaflets

6. Increased systolic motion of the interventricular septum and posterior left ventricular wall

Even when none of these features is found in the patient with mitral stenosis, the possibility of at least mild mitral regurgitation cannot be excluded.

Nonrheumatic Mitral Regurgitation

The appearance of the mitral valve in the chronic nonrheumatic conditions that cause mitral regurgitation often reflects the underlying etiology. Other causes, such as infective endocarditis, may produce only nonspecific findings caused by increased flow across the valve. One of the most common conditions is mitral prolapse, characterized by a distinctive posteriorly directed leaflet motion during ventricular systole. Calcification of the mitral valve annulus, chordal rupture, congestive cardiomyopathy, asymmetric septal hypertrophy, and papillary muscle dysfunction are other causes of mitral regurgitation.

MITRAL PROLAPSE

Confusion has arisen over the term "mitral prolapse." Edwards[59] has pointed out that mitral overshooting during left ventricular systole may be a result of one of two groups of anatomic abnormalities: (1) those states, such as chordal rupture, in which there is a loss of continuity of some portion of the mitral apparatus or (2) those in which continuity is maintained, such as mitral leaflet connective tissue degeneration. We have chosen to identify these two groups as "primary prolapse," when continuity is maintained, and "secondary prolapse," when there is discontinuity with prolapse when the leaflet supporting structures fail to function normally.

The two mitral leaflets normally bulge slightly into the left atrium during ventricular systole. This may be demonstrated on the cineangiogram and on the echocardiogram, with the mitral–aortic sweep. The systolic movement into the left atrium is normally less than 8 mm from the posterior aortic wall on the mitral–aortic sector scan recording.[58]

Primary Mitral Prolapse

Abnormal systolic protrusion of one or both mitral valve leaflets into the left atrium has become an increasingly important clinical entity in recent years. It is frequently identified in children,[51, 60] although most studies relate to adults. Such overshooting has been observed both as part of diseases in which there are generalized connective tissue disorders, such as Marfan's disease, and as an isolated phenomenon in individuals or in families. (It is possible, of course, that the latter, apparently isolated type actually represents a forme fruste of the connective tissue disorders, [61, 62] but because this has not been firmly established, they continue to be treated as clinically separate entities).

Mitral prolapse has been described under various names, including "Barlow's Syndrome,"[63] "floppy valve syndrome," "systolic click–late systolic murmur syndrome," "billowing posterior leaflet," and "myxomatous degeneration." It is not an uncommon finding. Pomerance et al. report that mucoid degeneration of the mitral leaflets may be seen in 1 percent of necropsies.[64] Kern et al. found severe myxoid changes of the mitral valve to be present in most patients with nonrheumatic mitral insufficiency.[65] Behar et al. detected prolapse in 6 percent of patients undergoing left ventricular cineangiography.[66]

The pathogenesis of mucoid degeneration is unresolved, although it is clear that genetic factors account for many cases, as familial occurrences have been well documented.[61,67–69] In a study of 130 patients with this syndrome, Pocock and Barlow concluded that the cause was unknown in 80 cases.[67] In 23 patients, a familial factor was recognized, and in 18 others there was an associated congenital defect, most often a secundum atrial septal defect. Weiss et al. found mitral prolapse in 47 percent of first-degree relatives, consistent with an autosomal dominant mode of inheritance.[69]

The clinician is often first led to suspect this entity by the presence of a systolic click followed by a systolic murmur. The murmur, while typically beginning in mid-systole,[70] may occur in early- or late-systole as well, and becomes earlier with amyl nitrite inhalation, the Valsalva maneuver, and the upright posture.[71] The click is particularly accentuated by the upright posture.[70] A distinctive complaint, although uncommon, is that the patient himself may hear a peculiar "whooping" sound intermittently emanating from his chest. Other symptoms sometimes include chest pain atypical of angina pectoris and effort-related dyspnea, palpitations, and even syncope.[61,68,70–73] Because these symptoms may occur in the absence of the classic auscultatory findings of a click and murmur, an echocardiogram is indicated in many patients with these complaints.[74] Frequently, however, the patient is asymptomatic.[61] Thoracic skeletal abnormalities, especially pectus excavation, straight thoracic spine, and scoliosis are common in these patients.[75,76]

The prolapse of the mitral leaflets in the majority of asymptomatic cases probably does not progress to significant clinical deterioration, although prospective long-term follow-up is not yet available. Although the prognosis may be quite good,[77] several complications have been described, including: (1) mitral regurgitation;[64,78] (2) bacterial endocarditis;[64] (3) serious arrhythmias, especially in the post-exercise state;[61,67,70,72,73,79–81] (4) chordal rupture;[64,77] (5) myocardial ischemia, usually of the inferolateral type;[61,63,66,67,70,80] and (6) sudden death.[68,82]

Echocardiographic Features

Normally, the two mitral leaflets move slowly anteriorly in parallel during left ventricular ejection as left ventricular volume is reduced.[83] Furthermore, during systole their echoes are clearly separated from those reflected from the adjacent posterior cardiac wall.

The left atrium lies posterior to the mitral valve echo when the transducer is angled slightly superiorly near the aortic root. When either or both of the leaflets appear to move posteriorly at any point after the C point, prolapse into the atrium must be suspected. While this has more often proved to be affecting the posterior leaflet in angiographic studies, it is sometimes not clear from the echocardiogram which of the two leaflets is prolapsing. It has recently been emphasized that incorrect transducer angulation can simulate mitral prolapse, particularly if the transducer is placed too high on the chest wall.[69] With correct transducer position, two echocardiographic patterns of prolapse, pan-systolic and mid-systolic, have been recognized.

In the case of pan-systolic prolapse, one or both valve leaflets continues to move posteriorly after the time of the C point, in general reaching the furthest posterior position in mid-systole rather than exhibiting the normal anterior excursion as systole begins (Figs. 4–24 and 4–25). The leaflet echoes may actually become buried within the posterior wall echoes. DeMaria et al. found pansystolic prolapse to be the more common form.[28] The "hammock-like" effect of multiple, parallel echoes is frequently seen in this form, and has a highly characteristic appearance.[84] This echo configuration apparently results from the redundant layers of the abnormal leaflet structure, each layer of which presents a reflecting surface for the ultrasound beam.[83]

In most series, mid-systolic prolapse is the form most commonly identified (Fig. 4–26). The posterior displacement of the leaflets occurs approximately 0.05 sec preceding the systolic click (Fig. 4–27).[85] The click is probably caused by a sudden tensing of the prolapsed leaflet, although it is possible that abrupt tightening of the chordae tendineae could also generate this sound.[86]

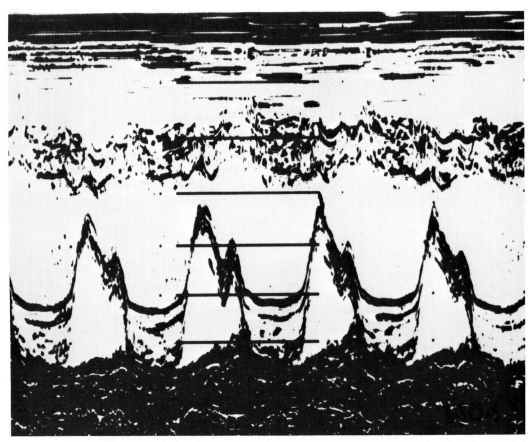

FIGURE 4–24. Pansystolic mitral valve prolapse. Part of the anterior leaflet echo is buried within the posterior wall echo throughout ventricular systole. Note the "hammock" effect of echoes from other portions of the redundant mitral leaflets. The maximal posterior displacement occurs in midsystole.

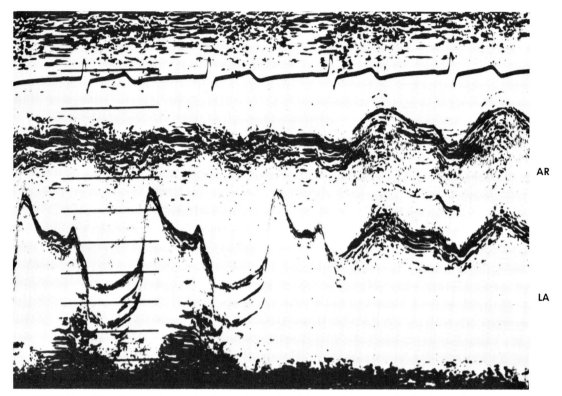

AR

LA

FIGURE 4-25. Pansystolic mitral valve prolapse. On this scan from the mitral valve to the aortic root (AR), the multiple leaflet echoes are displaced far into the left atrium (LA) during ventricular systole. The left atrium is dilated as a result of associated mitral regurgitation.

Mitral prolapse is sometimes best appreciated on the mitral–aortic sweep (see Fig. 4–25). The anterior leaflet normally moves no more than a few millimeters beyond the most posterior excursion of the aortic posterior wall. When during systole the anterior leaflet appears to move as far posteriorly as the left atrial wall, this may be regarded as strong evidence for prolapse.

As mentioned earlier, failure of the two leaflets to appear to come together ordinarily cannot be considered representative of true leaflet separation. In mitral prolapse, however, apparent diastolic divergence of the two leaflets probably does represent true leaflet separation, which in some cases causes mitral regurgitation (see Fig. 4–26)[55] leading to left atrial dilatation (see Fig. 4–25). In most cases of prolapse, however, significant mitral regurgitation is not present, and the left atrial dimension is normal.

It should be mentioned that while clinical diagnosis of mitral prolapse has emphasized the posterior leaflet, echocardiographic studies have demonstrated that both leaflets usually are involved. Spencer et al. found that 20 of 23 patients with prolapse showed abnormal motion involving both cusps of the mitral valve,[87] and Reinke et al. found that 49 of the 58 patients in their series exhibited prolapse of both cusps.[88]

Because some patients exhibit only equivocal findings of mitral prolapse, a simple provocative test utilizing amyl nitrite inhalation[78, 89] may be useful in defining the condition. Inhalation of amyl nitrite causes an increase in venous pooling, and the end-diastolic volume of the left ventricle becomes diminished, conceivably leaving the leaflets nearer a position of prolapse at end-diastole. Thus, earlier prolapse with increased mitral regurgitation will occur. For the same reasons, systolic clicks of mitral prolapse also tend to occur earlier in inspiration.[71] Fontana et al. have found that the upright posture increases the duration of the murmur as prolapse occurs earlier, again probably as a result of decreased venous return and end-diastolic left ventricular volume.[70] Thus, it is useful to make echocardiographic recordings in both the upright and the reclining positions in patients in whom prolapse is suspected. Premature ventricular systole also may accentuate the prolapse, a result of decreased ventricular volume at the time contraction begins (Fig. 4–28).

In some cases of severe prolapse, a mass of echoes resembling a protruding atrial tumor appears behind the mitral valve echo in diastole (Fig. 4–29; see also Fig. 6–10).[90, 91] These echoes probably are reflected from layers of redundant valve tissue.

The presence of an apical mid-systolic click without a murmur may occur inexplicably in patients without evidence of prolapse. While some such patients do have true intermittent prolapse that is not detected by echo,[74] we have found one in whom a sudden, short anterior displacement of the anterior leaflet coincided with a click (see Fig. 3–7).

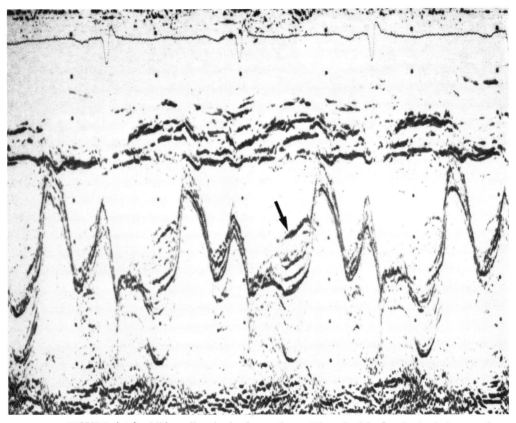

FIGURE 4–26. Midsystolic mitral valve prolapse. The mitral leaflets begin their normal anterior excursion after the C point, but this motion is interrupted in midsystole by an abrupt posterior motion at the time of prolapse. Both the anterior and the posterior leaflets probably prolapse in this case, although some portions of the anterior leaflet appear to continue their anterior excursion (arrow), with apparent leaflet divergence during the time of the prolapse.

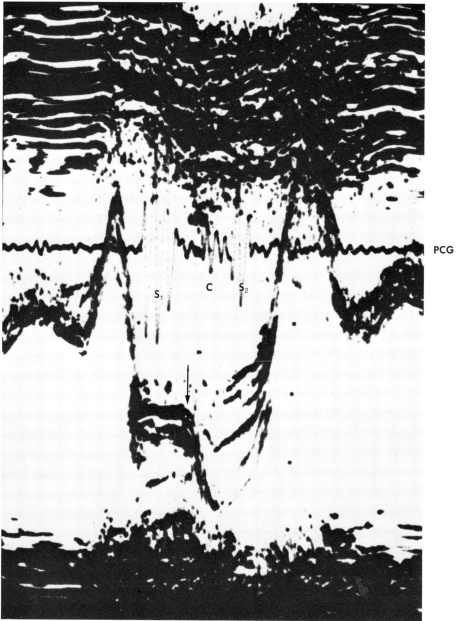

FIGURE 4-27. Midsystolic mitral valve prolapse. The posterior systolic excursion (arrow) begins slightly before the click (C) recorded on the phonocardiogram (PCG) (S_1 = first heart sound; S_2 = second heart sound).

Other valve tissue may be similarly affected. In some cases the tricuspid valve may show degenerative changes with prolapse.[92] In one case report,[93] a subaortic membrane and aortic regurgitation due to myxomatous degeneration of the aortic leaflets were seen in association with mitral prolapse.

Associated Disorders

Mitral valve changes that occur in patients with generalized disorders of connective tissue may be closely related to the syndrome of isolated mitral prolapse.[94] The most notable instance is Marfan's syndrome, in which mitral regurgitation due to mitral valve prolapse is well recognized (Fig. 4–29).[56, 62, 95] The Ehlers-Danlos syndrome is also associated with mitral prolapse.[56] Hemry et al. have reported the case of a patient with relapsing polychondritis, migratory polytendonitis, and mitral insufficiency.[96] This patient showed mid-systolic prolapse of the posterior mitral leaflet on echocardiography and had a mid-systolic click and a late-systolic murmur. Mitral valve prolapse has also been reported in association with pulmonary hypertension[90] and atrial septal defect.

Secondary Mitral Prolapse

Ruptured Chordae Tendineae

Despite the remarkable strength of the chordae tendineae, total severance is not a rare event. It may occur either as an acute isolated event or from multiple causes, which are usually long-standing before the rupture occurs.[59, 97–102]

Selzer has suggested that isolated chordal rupture is characterized clinically by (1) acute onset, (2) selective involvement of the chordae attached to the posterior leaflet, and (3) an otherwise virtually intact mitral valve with localized loss of chordal support.[97] Because chordal rupture is generally acute, the usual

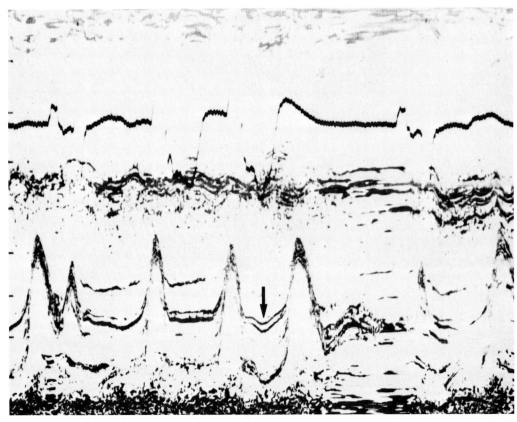

FIGURE 4–28. Mitral valve prolapse accentuated by premature ventricular systole. While only mild posterior excursion is observed after the first beat, the third beat occurs after a markedly abbreviated diastolic filling period and is associated with more obvious valve prolapse (arrow).

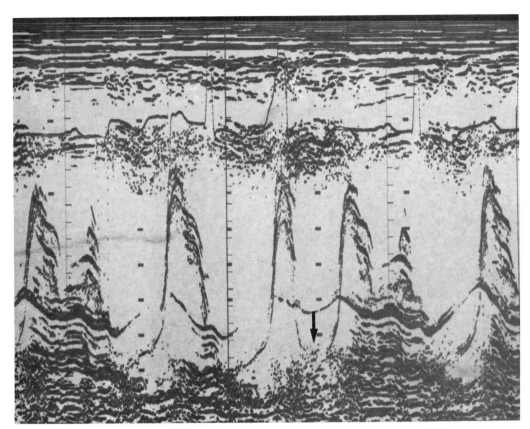

FIGURE 4-29. Mitral valve prolapse in Marfan's syndrome. The anterior mitral leaflet has markedly increased opening amplitude, in excess of 40 mm. The systolic prolapse is most evident during a premature beat (arrow). Note also the multiple echoes from redundant valve tissue best seen during mitral opening.

clinical signs of mitral regurgitation, i.e., dilatation of the left atrium and left ventricular hypertrophy, are absent. The most characteristic clinical feature is a murmur that bears a resemblance to the murmur heard in aortic stenosis.

Echocardiographic Features. The leaflet whose chordae have ruptured may be seen to prolapse into the left atrium throughout systole. In most cases it is the posterior leaflet that is affected. It appears as a fleeting echo within the left atrium during ventricular systole,[103, 104] and is similar in appearance to papillary muscle transection (see Figs. 14-1 and 14-2). A fluttering motion of the anterior leaflet during systole also may be observed (see Fig. 4-30).[104]

The effect of papillary muscle transection is equal to that of chordal rupture. Total transection is usually a complication of myocardial infarction.

Because of the increased flow across the mitral valve, the anterior leaflet will show greatly exaggerated motion in its opening. The increased left ventricular output is associated with enhanced systolic motion of the interventricular septum and the posterior left ventricular wall. The left atrial dimension remains normal or only slightly increased unless there has been prior disease.

Papillary Muscle Dysfunction

An intact papillary muscle may fail to maintain normal chordal tension during ventricular systole as a result of (1) abnormal papillary muscle contraction, a common occurrence in coronary artery disease; (2) adjacent myocardial wall dysfunction, i.e., infarction or fibrosis; and (3) left ventricular dilatation.

In the case of coronary disease, papillary muscle dysfunction may be intermittent, occurring only during ischemic episodes,[105, 106] or persistent, probably a result of fibrosis of the papillary muscle itself or the adjacent wall of the left ventricle.[107]

While coronary disease is easily the most common cause of papillary muscle dysfunction, other etiologies must be considered when it is detected.[4] For example, congenital malformations of the aortic valve often are associated with papillary muscle dysfunction. Cardiomyopathy, myocardial infiltrative diseases, and endocardial fibroelastosis may cause this syndrome both by direct papillary muscle involvement and by disease of the adjacent left ventricular wall.

Severe left ventricular dilatation, regardless of etiology, causes a displacement of the papillary muscle to a more distant position from the mitral leaflets. This may create undue tension on the chordae and prohibit mitral leaflet coaptation during ventricular systole.[4, 108, 109]

Echocardiographic Features.   When the papillary muscle dysfunction is sufficiently severe, systolic prolapse may be observed.[110] This form of prolapse may be differentiated from myxomatous degeneration in that the leaflets characteristically have normal or reduced opening amplitude.

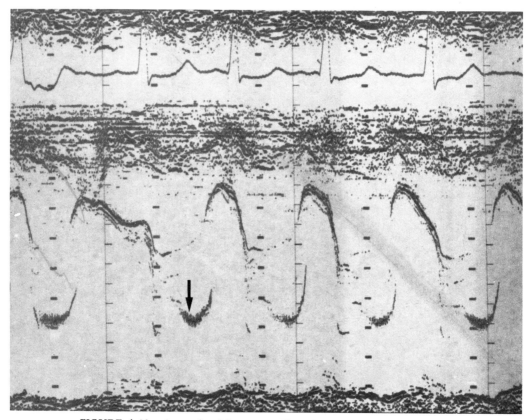

FIGURE 4–30.   Acute chordal rupture. The mitral valve diastolic opening amplitude is increased to 45 mm. During ventricular systole a rapid fluttering motion (arrow) occurs.

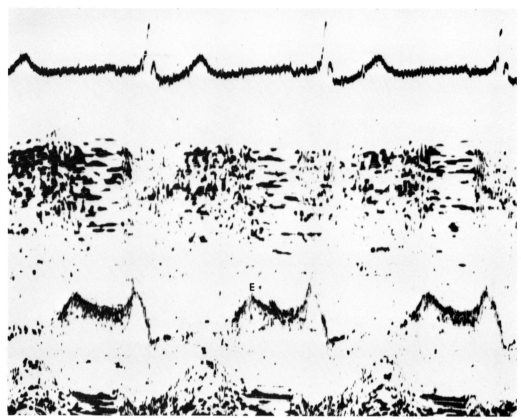

FIGURE 4-31. Papillary muscle dysfunction. The E point of the anterior leaflet is obscure, and there is a fine leaflet fluttering throughout diastole.

Usually the changes in the mitral valve motion are nonspecific and consist of a blunted E point and diastolic leaflet fluttering (Fig. 4-31). The blunted E point is probably related to reduced left ventricular compliance and in some cases to elevated end-systolic pressure in the left ventricle. The diastolic fluttering of the leaflets may be a result of the failure of the chordae to maintain tension when the leaflets are in their open position. When the left ventricle is large, similar fluttering is seen, and in the case of left ventricular failure the typical low-flow "fishmouth" appearance is seen (Fig. 4-32; see also Figs. 8-11 and 8-13).

Differentiation of the leaflet fluttering due to papillary muscle dysfunction from aortic regurgitation is difficult solely on echocardiographic grounds, necessitating other clinical information in most cases. Similar fluttering has also been observed in patients with ventricular septal defects.[111]

MITRAL VALVE VEGETATIONS

One of the prime indications for the performance of echocardiography is suspected or proved arterial embolism. In this condition the echocardiogram may be useful in the detection of left atrial myxoma, unsuspected mitral stenosis with thrombus formation, or mitral leaflet vegetations.

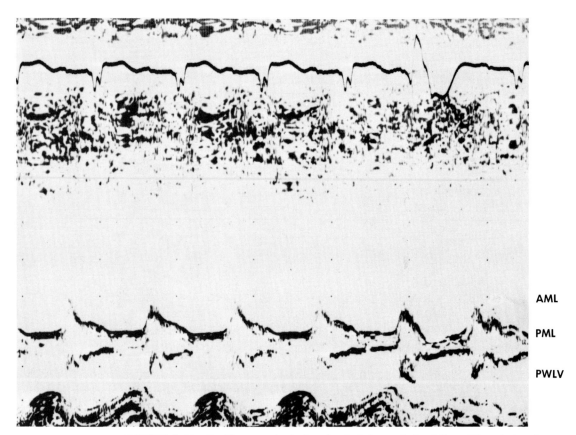

AML

PML

PWLV

FIGURE 4-32. Papillary muscle dysfunction in left ventricular failure. There is fine fluttering of both the anterior and the posterior mitral leaflets, with reduced opening and displacement of the valve from the posterior wall of the enlarged left ventricle (PWLV).

The most common mitral vegetation to result in peripheral embolism is infective endocarditis. This may occur on either the aortic valve or the mitral valve, and in either instance it may be detected echocardiographically.[112] Primary infective endocarditis of the aortic valve, with secondary infection of the mitral valve and resultant mitral insufficiency, may also occur.[113]

In a series of eight cases, Dillon et al. determined that such vegetations must exceed 2 mm in diameter before they can be detected on the echocardiogram.[112] Vegetations appear as shaggy, nonuniform valvular thickening, with no limitation of leaflet motion.

ABNORMALITIES OF THE MITRAL ANNULUS

The Thickened Annulus

Calcification of the mitral ring commonly occurs with increasing age.[114, 115] On postmortem examination, Pomerance found annulus calcification in 8.5 percent of patients over 50 years of age.[116] Calcification was twice as frequent among women as men, and systolic murmurs were present in many prior to death. About one third of these patients also had calcification of the aortic valve.

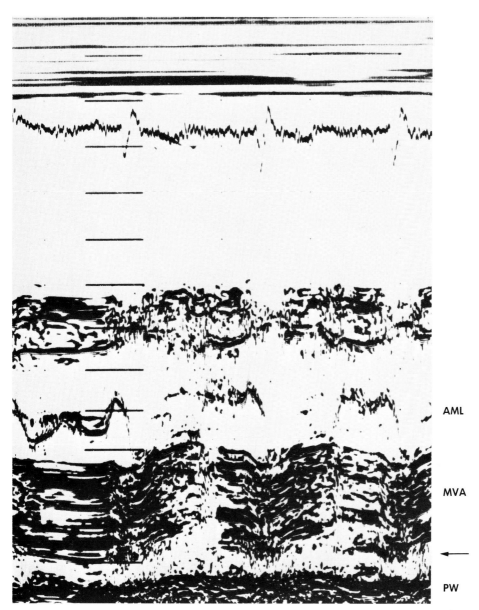

FIGURE 4-33. Calcified mitral annulus (MVA). The annulus measures approximately 25 mm in thickness and creates a false impression of a pericardial effusion (arrow) (AML = anterior mitral leaflet; PW = posterior wall).

The etiology of these changes is unknown. The murmur in the presence of annular calcification has been associated with impingement of calcific spurs upon the posterior mitral leaflet. These spurs project into the left atrium, and when the overlying endocardium becomes ulcerated secondarily, thromboses and infective endocarditis may supervene.[64, 117, 118] The process may also result in conduction abnormalities, presumably as a result of involvement of the bundle of His and the bundle branches, which lie within the interventricular septum at the junction of the mitral cusps.

The mitral annulus normally is only a few millimeters in thickness, and annulus calcification may result in thickening up to several centimeters. The condition may be associated with mitral regurgitation.[119] As has been described in pathologic studies, such thickening is particularly common in elderly persons, and may account for an otherwise unresolved murmur in such patients.[116, 120]

In many cases, the thickened mitral annulus may also account for an abnormal echo paralleling the posterior left atrial wall (see Chapter 6). On the echocardiogram, the calcified annulus may be mistaken for the posterior left ventricular wall, giving the appearance of a pericardial effusion (Fig. 4–33).[120]

Dilatation of the Annulus

Whether the annulus truly dilates under certain conditions is controversial. Bulkley and Roberts have reported that annulus dilatation is sufficient to cause mitral regurgitation only in patients with connective tissue disorders affecting the cardiac fibrous skeleton, such as Marfan's disease.[121] Millward has provided echocardiographic evidence in patients with congestive cardiomyopathy that mitral regurgitation occurs as a result of systolic leaflet separation or prolapse.[108] This has been suggested as indirect evidence that papillary muscle dysfunction rather than annulus dilatation is the cause of mitral regurgitation in these cases.

References

1. Brock RC: The surgical and pathological anatomy of the mitral valve. Br Heart J 14:489–513, 1952.
2. Edwards JE: Pathologic aspects of cardiac valvular insufficiencies. Arch Surg 77:634–649, 1958.
3. Lam JCH, Ranganathan N, Wigle ED, and Silver MD: Morphology of the human mitral valve: I. Chordae tendineae: A new classification. Circulation 41:449–458, 1970.
4. Roberts WC, and Cohen LS: Left ventricular papillary muscles: Description of the normal and a survey of conditions causing them to be abnormal. Circulation 46:138–154, 1972.
5. Kerber RE: Errors in performance and interpretation of echocardiograms. J Clin Ultrasound 1:330–343, 1971.
6. Pohost GM, Dinsmore RE, Rubenstein JJ, O'Keefe DD, Grantham RN, Scully HE, Beierholm EA, Frederiksen JW, Wiesfeldt ML, and Daggett WM: The echocardiogram of the anterior leaflet of the mitral valve: Correlation with hemodynamic and cineroentgenographic studies in dogs. Circulation 51:88–97, 1975.
7. Rubenstein JJ, Pohost GM, Dinsmore RE, and Harthorne JW: The echocardiographic determination of mitral valve opening and closure: Correlation with hemodynamic studies in man. Circulation 51:98–103, 1975.
8. Zaky A, Steinmetz E, and Feigenbaum H: Role of atrium in closure of mitral valve in man. Am J Physiol 217:1652–1659, 1969.
9. Bonanno JA, Lies JE, DeMaria A, and Mason DT: Origin of the first heart sound: Its relation to mitral and aortic valve mechanics assessed by echocardiography (Abstr). Circulation (Suppl IV) 7,8:147, 1973.
10. Parisi AF, and Milton BG: Relation of mitral valve closure to the first heart sound in man: Echocardiographic and phonocardiographic assessment. Am J Cardiol 32:779–782, 1973.
11. Zaky A, Nasser WK, and Feigenbaum H: A study of mitral valve action recorded by reflected ultrasound and its application in the diagnosis of mitral stenosis. Circulation 37:789–799, 1968.
12. Stanton PN, Sewell HD Jr., Fisher RD, and Morrow AG: The influence of atrial contraction and mitral valve mechanics on ventricular filling. Am Heart J 77:784–791, 1969.

13. Edler I, Gustafson A, Karlefors T, and Christensson B: Ultrasoundcardiography. Acta Med Scand *170*: (Suppl) 370:1, 1961.

14. Gabor GE, and Winsberg F: Motion of mitral valves in cardiac arrythmias (sic): Ultrasonic cardiographic study. Invest Radiol *5*:355–360, 1970.

15. Zaky A, Grabhorn L, and Feigenbaum H: Movement of the mitral ring: A study in ultrasound cardiography. Cardiovasc Res *1*:121–131, 1967.

16. Chakhorn SA, Siggers DC, Wharton CFP, and Deuchar DC: Study of normal and abnormal movements of mitral valve ring using reflected ultrasound. Br Heart J *34*:480–486, 1972.

17. Dayem MKA, Oakley CM, Preger L, and Steiner RE: Movements of the mitral valve annulus. Cardiovasc Res *1*:116–120, 1967.

18. Ferencz C, Johnson AL, and Wiglesworth FW: Congenital mitral stenosis. Circulation *9*:161–179, 1954.

19. Friedberg CK: Diseases of the Heart. Philadelphia, W. B. Saunders Company, 1966.

20. Selzer A, and Cohn KE: Natural history of mitral stenosis: A review. Circulation *45*:878–890, 1972.

21. Dexter L: Physiologic changes in mitral stenosis. N Engl J Med *254*:829–830, 1956.

22. Duchak JM Jr., Chang S, and Feigenbaum H: The posterior mitral valve echo and the echocardiographic diagnosis of mitral stenosis. Am J Cardiol *29*:628–632, 1972.

23. Joyner CR Jr., Reid JM, and Bond JP: Reflected ultrasound in the assessment of mitral valve disease. Circulation *27*:503–511, 1963.

24. Segal BL, Likoff W, and Kingsley B: Echocardiography: Clinical application in mitral stenosis. JAMA *195*:99–104, 1966.

25. Gustafson A: The correlation between ultrasoundcardiography, hemodynamics and surgical findings in mitral stenosis. Am J Cardiol *19*:32, 1967.

26. McLaurin LP, Gibson TC, Waider W, Grossman W, and Craige E: An appraisal of mitral valve echocardiograms mimicking mitral stenosis in conditions with right ventricular pressure overload. Circulation *43*:801–809, 1973.

27. Wharton CFP, and Bescos LL: Mitral valve movement: A study using an ultrasound technique. Br Heart J *32*:344–349, 1970.

28. DeMaria AN, King JF, Bogren HG, Lies JE, and Mason DT: The variable spectrum of echocardiographic manifestations of the mitral valve prolapse syndrome. Circulation *50*:33–41, 1974.

29. Effert S: Pre- and postoperative evaluation of mitral stenosis by ultrasound. Am J Cardiol *19*:59–65, 1967.

30. Winters WL, Riccetto A, Gimenez J, McDonough M, and Soulen R: Reflected ultrasound as a diagnostic instrument in study of mitral valve disease. Br Heart J *29*:788–800, 1967.

31. Edler I: Ultrasoundcardiography in mitral valve stenosis. Am J Cardiol *19*:18–31, 1967.

32. Cope GD, Kisslo JA, Johnson ML, and Behar VS: A reassessment of the echocardiogram in mitral stenosis. Circulation *52*:664–670, 1975.

33. Friedman NJ: Echocardiographic studies of mitral valve motion. Genesis of the opening snap in mitral stenosis. Am Heart J *80*:177–187, 1970.

34. Oriol A, Palmer WH, Nakhjavan F, and McGregor M: Prediction of left atrial pressure from the second sound–opening snap interval. Am J Cardiol *16*:184–188, 1965.

35. Levisman JA, Abbasi AS, and Pearce ML: Posterior mitral leaflet motion in mitral stenosis. Circulation *51*:511–514, 1975.

36. Flaherty JT, Livengood S, and Fortuin NJ: Atypical posterior leaflet motion in echocardiogram in mitral stenosis. Am J Cardiol *35*:675–678, 1975.

37. Wynn A: Gross calcification of the mitral valve. Br Heart J *15*:214–220, 1953.

38. ten Cate FJ, Kloster FE, van Dorp WG, Meester GT, and Roelandt J: Dimensions and volumes of left atrium and ventricle determined by single beam echocardiography. Br Heart J *36*:737–746, 1974.

39. Jordan RA, Scheifley CH, and Edwards JE: Mural thrombosis and arterial embolism in mitral stenosis: A clinico-pathologic study of fifty-one cases. Circulation *3*:363–367, 1951.

40. Kasalicky H, Hurych J, Widinský J, Dejdar R, Metyš R, and Staněk V: Left heart haemodynamics at rest and during exercise in patients with mitral stenosis. Br Heart J *30*:188–195, 1968.

41. Heller SJ, and Carleton RA: Abnormal left ventricular contraction in patients with mitral stenosis. Circulation *42*:1099–1110, 1970.

42. Curry GC, Elliott LP, and Ramsey HW: Quantitative left ventricular angiocardiographic findings in mitral stenosis: Detailed analysis of the anterolateral wall of the left ventricle. Am J Cardiol *29*:621–627, 1972.

43. Lewis BM, Gorlin R, Houssay HE, Haynes FW, and Dexter L: Clinical and physiological correlations in patients with mitral stenosis. V. Am Heart J *44*:2–26, 1952.

44. Segal BL, Likoff W, and Kaspar AJ: "Silent" rheumatic aortic regurgitation. Am J Cardiol *14*:628–632, 1964.

45. Zitnick RS, Piemme TE, Messer RS, et al.: The masking of aortic stenosis by mitral stenosis. Am Heart J *69*:22–30, 1965.

46. Joyner CR Jr., Hey EB Jr., Johnson J, and Reid JM: Reflected ultrasound in the diagnosis of tricuspid stenosis. Am J Cardiol *19*:69–73, 1967.

47. Segal BL, Likoff W, and Kingsley B: Echocardiography: Clinical application in combined mitral stenosis and mitral regurgitation. Am J Cardiol *19*:42–49, 1967.
48. Gramiak R, Nanda NC, and Shah PM: Echocardiographic detection of the pulmonary valve. Radiology *102*:153–157, 1972.
49. Nanda NC, Gramiak R, Robinson TL, and Shah PM: Echocardiographic evaluation of pulmonary hypertension. Circulation *50*:575–581, 1974.
50. Weyman AE, Dillon JC, Feigenbaum H, and Chang S: Echocardiographic patterns of pulmonic valve motion with pulmonary hypertension. Circulation *50*:905–910, 1974.
51. Vlad P: Mitral valve anomalies in children (Editorial). Circulation *43*:465–466, 1971.
52. Lundström N-R: Echocardiography in the diagnosis of congenital mitral stenosis and in evaluation of the results of mitral valvotomy. Circulation *46*:44–54, 1972.
53. Braunwald E: Mitral regurgitation: Physiologic, clinical and surgical consideration. N Engl J Med *281*:425–433, 1969.
54. Steinfeld L, Dimich I, Rappaport H, and Baron M: Late systolic murmur of rheumatic mitral insufficiency. Am J Cardiol *35*:397–401, 1975.
55. Burgess J, Clark R, Kamigaki M, and Cohn K: Echocardiographic findings in different types of mitral regurgitation. Circulation *48*:97–106, 1973.
56. Segal BL, Likoff W, and Kingsley B: Echocardiography: Clinical application in mitral regurgitation. Am J Cardiol *19*:50–58, 1967.
57. Winters WL Jr., Hafer J, and Soloff LA: Abnormal mitral valve motion as demonstrated by the ultrasound technique in apparent pure mitral insufficiency. Am Heart J *77*:196–205, 1969.
58. Johnson ML, Holmes JH, Spangler RD, and Paton BC: Usefulness of echocardiography in patients undergoing mitral valve surgery. J Thorac Cardiovasc Surg *64*:922–934, 1972.
59. Edwards JE: Mitral insufficiency resulting from "overshooting" of leaflets. Circulation *43*:606–612, 1971.
60. Schwartz DC, Kaplan S, and Meyer RA: Mitral valve prolapse in children: Clinical, echocardiographic, and cineangiographic findings in 81 cases (Abstr). Am J Cardiol *35*:169, 1975.
61. Rizzon P, Biasco G, Brindicci G, and Mauro F: Familial syndrome of midsystolic click and late systolic murmur. Br Heart J *35*:245–259, 1973.
62. Read RC, Thal AP, and Wendt VE: Symptomatic valvular myxomatous transformation (the floppy valve syndrome): A possible *forme fruste* of the Marfan syndrome. Circulation *32*:897–910, 1965.
63. Barlow JB, and Bosman CK: Aneurysmal protrusion of the posterior leaflet of the mitral valve: An auscultatory-electrocardiographic syndrome. Am Heart J *71*:166–178, 1966.
64. Pomerance A: Pathology and valvular heart disease. Br Heart J *34*:437–443, 1972.
65. Kern WH, and Tucker BL: Myxoid changes in cardiac valves: Pathologic, clinical, and ultrastructural studies. Am Heart J *84*:294–301, 1972.
66. Behar VS, Whalen RE, and McIntosh HD: The ballooning mitral valve in patients with the "precordial honk" or "whoop." Am J Cardiol *20*:789–795, 1967.
67. Pocock WA, and Barlow JB: Etiology and electrocardiographic features of the billowing posterior mitral leaflet syndrome: Analysis of a further 130 patients with a late systolic murmur or nonejection systolic click. Am J Med *51*:731–739, 1971.
68. Shappell SD, Marshall CE, Brown RE, and Bruce TA: Sudden death and the familial occurrence of mid-systolic click, late systolic murmur syndrome. Circulation *48*:1128–1134, 1973.
69. Weiss AN, Mimbs JW, Ludbrook PA, and Sobel BE: Echocardiographic detection of mitral valve prolapse: Exclusion of false positive diagnosis and determination of inheritance. Circulation *52*:1091–1096, 1975.
70. Fontana ME, Peuce HL, Leighton RF, and Wooley CF: The varying clinical spectrum of the systolic click–late systolic murmur syndrome. Circulation *41*:807–816, 1970.
71. Hutter AM, Dinsmore RE, Willerson JT, and DeSanctis RW: Early systolic clicks due to mitral valve prolapse. Circulation *44*:516–522, 1971.
72. Rizzon P, Biasco G, and Maselli-Campagna G: The praecordial honk. Br Heart J *33*:707–715, 1971.
73. Gooch AS, Vincencio F, Maranhao V, and Goldberg H: Arrhythmias and left ventricular asynergy in the prolapsing mitral leaflet syndrome. Am J Cardiol *29*:611–620, 1972.
74. Jeresaty RM, Landry AB, and Liss JP: "Silent" mitral valve prolapse. Analysis of 32 cases (Abstr). Am J Cardiol *35*:146, 1975.
75. Bon Tempo CP, Ronan JA Jr., deLeon AC Jr., and Twigg HL: Radiographic appearance of the thorax in systolic click–late systolic murmur syndrome. Am J Cardiol *36*:27–31, 1975.
76. Solomon J, Shah PM, and Heinle RA: Thoracic skeletal abnormalities in idiopathic mitral valve prolapse. Am J Cardiol *36*:32–36, 1975.
77. Goodman D, Kimbiris D, and Linhart JW: Chordae tendineae rupture complicating the systolic click–late systolic murmur syndrome. Am J Cardiol *33*:681–684, 1974.
78. Dillon JC, Haine CL, Chang S, and Feigenbaum H: Use of echocardiography in patients with prolapsed mitral valve. Circulation *49*:428, 1974.
79. Pocock WA, and Barlow JB: Postexercise arrhythmias in the billowing posterior mitral leaflet syndrome. Am Heart J *80*:740–745, 1970.

80. Sloman G, Wong M, and Walker J: Arrhythmias on exercise in patients with abnormalities of the posterior leaflet of the mitral valve. Am Heart J *83*:312–317, 1972.

81. Winkle RA, Lopes MG, Fitzgerald JW, Goodman DJ, Schroeder JS, and Harrison DC: Arrhythmias in patients with mitral valve prolapse. Circulation *52*:73–81, 1975.

82. Shappell SD, and Marshall CE: Ballooning posterior leaflet syndrome: Syncope and sudden death. Arch Intern Med *135*:664–667, 1975.

83. Popp RL, Brown OR, Silverman JF, and Harrison DC: Echocardiographic abnormalities in the mitral valve prolapse syndrome. Circulation *49*:428–433, 1974.

84. Shah PM, and Gramiak R: Echocardiographic recognition of mitral valve prolapse (Abstr). Circulation (Suppl III) *42*:45, 1970.

85. Kerber RE, Isaeff CM, and Hancock EW: Echocardiographic patterns in patients with the syndrome of stystolic click and late systolic murmur. N Engl J Med *284*:691–693, 1971.

86. Lewis HP: Midsystolic clicks and coronary heart disease (Editorial). Circulation *44*:493–494, 1971.

87. Spencer WH III, Behar VS, and Orgain ES: Apex cardiogram in patients with prolapsing mitral valve. Am J Cardiol *32*:276–283, 1973.

88. Reinke R, Higgins C, Gosink B, and Leopold G: Significance of mitral valve prolapse (Abstr). Circulation (Suppl III) *49,50*:76, 1974.

89. Winkle RA, Goodman DJ, and Popp RL; Simultaneous echocardiographic-phonocardiographic recordings at rest and during amyl nitrite administration in patients with mitral valve prolapse. Circulation *51*:522–529, 1975.

90. Phillips B, Diethrich EB, Friedewald VE, and Ellis J: Calcified intra-atrial mass detected by M-mode echocardiography and multi-head transducer scanning. A case report. *In* White D (Ed.): Ultrasound in Medicine, New York, Plenum Press, 1975, p. 49.

91. Watts LE, Nomeir AM, and DeMelo RA: Echocardiographic findings in patients with mitral valve prolapse mimicking left atrial tumor (Abstr). *In* White D (Ed.): Ultrasound in Medicine, New York, Plenum Press, 1975, p. 100.

92. Spangler RD, Okin JT, and Blount SG: Echocardiography in connective tissue disorders (CTD) (Abstr). Am J Cardiol *31*:159, 1973.

93. Chandraratna PAN, Lopez JM, Fernandez JJ, and Cohen LS: Diagnosis of tricuspid valve prolapse by echocardiography (Abstr). *In* White D (Ed.): Ultrasound in Medicine, New York, Plenum Press, 1975, p. 97.

94. Jamshidi A, and Klein-Robbenhaar J: Myxomatous transformation of the aortic and mitral valve with subaortic "sail-like" membrane. Am J Med *49*:114–117, 1970.

95. Brown OR, DeMots H, Kloster FE, Roberts A, Menashe VD, and Beals RK: Aortic root dilatation and mitral valve prolapse in Marfan's syndrome. Circulation *52*:651–657, 1975.

96. Hemry DA, Moss AJ, and Jacox RF: Relapsing polychondritis, a "floppy" mitral valve, and migratory polytendonitis. Ann Intern Med *77*:576–580, 1972.

97. Selzer A, Kelly JJ Jr., Vannitamby M, Walker P, Gerbode F, and Kerth WJ: The syndrome of mitral insufficiency due to isolated rupture of the chordae tendineae. Am J Med *43*:822–836, 1967.

98. Sanders CA, Austen GA, Harthorne JW, Dinsmore RE, and Scannell JG: Diagnosis and surgical treatment of mitral regurgitation secondary to ruptured chordae tendineae. N Engl J Med *276*:943–949, 1967.

99. Childress RH, Maroon JC, and Genovese PD: Mitral insufficiency secondary to ruptured chordae tendineae. Ann Intern Med *65*:232–244, 1966.

100. Caves PK, and Paneth M: Acute mitral regurgitation in pregnancy due to ruptured chordae tendineae. Br Heart J *34*:541–544, 1972.

101. Schroeder JS, Stinson EB, Bieber CP, Wexler L, Shumway NE, and Harrison DC: Papillary muscle dysfunction due to non-penetrating chest trauma: Recognition in a potential cardiac donor. Br Heart J *34*:645–647, 1972.

102. Luther RR, and Meyers SN: Acute mitral insufficiency secondary to ruptured chordae tendineae. Arch Intern Med *134*:568–578, 1974.

103. Sweatman T, Selzer A, Kamagaki M, and Cohn K: Echocardiographic diagnosis of mitral regurgitation due to ruptured chordae tendineae. Circulation *46*:580–586, 1972.

104. Giles TD, Burch GE, and Martinez EC: Value of exploratory "scanning" in the echocardiographic diagnosis of ruptured chordae tendineae. Circulation *49*:678–681, 1974.

105. Brody W, and Criley JM: Intermittent severe mitral regurgitation: Hemodynamic studies in a patient with recurrent acute left-sided heart failure. N Engl J Med *283*:673–676, 1970.

106. Cheng TO: Some new observations on the syndrome of papillary muscle dysfunction. Am J Med *47*:924–945, 1969.

107. Burch GE, DePasquale NP, and Phillips JH: Clinical manifestations of papillary muscle dysfunction. Arch Intern Med *112*:112–117, 1963.

108. Millward DK, McLaurin LP, and Craige E: Echocardiographic studies of the mitral valve in patients with congestive cardiomyopathy and mitral regurgitation. Am Heart J *85*:413–421, 1973.

109. DeBusk RF, and Harrison DC; The clinical spectrum of papillary-muscle disease. N Engl J Med *281*:1458–1467, 1969.

110. Machado H, Aranda J, Befeler B, Embi A, and Lazarra R: Mitral valve prolapse and coronary artery disease: Clinical, hemodynamic and angiographic correlations (Abstr). Am J Cardiol *35*:154, 1975.
111. Meyer R, Bloom K, Schwartz D, and Kaplan S: Mitral flutter without aortic incompetence (Abstr). Circulation (Suppl IV) *7,8*:81, 1973.
112. Dillon JC, Feigenbaum H, Konecke LL, Davis RH, and Chang S: Echocardiographic manifestations of valvular vegetations. Am Heart J *86*:698–704, 1973.
113. Edwards JE: Mitral insufficiency secondary to aortic valvular bacterial endocarditis. Circulation *46*:623–626, 1972.
114. Sell S, and Scully RE: Aging changes in the aortic and mitral valves. Histologic and histochemical studies, with observations on the pathogenesis of calcific aortic stenosis and calcification of the mitral annulus. Am J Pathol *46*:345–355, 1965.
115. Korn D, DeSanctis RW, and Sell S: Massive calcification of the mitral annulus: A clinicopathological study of fourteen cases. N Engl J Med *267*:900–909, 1962.
116. Pomerance A: Pathological and clinical study of calcification of the mitral valve ring. J Clin Pathol *23*:354–361, 1970.
117. Burnside JW, and DeSanctis RW: Bacterial endocarditis on calcification of the mitral anulus fibrosus. Ann Intern Med *76*:615–618, 1972.
118. Weinstein L: Case Records of the Massachusetts General Hospital, Case 5–1975. N Engl J Med *292*:255–260, 1975.
119. Burgess J, Clark R, and Kamigaki M: Echocardiographic findings in different types of mitral regurgitation. Circulation *48*:97–106, 1973.
120. Hirschfeld DS, and Emilson BB: Echocardiogram in calcified mitral anulus. Am J Cardiol *36*:354–356, 1975.
121. Bulkley BH, and Roberts WC: Dilatation of the mitral annulus: A rare case of mitral regurgitation. Am J Med *59*:457–463, 1975.

5

The Aortic Valve and Aortic Root

The clinical value of echocardiography in the diagnosis of abnormalities of the aortic valve has been overshadowed by its many other applications. This has been due in part to the difficulties inherent in the recording of the aortic valve leaflets, particularly when they are diseased. It is important to recognize, however, that the aortic root walls are among the easiest structures to record consistently throughout the cardiac cycle and that wall echoes serve as excellent technical landmarks, especially important when the mitral anterior leaflet is not located at the outset of the echocardiographic examination. In the majority of instances, once the walls have been located, the leaflets themselves can be visualized.

Furthermore, the echocardiographic appearance of the left heart structures other than the aortic valve may reveal abnormalities secondary to diseases of the aortic valve and aortic root and sometimes primary concomitant pathologies of these nonaortic structures. This application is most significant in the case of coexisting chronic rheumatic mitral valve disease which might go unnoticed in the presence of known dominant aortic valvular disease.[1] Conversely, disease of the mitral valve can mask coexisting aortic disease as well.[2, 3].

NORMAL ANATOMY

The root of the aorta, also known as the proximal ascending thoracic aorta, is composed of (1) the aortic sinuses of Valsalva, (2) the valve cusps, (3) the coronary artery ostia, (4) the aortic annulus, and (5) the walls of the aorta.[4]

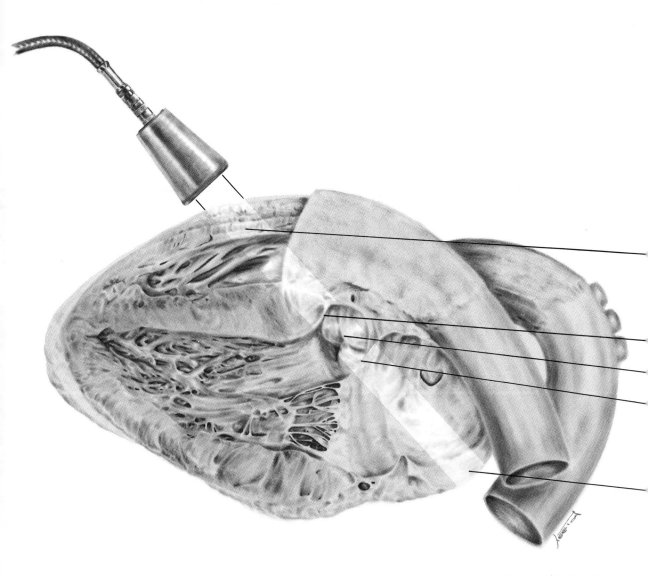

FIGURE 5-1.   Ultrasonic beam through the heart, viewed from the left lateral projection. Key: AWRV = Anterior wall of right ventricle. AAR = Anterior aortic root wall. AV = Aortic valve. PAR = Posterior aortic root wall. PWLA = Posterior wall of left atrium.

The vessel originates approximately at the level of the third costal cartilage behind the left half of the sternum, and it is oriented anteriorly, superiorly, and to the right. This position places its axis perpendicular to the beam of a transducer placed at the fourth intercostal space and angled slightly superiorly and medially (Fig. 5–1). The entire ascending aorta is about 5 cm in length, but in most cases only the most proximal portion is recorded by ultrasound.

Immediately anterior to the aortic root is the pulmonary outflow tract (*conus arteriosus*). Posterior to the aorta is the chamber of the left atrium. The right atrium is to the right of the aortic root and the pulmonary trunk is to the left.

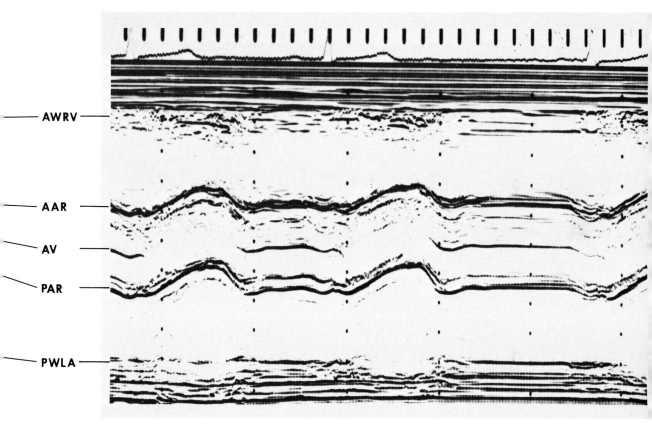

AWRV

AAR

AV

PAR

PWLA

FIGURE 5-1. Continued.

The aortic valve is composed of three semilunar leaflets attached to the annulus: the left coronary cusp, situated laterally and somewhat anteriorly within the aortic root; the right coronary cusp, located anteriorly and slightly to the right; and the noncoronary cusp, which has the posterior position. The left and right cusps lie immediately inferior to the ostia of the left main and right coronary arteries and their respective sinuses of Valsalva. The noncoronary cusp lies below the false sinus.

ECHOCARDIOGRAPHIC FEATURES

To record the aortic root, it is best first to locate the anterior mitral valve leaflet.[4] Once this has been accomplished, the transducer is rotated superiorly

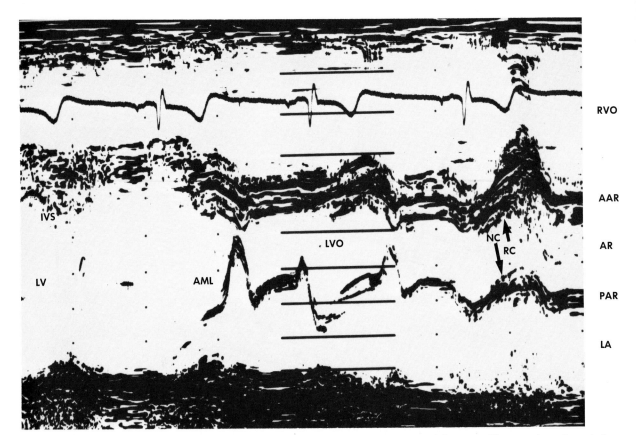

FIGURE 5–2. Scan from the left ventricle to the root of the aorta. The transducer is angled superiorly and medially from the body of the left ventricle (LV), to the left ventricular outflow tract (LVO), to the aortic root (AR). The right coronary (RC) and noncoronary (NC) aortic valve leaflets are also apparent. The anterior mitral valve leaflet (AML) projects into the left ventricular outflow tract and is continuous with the posterior wall of the aorta (PAR). The interventricular septum (IVS) is continuous with the anterior wall (AAR). The right ventricular outflow tract (RVO) lies anterior, and the left atrium (LA) posterior, to the aortic root.

and medially (Fig. 5–2). The mitral leaflet is contiguous with the posterior wall of the aorta root, and the interventricular septum merges into the anterior aortic root wall. (The tricuspid valve, though less often visualized, also is continuous with the anterior aortic wall from its inferior and medial position.) The A-mode appearance of the parallel-moving double echoes of the aortic root is among the most characteristic of all patterns seen on the echocardiogram.

The aortic root can also be visualized from both the suprasternal[5] and the subxiphoid[6] transducer positions.

Aortic Root Walls

The motion of the aortic root is the same as that of the other components of the cardiac skeleton, i.e., anterior in direction during ventricular systole and posterior during diastole (Fig. 5–3).[4] At the time of mitral closure, during the QRS complex of the electrocardiogram, the aortic root wall is maximally posterior, and at that time it begins its anterior excursion, shortly before aortic valve opening. The anterior movement continues during aortic valve opening and after closure, and it does not reverse until after the pressures in the aorta and the left ventricle are equal.[7] The echocardiographic appearance of anterior displacement varies with transducer angulation and is maximal when the beam intersects the aortic root at a 90-degree angle. The degree of anterior motion during systole also appears to be influenced by the stroke volume of the left ventricle. Posterior movement occurs at a rate approximately equal to the anterior rate until mid-diastole, when no motion is apparent. Coincident with the beginning of the P wave of the electrocardiogram, there occurs a posterior motion that coincides with left atrial systole. The cycle is then repeated.

The characteristic motion of the aortic root is probably a result of a multiplicity of interacting events effected principally by the activity of the contractile structures of the heart.[4] Myocardial fibers of the four cardiac chambers are attached to the fibrous cardiac skeleton, of which the aortic annulus is an integral part. The anterior motion during systole appears to occur as a result of the counterclockwise twisting motion of the left ventricle, with subsequent anterior displacement of the entire heart and the great vessels; this motion is then reversed with myocardial relaxation. The late-diastolic, small-amplitude posterior motion may occur with contraction of the left atrium.

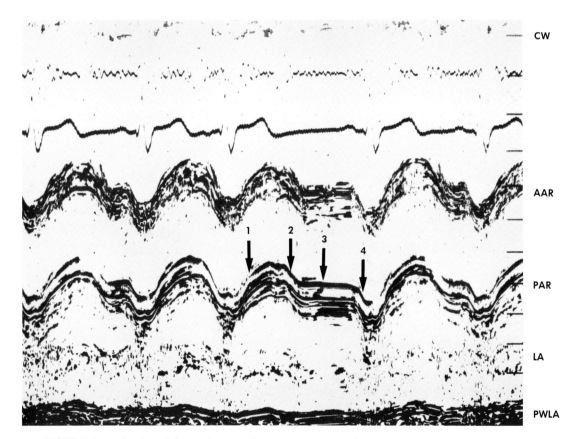

FIGURE 5-3. Motion of the aortic root. The anterior (AAR) and posterior (PAR) aortic root echoes move in parallel, anteriorly in systole (1) and posteriorly following the completion of ventricular systole (2). Depending on the cycle length (compare beat 1 to beat 3 which follows a premature atrial contraction), the position of the aorta remains relatively fixed during diastole (3) until atrial systole, when an abrupt posterior displacement occurs (4) (CW = chest wall; LA = left atrium; PWLA = posterior wall of left atrium).

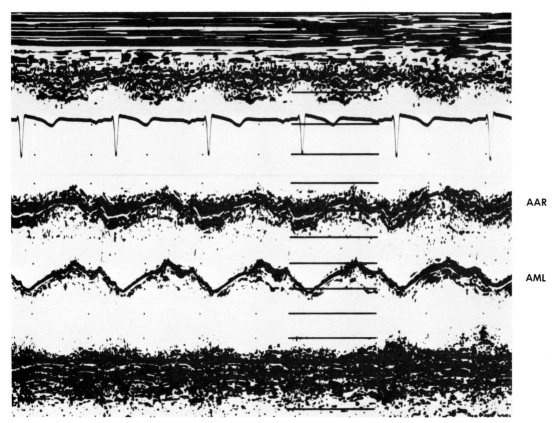

FIGURE 5-4.   As a result of improper positioning of the transducer, the base of the anterior mitral leaflet (AML) may be mistaken for the posterior aortic wall. The transducer has been placed high and angled inferiorly. The anterior leaflet may be identified by its E and A waves. The apparent "root" dimension is narrowed, and the excursion of the anterior wall (AAR) is delayed and diminished in amplitude.

The dimension of the aortic root varies from individual to individual in proportion to body size. In any case, when the echocardiographic recording is made immediately above the fibrous skeleton, the aortic root diameter may be observed to change as a gross function of cardiac output. It must be emphasized that when the echo beam transects the aortic root off-center, the recorded dimension will be significantly smaller than the actual diameter of the structure. This should be considered if the root walls appear unusually thick. If the beam is oriented on the long axis of the aorta, an erroneously large dimension will be recorded. This error, however, is probably less common. Another error is to simulate the echocardiographic appearance of the aorta by placing the transducer too high and directing the beam inferiorly, such that the anterior aortic wall is recorded together with the anterior mitral leaflet. On such a recording, the base of the anterior mitral leaflet may be mistaken for the posterior aortic wall (Fig. 5-4).

Normal values for the aortic root dimension vary with the technique adopted for calculating this measurement. Furthermore, this dimension changes according to the phase of the cardiac cycle in which the recording is made. The largest aortic dimension is recorded at the time of maximal anterior displacement, probably as a result of the transient aortic expansion that occurs in order to accommodate the blood entering from the left ventricle. The narrowest recorded dimension occurs immediately preceding ventricular systole at the commencement of the QRS complex of the electrocardiogram. The latter is the single most reproducible measurement because it is least affected by stroke volume and it is taken at a fixed point in the cardiac cycle with reference to the electrocardiogram.

There is also a dimensional variability according to the portion of the wall echo that is used for measurement. The distance between the anterior edge of the anterior wall and the posterior edge of the posterior wall is probably most often used, although the distance between the anterior edges of both walls is also an accepted parameter.

The thickness of both walls of the aorta can also be determined from the echocardiogram. This measurement is especially useful in the diagnosis of aortic dissection.[9-11]

Aortic Valve Leaflets

During diastole the echoes of the normal aortic valve leaflets are recognized most commonly as a single echo or as a thin band of echoes approxi-

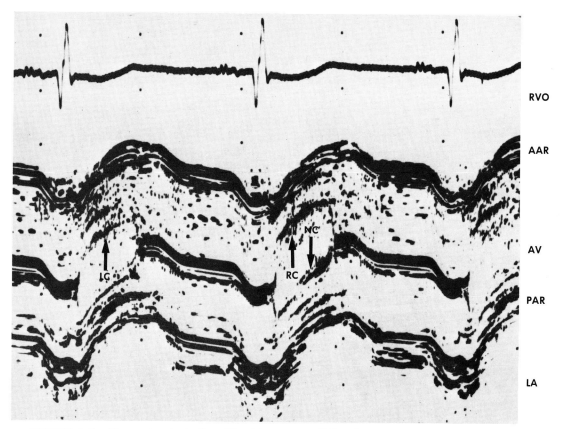

FIGURE 5–5. The aortic valve leaflets. The right coronary (RC) and noncoronary (NC) leaflets are best seen in their fully open position during ventricular systole. The left coronary leaflet (LC) is less distinct. Note that all three leaflets merge approximately in the center of the aorta during diastole, but some separation of the echoes in diastole is a normal finding. During diastole, the motion of the closed leaflets parallels that of the aortic wall (RVO = right ventricular outflow tract; AAR = anterior aortic root wall; AV = aortic valve; PAR = posterior aortic root wall; LA = left atrium).

mately in the center of the root of the aorta (Fig. 5–5). When viewed in systole, an anterior leaflet and a posterior leaflet are each seen as single thin echoes adjacent to and parallel with the aortic walls. With careful machine adjustment and transducer angulation, aortic valve leaflet motion can usually be recorded throughout both systole and diastole. Hernberg and associates[7] demonstrated some portion of aortic leaflet motion in 70 percent of cases in which the mitral valve could be recorded. Nevertheless, aortic leaflet recording is often difficult, primarily because the leaflets present a relatively small target for the ultrasound beam. Furthermore, the aortic valve leaflets are truly perpendicular to the ultrasound beam only when they are fully open. Finally, recalling that the chambers separated by the aortic valve are characterized by rapid, high-pressure changes, the valve leaflets move with great rapidity, which makes their recording difficult during the short opening and closing movements. Aortic valve opening occurs in 20 msec, twice as quickly as mitral and tricuspid valve opening.[7] It is particularly difficult to record the diseased aortic valve, which often shows no discrete leaflet motion because it is calcified and fibrotic. Leaflet retraction due to scarring may compound the problem further. Also, left ventricular dilatation in advanced aortic valve abnormalities may result in cardiac rotation, which causes displacement of the aortic valve from its usual position.[7] Added to these problems is the fact that the structure is a three-leaflet, semilunar valve, and as the leaflets separate during valve opening, even excellent recordings usually show the motion of only two of the leaflets.

When in their closed position during ventricular diastole, the leaflets form roughly a single plane parallel to the ultrasound beam; the result is a thin band of echoes in approximately the center of the aortic root, with motion that parallels that of the aortic walls. With the onset of left ventricular systole, the three leaflets diverge onto three separate planes as the valve opens. The posterior or noncoronary cusp moves away from the ultrasound transducer into a perpendicular position parallel and adjacent to the posterior wall of the ascending aorta.

The opening positions of the right and left coronary cusps relative to the ultrasound beam have been the subject of some controversy. While some investigators have felt that the left coronary cusp moves anteriorly in systole,[7] others maintain that its opening is directed more laterally.[12] The latter assumption is probably true, and as a result the left coronary leaflet is seldom identified because (1) in the open position, the broad plane of this leaflet is parallel to the echo beam; (2) its lateral motion carries the leaflet out of the beam target area; and (3) there is only minimal or absent anterior–posterior (perpendicular) motion relative to the transducer. Consequently, when it is recorded during ventricular systole, the left coronary leaflet appears as a slightly off-center echo within the aorta. The right coronary cusp, however, opens anteriorly and its echo appears adjacent to the anterior aortic wall during systole.

Although in some cases all three leaflets may be recorded simultaneously, only one of the three (Fig. 5–6) or any combination of two of the three may be seen in other instances. The right coronary leaflet is the easiest and most frequently recorded, followed by the noncoronary, and then the left coronary.

Following the beginning of the QRS complex of the electrocardiogram, the mitral valve closes and ventricular pressure begins to rise. When the intraventricular pressure exceeds the aortic pressure, the aortic valve leaflets open. The period from the beginning of the QRS complex of the electrocardio-

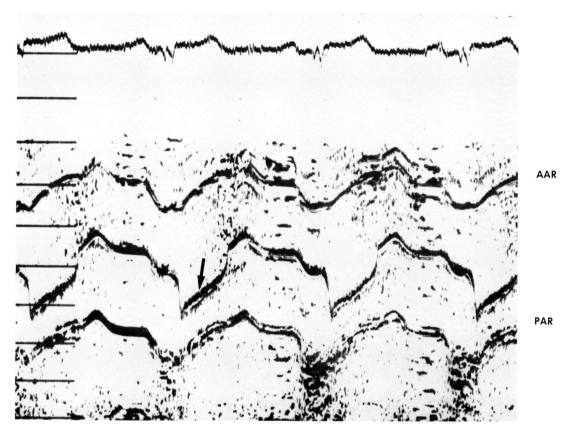

AAR

PAR

FIGURE 5-6. Normal aortic valve. In this example only a strong, posteriorly moving leaflet (arrow) can be seen within the aortic root, and this probably is the noncoronary leaflet. Note that the leaflet motion in diastole parallels that of the aortic walls (AAR = anterior aortic root wall; PAR = posterior aortic root wall).

gram to the opening of the aortic valve is the "pre-ejection period," and the 4 to 8 msec immediately preceding the valve opening, during which both the mitral and the aortic valves are closed, is the "isovolumetric contraction period" of the left ventricle. During this time the aortic root begins its anterior excursion.

As a result of the rapidly rising intraventricular pressure, the aortic valve opens quickly and remains in a fully open position until the intraventricular pressure falls below the pressure within the aorta. While it is open, the separation between the right coronary and posterior leaflets remains constant. (In adults this separation ranges from 1.7 to 2.1 cm.) Normal aortic leaflets may sometimes exhibit fine oscillations during systole (Fig. 5–7). During systolic opening the leaflets continue to move anteriorly in concert with the entire aortic root.

The duration of aortic valve opening, or the left ventricular ejection time, is determined by multiple factors, including the length of time allowed for ventricular filling prior to systole. Among normal persons this is primarily a function of heart rate. This calculation has been shown to have an excellent correlation with similar measurements of systolic time intervals using indirect carotid pulse tracing measurements.[13] As depicted in Figure 5–8, ejection time indices can be determined from the echocardiogram, provided at least one of the aor-

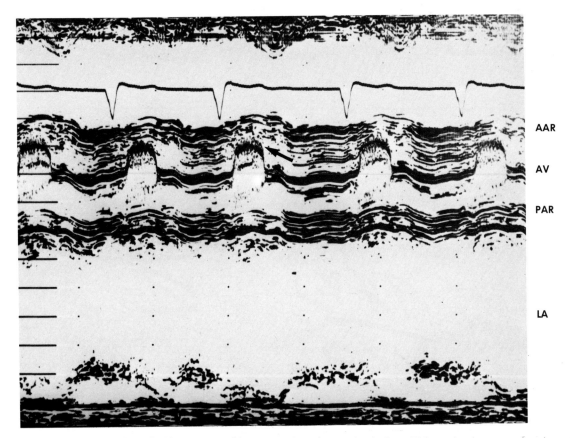

FIGURE 5-7. Sawtooth appearance of aortic valve leaflets. This motion is a normal variant and here is seen best in the right coronary leaflet (arrow). The left atrium (LA) is mildly dilated and the aortic walls are thickened. (AAR = anterior aortic root wall; AV = aortic valve; PAR = posterior aortic root wall).

tic valve leaflets is satisfactorily recorded. Patients with varying R-R intervals, such as occur in atrial fibrillation and premature contractions, will show corresponding variations of ventricular ejection after longer diastolic filling periods (Fig. 5–9). During a premature ventricular contraction, the aortic valve may fail to open at all, or more frequently, it will exhibit only abbreviated opening. The first beat after the premature ventricular contraction will then show a longer ejection time.

Aortic valve closure is rapid and may be difficult to record. It occurs while the aortic root is moving anteriorly. Leaflet closure on the echocardiogram actually precedes the aortic component of the second heart sound by about 10 msec, which suggests that the aortic second sound does not originate from leaflet coaptation.[14-16]

DISEASES OF THE AORTIC VALVE AND AORTIC ROOT

Among persons with aortic valve abnormalities who are beyond the pediatric age, the overwhelming majority have as the etiology either rheumatic

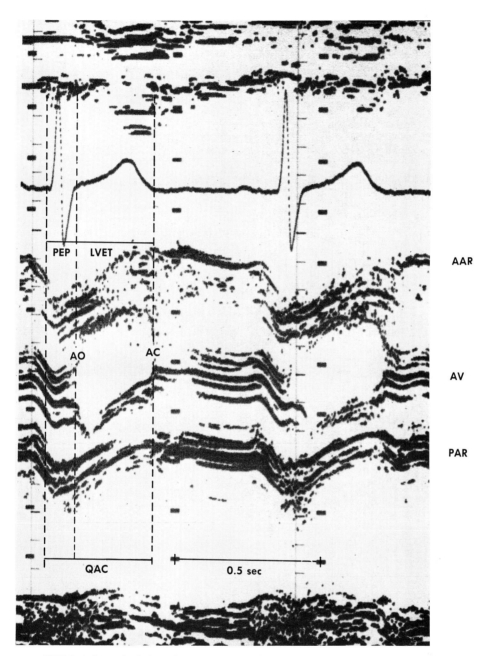

FIGURE 5–8. Calculation of ejection time indices. The interval (QAC) from the beginning of the QRS complex to aortic valve closure (AC) is the time of total electromechanical systole. The pre-ejection period (PEP) is the time from the initiation of electrical systole until aortic valve opening (AO). The left ventricular ejection time (LVET) is the duration of actual ejection from the left ventricle (AAR = anterior aortic root wall; AV = aortic valve; PAR = posterior aortic root wall).

valvulitis or congenital malformation (usually bicuspid aortic valve). Regardless of the etiology, the deformity may result in (1) stenosis of the valve, with increased pressure work imposed on the left ventricle; (2) regurgitation, with increased left ventricular volume loads; or (3) a combination of the two.[31]

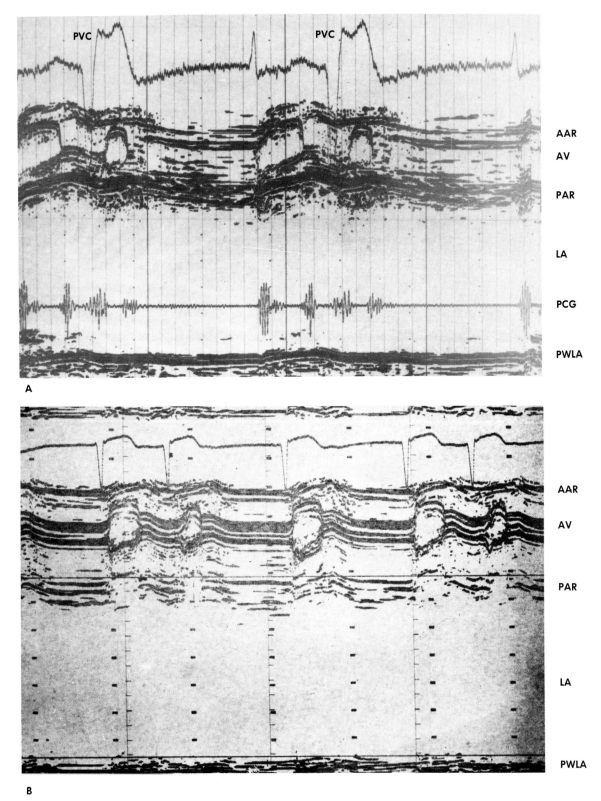

FIGURE 5-9. Effect of varying cardiac cycle intervals on the duration of aortic valve opening. *A*, Premature ventricular contractions (PVC's). The first and third beats have normal aortic valve opening. The second and fourth beats are PVC's with markedly abbreviated duration of opening. *B*, Atrial fibrillation. The aortic valve opening time is proportional to the duration of the previous diastolic period (AAR = anterior aortic root wall; AV = aortic valve; PAR = posterior aortic root wall; LA = left atrium; PCG = phonocardiogram; PWLA = posterior wall of the left atrium).

In addition to abnormalities of the aortic valve leaflets themselves, there are other anatomical derangements that may also affect their performance. A prime example is the valvular incompetence that occurs secondary to aneurysmal dilatation of the ascending aorta. Furthermore, obstruction of the left ventricular ejection of blood into the aorta can occur at sites other than those involving the valves, and the echocardiogram is useful in the differentiation of these abnormal states as well.

Aortic Stenosis

Obstruction to left ventricular outflow is classified according to the site of the anatomical derangement as subvalvular aortic stenosis, valvular aortic stenosis, or supravalvular aortic stenosis.

Subvalvular Aortic Stenosis

At the subvalvular level, stenosis may occur either as a fixed obstruction, usually as a discrete membranous ring, or as the variable obstruction of asymmetric septal hypertrophy (ASH).[17] Because of the importance of echocardiography in the diagnosis of the hypertrophic form of stenosis, it is discussed in depth in Chapter 13.

Membranous subaortic stenosis may not become clinically apparent until adulthood, and clinically it may be difficult to differentiate from valvular and supravalvular stenosis.[18] It is often associated with pulmonic stenosis.

On the echocardiogram the left ventricular outflow tract appears narrowed on the scan from the mitral valve to the aortic root. This abnormal systolic narrowing is seen high in the outflow tract where the mitral valve echo merges into the posterior aortic wall echo, and this area may actually be filled in with echoes.[19] A thin echo considered to be from the subaortic membrane has also been described in one case to move in a manner opposite to that of the mitral valve.[19] In another study involving two cases of membranous subaortic stenosis, a fine echo was also observed, but its motion was similar to that of the mitral valve.[20] The authors attributed the motion of this echo to the fact that the subaortic membrane usually attaches to the anterior mitral leaflet and thus actually resembles the motion of mitral stenosis. There have been additional reports of an abnormal subvalvular echo in such patients.[21–23] Contrasted to the hypertrophic form of obstruction, the ratio of septal–posterobasal left ventricular wall thickness is normal (less than 1.3:1) in patients with membranous subaortic stenosis.

The aortic valve often exhibits an abnormal motion in the presence of membranous subaortic stenosis (Fig. 5–10).[19, 21, 22, 24] The aortic valve leaflets may open rapidly at the onset of systole and then partially close either only transiently or for the remainder of systole.[19, 22, 24] (This is similar to a pattern frequently seen in obstructive asymmetric septal hypertrophy, although with that condition the leaflets characteristically completely reopen in mid- to late-systole.) A variation of this abnormal valve motion involves normal initial separation of the leaflets, but before the full open position is reached, the opening rate slows.[21] The leaflets then proceed to reach full separation, where they

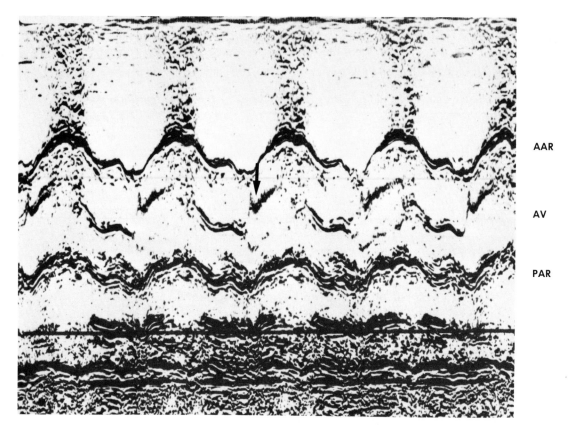

FIGURE 5-10. Aortic valve motion in a case of discrete subaortic stenosis. Normal initial leaflet opening is followed by premature partial closure (arrow) for the duration of ventricular systole (AAR = anterior aortic root wall; AV = aortic valve; PAR = posterior aortic root wall). (Courtesy of M. Johnson, M.D., Duke University Medical Center, Durham, North Carolina. Printed with permission.)

remain for the duration of systole. The valve leaflets may also exhibit a coarse fluttering motion that is much more marked than that normally seen.[22]

The rapid jet of blood onto the aortic valve leaflets subjects them to trauma that may result in leaflet deformity with calcification and fibrosis.[25] A mild degree of aortic insufficiency is common, so mitral valve fluttering is to be expected in some cases.

It is also important to recognize that congenital deformities of the aortic valve leaflets, as well as a variety of other congenital anomalies, are frequent among patients with subvalvular stenosis.[26] Included among these associated anomalies are many that also can be suspected echocardiographically, such as valvular aortic stenosis, pulmonic stenosis, and the hypoplastic left heart syndrome.

Valvular Aortic Stenosis

Valvular aortic stenosis is characterized by a systolic pressure gradient across the aortic valve. While this gradient may range from only a few millimeters of mercury to over 150 mm Hg, symptoms only rarely occur solely as a result of obstruction when the gradient is less than 40 mm Hg.[18]

The most common echocardiographic finding in aortic stenosis is an increased number of echoes from the region of the aortic valve, with the density generally increasing in proportion to the degree of obstruction. These abnormal echoes are due to calcification and fibrosis of the valve leaflets and annulus. The normal aortic valve reflects three or fewer echoes in diastole, and these echoes are less intense than those of the walls of the aorta.[12] In mild aortic stenosis, the number of diastolic echoes is increased (Fig. 5–11), and the valve leaflets lose their thin, delicate appearance. In the absence of significant obstruction, one or both leaflets may appear thickened, with preservation of their normal separation during the period of valve opening. As the severity of stenosis increases, these echoes increase in density until, at the most severe extreme, the entire aortic root is filled with an almost continuous band of echoes paralleling the normal movements of the aorta (Fig. 5–12). The phenomenon of dense aortic root echoes is a remarkably constant finding. Also, when calcium is present in the aortic valve, stronger echoes, denser even than the aortic wall signal, are generally detected.[12] In 162 patients with isolated valvular stenosis, Roberts[27] found at autopsy that 159 had significant calcification of the aortic valve; this was heaviest in the bicuspid and tricuspid valves, but was also present in all patients with the unicommissural type of valvular stenosis. Calcification of the postinflammatory (usually rheumatic) type of aortic stenosis is almost invariably present in afflicted patients over 35 years of age.[28]

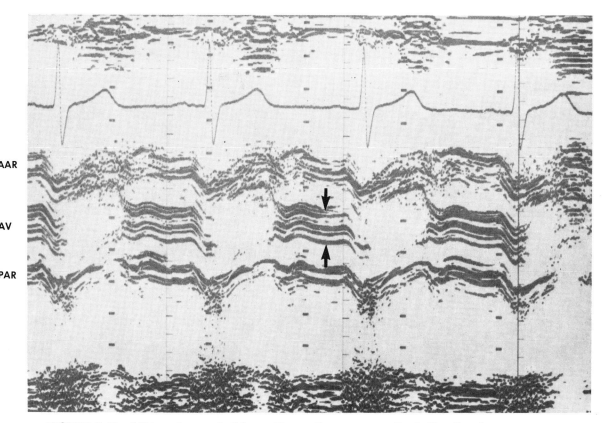

FIGURE 5-11. Mild aortic stenosis (15 mm Hg systolic pressure gradient). The diastolic leaflet echoes (arrows) are increased although systolic leaflet separation appears normal (AAR = anterior aortic root wall; AV = aortic valve; PAR = posterior root wall).

Alteration in the motion of the valve leaflets occurs primarily in the form of restriction of the separation of the leaflets in systole (Fig. 5–13). The normal separation of 1.7 to 2.1 cm varies little among normal adult persons; thus, smaller separation is a significant finding. Yeh et al.[29] have correlated the aortic valve orifice measured on the echocardiogram with the peak systolic gradient and with the hemodynamically estimated valve area in patients with aortic stenosis. The correlation was best when the orifice dimension was smaller than 1.0 cm. From a practical standpoint, precise orifice measurements are very difficult to obtain in high-grade stenosis when one deals with the multitude of echoes recorded in such cases,[12] but the correlation does emphasize the general implication of restricted leaflet separation.

In the mild and moderate forms of aortic stenosis, the diminished leaflet excursion may be equivocal and limited to only one leaflet (Fig. 5–14). This finding is especially suggestive of a bicuspid aortic valve in which the two leaflets are usually of unequal size.[30] As a result, an eccentric location of leaflet echoes is seen, with one leaflet showing only slight systolic opening; the other leaflet may have normal or increased excursion. Typically, the position of the bicuspid leaflets at the time of valvular closure in diastole is also off-center, and multiple echoes caused by valve redundancy as well as calcification and fibrosis are observed during the diastolic phase of the cardiac cycle (Fig. 5–15). As the disease progresses, however, all evidence of distinct leaflet motion may be lost as the

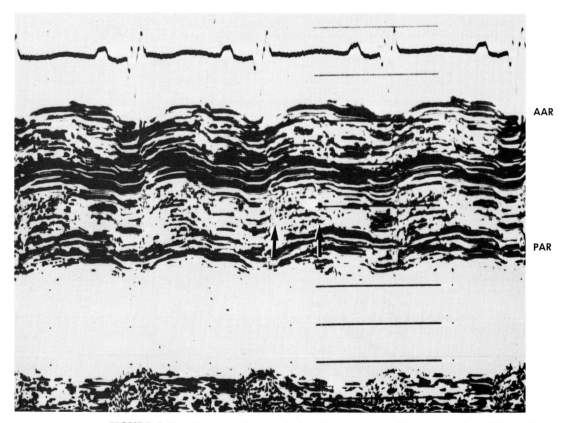

FIGURE 5–12. Severe aortic stenosis (systolic pressure gradient greater than 150 mm Hg). The entire aortic root is a mass of heavy echoes, with only faintly discernible valvular systolic opening and closure (arrows) (AAR = anterior aortic root wall; PAR = posterior aortic root wall).

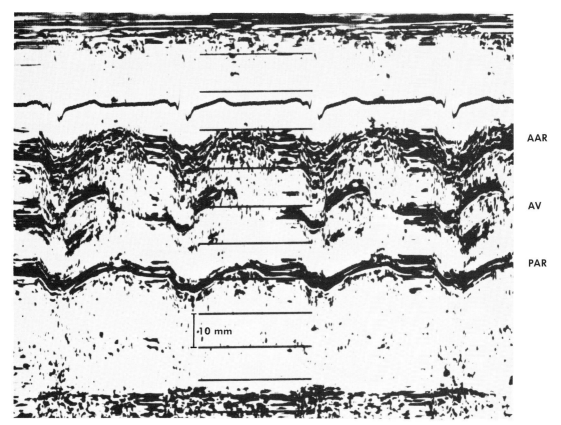

FIGURE 5–13. Moderate aortic stenosis. The leaflets are slightly thickened and are restricted in their systolic separation (arrows) (approximately 10 mm) (AAR = anterior aortic root wall; AV = aortic valve; PAR = posterior aortic root wall).

valve becomes rigid. When this occurs, only an apparent "clearing" of echoes with poorly discernible leaflet echoes may be seen in systole (Figs. 5–16 and 5–17). Ultimately, in the most severe cases, only a solid band of echoes, unchanging from systole to diastole, can be recorded. At this point, the valve commissures have become completely fused. Gramiak and Shah[12] correlated the finding of thick echoes that were unbroken in systole with pressure gradients exceeding 75 mm Hg.

Associated Findings. The etiology of the aortic stenosis may be suggested by careful echocardiographic analysis of the mitral valve. Patients with rheumatic aortic valvular disease usually have disease of the mitral valve as well, whereas the congenital form of the disease only rarely is associated with primary mitral involvement.[27] Mitral rheumatic valve disease (see Chapter 4) is usually manifested as stenosis.

In the case of aortic stenosis without mitral disease, reduction of the EF slope of the mitral valve is often observed. This reduction in slope occurs because the aortic stenosis imposes a greater work load on the left ventricle, resulting eventually in left ventricular hypertrophy and decreased ventricular compliance. For this reason, special care must be taken to avoid mistaking a normal mitral valve with reduced left ventricular compliance for a truly stenotic mitral valve.

A third type of abnormal mitral valve motion found in association with aortic stenosis is aortic regurgitation, which is characterized by high-frequency oscillations of the mitral leaflets. (See "Aortic Regurgitation.")

The characteristic response of the left ventricle to aortic stenosis is hypertrophy of the myocardium, which occurs as ventricular workload increases. The hypertrophy is concentric (as opposed to the left ventricular outflow obstruction of ASH), with both the septum and posterobasal wall proportionately increasing in thickness. Bloom et al.[32] have pointed out that a secondary type of dynamic left ventricular outflow obstruction may also result from the septal hypertrophy. This should be suspected when there is evidence of fixed obstruction (valvular, subvalvular, or supravalvular), concentric hypertrophy, and systolic anterior mitral leaflet motion (SAM). Actual dilatation of the internal dimension of the ventricle does not occur until the point of ventricular failure is reached, unless significant aortic regurgitation is also present.

The interventricular septum may also show abnormal motion. Paradoxical septal movement would be expected in left bundle branch block, a common conduction defect in the presence of aortic stenosis. Another cause of abnormal septal motion is infarction of the septum, which may be due to coronary embolism or coronary atherosclerosis, both of which appear to occur with increased frequency among patients with aortic stenosis.

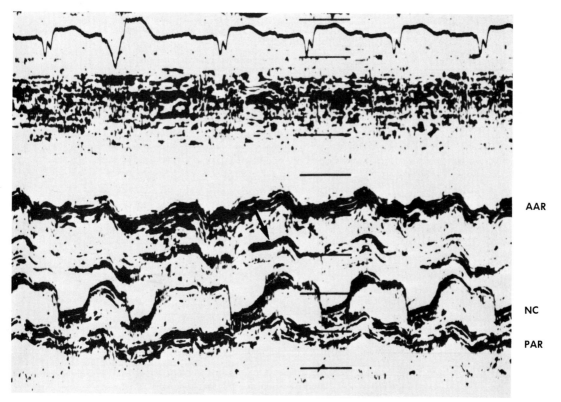

FIGURE 5-14.   Moderate aortic stenosis. The noncoronary leaflet (NC) is thickened and exhibits the only visible systolic leaflet opening. The echo anterior to it (arrow) is from an immobile right coronary leaflet. Note the slightly prolonged valve opening (third beat) after the premature beat and the compensatory pause (AAR = anterior aortic root wall; PAR = posterior aortic root wall).

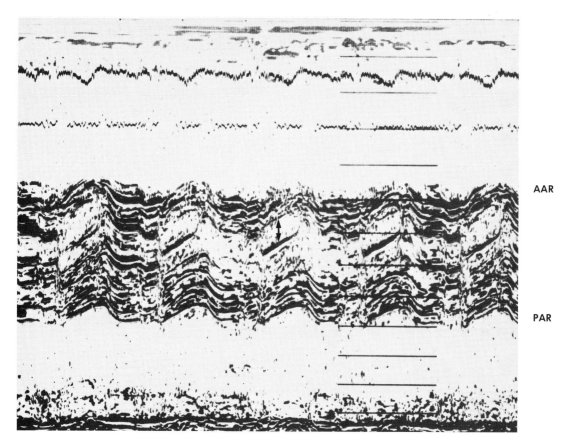

FIGURE 5-15. Congenital aortic stenosis. The aortic valve leaflets (arrows) are eccentrically located within the mass of echoes reflected from the calcium and fibrous tissue (AAR = anterior aortic root wall; PAR = posterior aortic root wall).

Dilatation of the left atrium[33, 34] and right ventricle occurs as left ventricular filling pressure increases, initially as a result of reduced compliance, and later as a consequence of left ventricular failure.

Post-stenotic dilatation of the aortic root may be detected by echocardiography, but frequently it is not apparent because the echo beam does not traverse the aorta high enough above the aortic valve to detect the change. The amplitude of aortic root wall motion and the rate of systolic movement, however, may be diminished in aortic stenosis.[12]

Supravalvular Stenosis

Congenital narrowing of the ascending aorta may be diffuse, as part of the syndrome of aortic atresia and hypoplastic left ventricle, or it may occur in a segmental fashion.[35] To detect supravalvular aortic stenosis, the transducer must scan the aorta superior to the valve.

Bolen and associates[70] have studied six children with supravalvular stenosis and have found that significant narrowing is seen in the ascending aorta as the transducer scans superiorly and medially above the aortic valve. Usher et al.,[37] in a single case of the segmental form of supravalvular stenosis, found narrowing followed by a widening of the aorta above the aortic valve.

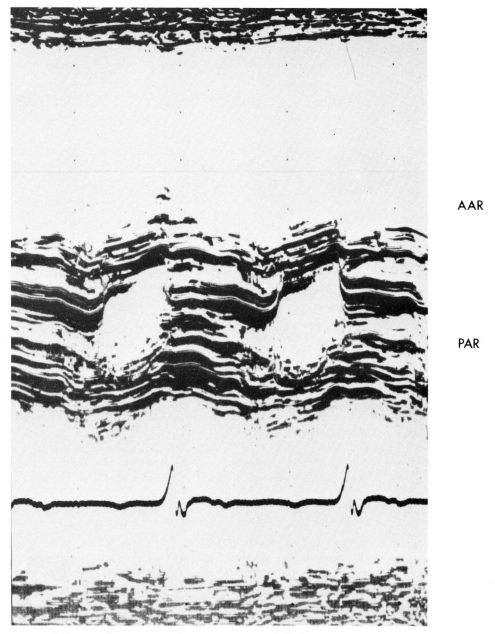

FIGURE 5-16. Severe aortic stenosis. Discernible leaflet separation is present in systole, but the aortic root is filled with echoes during diastole (AAR = anterior aortic root wall; PAR = posterior aortic root wall).

In the diffuse or hypoplastic form of this anomaly, the aorta above the valve is narrowed and may be difficult to record. The left ventricle is often hypoplastic as well, and as a result, a single, anterior ventricle with a single atrioventricular valve and a very small posterior (left ventricular) chamber is recorded.[36]

Among the cardiac abnormalities associated with supravalvular aortic stenosis are adhesions of the aortic valve cusps to the deformed aorta, and pulmonary artery stenosis. In addition, the mitral valve may exhibit prolapse, as it has been noted to be thickened and hooded in a few cases.[38]

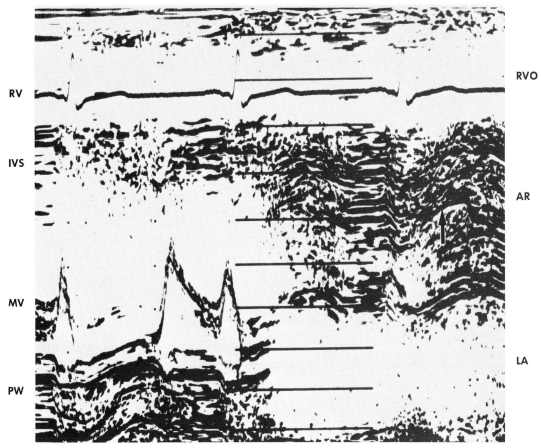

FIGURE 5-17. Sector scan from a normal mitral valve (MV) to a heavily calcified and fibrotic aortic valve. A faint aortic leaflet can be seen in systole (arrow) (RV = right ventricle; IVS = interventricular septum; PW = posterior wall; RVO = right ventricular outflow tract; AR = aortic root; LA = left atrium).

Aortic Regurgitation

Incompetency of the aortic valve may be due to disease of the valve tissue itself (Fig. 5–18) or to pathology of the walls of the ascending aorta (Fig. 5–19).[39] Aortic regurgitation can also be either acute or chronic, with vastly different clinical presentations and echocardiographic patterns, depending on the rapidity of onset.

Chronic Aortic Regurgitation

In all types of aortic insufficiency without significant concomitant stenosis, the aortic valve may appear entirely normal.[12] The valve usually exhibits normal pliability when it can be recorded, but frequently it is not seen at all, leaving an "empty root," sometimes with wall thickening. The difficulty in recording the valve in aortic insufficiency is probably a result of two factors: (1) leaflet retraction, which occurs in the chronic scarring process, and (2) a rotational effect on the aortic root caused by left ventricular dilatation and rotation of the heart itself; this may displace the leaflets from the beam target area. The fail-

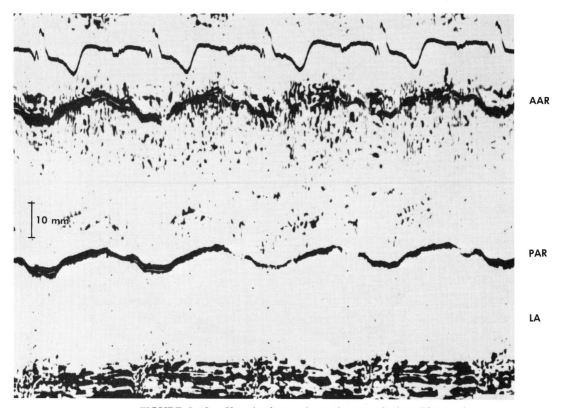

FIGURE 5-18. Chronic rheumatic aortic regurgitation. The aortic root appears "empty" with no definite leaflet echoes seen and is mildly dilated in comparison to the left atrial dimension (AAR = anterior aortic root wall; PAR = posterior aortic root wall; LA = left atrium).

ure of the leaflets to coapt in diastole cannot be diagnosed reliably by the echocardiogram because the broad leaflet surfaces lie in a plane parallel to the echo beam in diastole. Thus, while the leaflet *echoes* may merge, in actual fact the leaflet edges may only be partially coapted. Conversely, distinct separation of the leaflet echoes may be seen in diastole in normal persons. These echoes are reflected from regions of the leaflets removed from the coapting edges, and this finding does not connote aortic regurgitation (see Fig. 5–5).

In addition to rheumatic and congenital valve deformities, other less common causes of aortic regurgitation include valvular infection, excessive valvular tissue, ventricular septal defect, and prolapse of the valve leaflets, which may occur in trauma.[40] Chandraratna and associates[71] have reported a single case of "floppy" aortic valve in which marked diastolic leaflet fluttering was observed. (In rare instances echocardiographic recording of the high left ventricular outflow tract may show one of the aortic valve leaflets to be immediately anterior to the anterior mitral valve leaflets in diastole. This is an unusual finding, however, and does not necessarily imply aortic leaflet prolapse. It can be simulated when the transducer is placed too high and angled inferiorly at the time of mitral valve recording.)

Calcification of the aortic valve in regurgitation alone is unusual, but with combined regurgitation and stenosis, it occurs in almost 75 per cent of cases.[41] Gramiak and Shah[12] found that two of nine patients with pure aortic insuf-

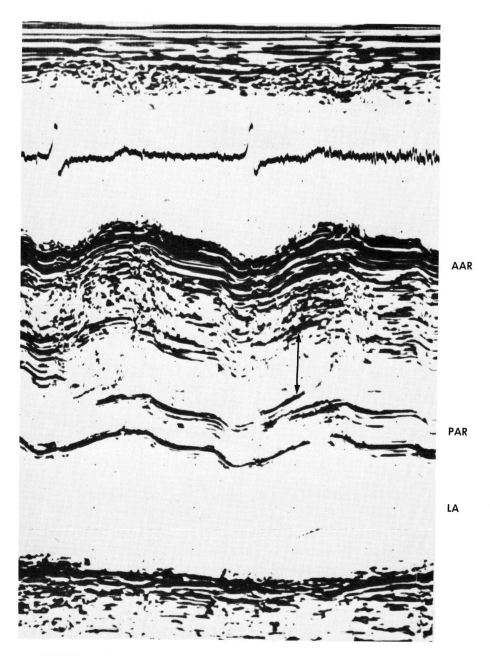

FIGURE 5-19. Aortic regurgitation secondary to luetic aortitis. The aortic walls (AAR, PAR) are thickened, and the aortic dimension is increased in comparison to the left atrial dimension. Faint aortic valve leaflet motion is discernible (arrows) (LA = left atrium).

ficiency had greater echo intensity from the cusps than from the aortic wall, but that seven of nine patients with aortic stenosis and aortic insufficiency (AS-AI) had increased cusp echoes. We have made similar observations in our laboratory, where seven of eleven cases of pure aortic insufficiency were observed to have normal or decreased echoes from the aortic root. In only one case was the number of aortic root echoes considered to be abnormally increased, whereas in seven of eight cases of AS-AI the echoes from within the root were increased in number and intensity. It would appear, therefore, that an increase in echoes

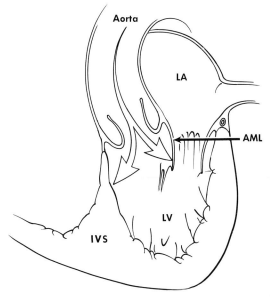

FIGURE 5-20. The regurgitant stream of aortic insufficiency may strike either or both the interventricular septum (IVS) and the mitral valve leaflets. (LA = left atrium; AML = anterior mitral leaflet; LV = left ventricle)

within the aortic root in the presence of aortic insufficiency usually connotes concomitant stenosis and that normal or diminished aortic echoes indicate that stenosis does not accompany the insufficiency.

The aortic root dimension may increase in chronic aortic regurgita-

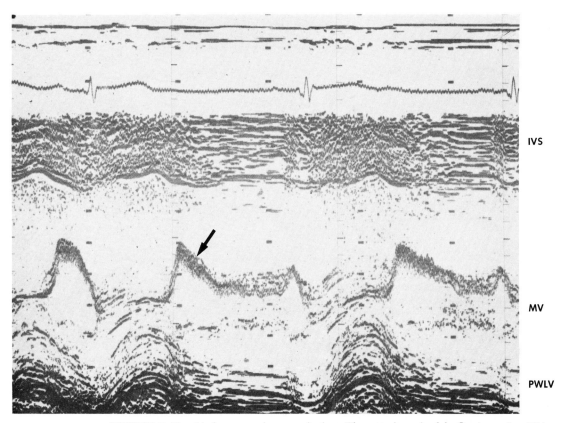

FIGURE 5-21. Moderate aortic regurgitation. The anterior mitral leaflet (arrow) exhibits fine oscillations, but the posterior leaflet is poorly visualized. The interventricular septum (IVS) is hypertrophied (MV = mitral valve; PWLV = posterior wall of the left ventricle).

tion, but this is an inconsistent finding dependent on the technical success with which the supravalvular aorta can be recorded. Gramiak and Shah[12] found the aortic root to be dilated an average of 5 mm from normal in cases of aortic insufficiency. They also found the amplitude of motion to be reduced from normals. Much more severe dilatation may be expected when aortic insufficiency is secondary to aneurysm of the ascending aorta.

Associated Findings.   The regurgitant flow of blood through an incompetent aortic valve may strike either the anterior mitral valve leaflet or the interventricular septum (Fig. 5–20).[42] This results in the phenomenon known as the "jet lesion," which consists of an area of fibrosis on either or both of these structures. High-frequency oscillations of the mitral valve may be detected in many of these patients (Figs. 5–21 to 5–23).[43–45] Winsberg et al.[45] found 11 of 35 patients to exhibit such vibrations, and five additional cases demonstrated equivocal fluttering of the mitral valve. In a series of 29 patients, we found 22 to have mitral valve motion characteristic of aortic regurgitation.

The presence or absence or the degree of mitral fluttering is of no predictive value in the quantification of the regurgitant flow in aortic insufficiency.[46] No doubt this is at least partially because the direction, rather than the severity, of regurgitation dictates whether the flow strikes the mitral valve. Furthermore, it should be noted that these oscillations may also be seen from the posterior leaflet. When mitral stenosis is present, fluttering is less likely to be seen. The

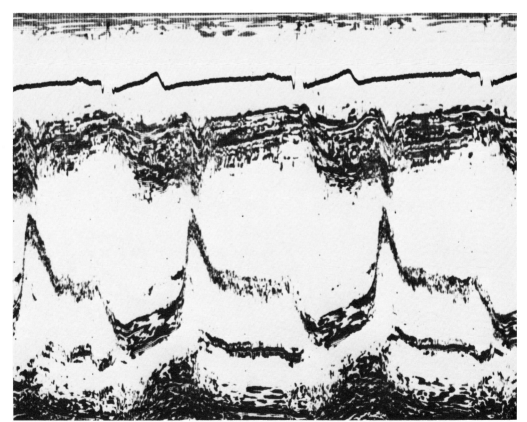

AML

PML

FIGURE 5–22.   Moderate aortic insufficiency with fine anterior (AML) and posterior (PML) mitral leaflet oscillations.

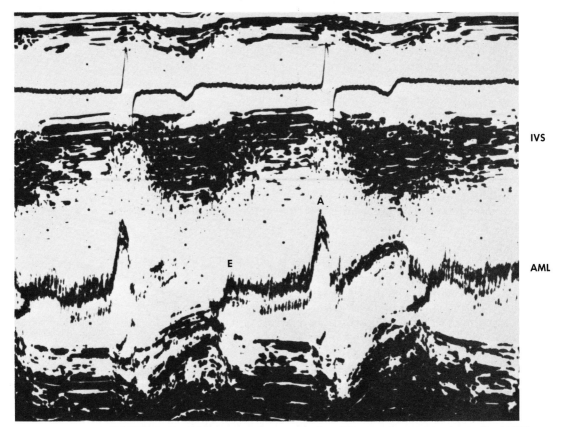

FIGURE 5-23. Moderate aortic regurgitation. The anterior mitral valve leaflet (AML) exhibits marked fluttering, and the E point is blunted; the A wave has become the dominant opening. The septal systolic motion is accentuated.

mitral leaflets also may appear thickened if jet impact has caused fibrosis on the ventricular surface of the anterior leaflet and on the atrial surface of the posterior leaflet.

In aortic insufficiency, the amplitude of mitral valve opening in early diastole (E-wave amplitude) may be reduced (Fig. 5–23) for any of several reasons: (1) the regurgitant flow limits valve opening; (2) the end-systolic volume is increased in severe AI; or (3) the end-systolic pressure may be increased. The possibility of mitral stenosis should also be considered if the opening amplitude is restricted. For the same reasons that the opening amplitude of the mitral valve is reduced and also because the left ventricular ejection time is prolonged in aortic insufficiency, mitral opening may be delayed.

The diastolic closure rate (EF slope) in chronic aortic insufficiency is usually normal or increased.[43] In the event that the E wave is markedly reduced, as in Figure 5–23, the EF slope is not a valid measurement. When the EF slope is reduced, mitral scarring due to rheumatic disease (mitral stenosis) or from the trauma of the regurgitant stream should be suspected (Figs. 5–24 to 5–26). The EF slope of mitral stenosis in the presence of aortic insufficiency is not, however, a good indicator of the degree of stenosis. Other causes of EF-slope reduction include decreased compliance (as with prior or simultaneous aortic stenosis) and increased end-systolic volume of the left ventricle.

The interventricular septum (membranous and high muscular portions) forms one of the borders of the left ventricular outflow tract. When the regurgitant flow of aortic insufficiency is intercepted by the septum, as occurs in about 50 percent of patients in our series, oscillations similar to those of the mitral valve can be recorded (Figs. 5–25 and 5–26).[47] Cope and associates[48] observed septal oscillations in 17 of 46 patients with aortic insufficiency. We have found that these movements are best seen in the upper septum immediately before the peak of the E wave of the mitral valve. They usually continue during most of diastole and bear a striking resemblance to the oscillations of the mitral valve leaflets when the valve and septum are seen together. The presence of septal oscillations does not correlate with the volume of regurgitant flow and is probably determined primarily by the direction of flow. In compensation for the aortic regurgitant flow, the septum also characteristically exhibits an increased amplitude of systolic motion as the stroke volume increases (Figs. 5–23, 5–24, 5–27, and 5–28).

The increased volume imposed on the left ventricle in chronic regurgitation is manifested by dilatation of that chamber many years before actual failure occurs. In general, the degree of left ventricular enlargement correlates with the amount of blood reflux through the incompetent aortic valve. As long

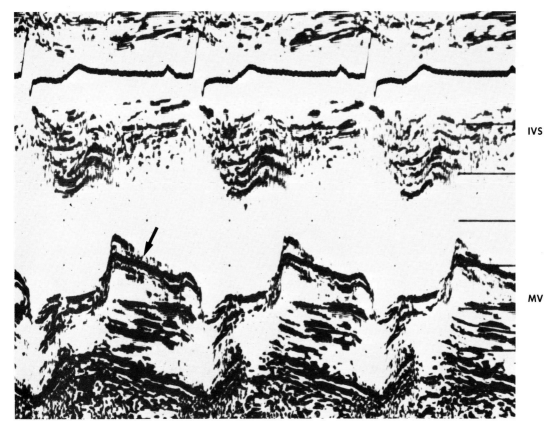

FIGURE 5-24. Severe aortic regurgitation. The mitral EF slope is reduced, with leaflet thickening, but no mitral gradient is present. Aortic insufficiency is suggested by the fine fluttering of the mitral leaflet (arrow). Note also the exaggerated septal (IVS) motion. The thickening of the mitral leaflets could be due to scarring either from previous rheumatic disease or from the chronic trauma imposed by the aortic regurgitant stream (IVS = interventricular septum; MV = mitral valve).

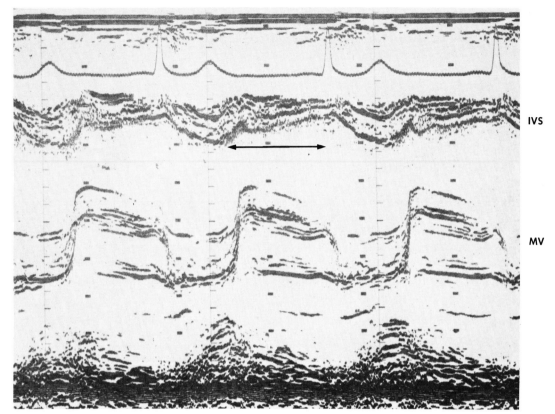

FIGURE 5–25. Moderate aortic regurgitation and mitral stenosis. The mitral EF slope is reduced with leaflet thickening, and exhibits a fine flutter. The interventricular septum (IVS) also has a fine flutter, principally on its left ventricular surface, beginning just before mitral opening and extending until the end of diastole (arrows) (MV = mitral valve).

as the left ventricle remains compensated, the end-diastolic dilatation is disproportionately greater than the systolic volume. This occurs because the end-diastolic volume is equal to that amount of blood regurgitated, plus the effective stroke volume (i.e., the amount delivered to the tissues), plus a small amount of nonejected blood. Provided that the effective cardiac output remains normal, the volume ejected is necessarily equal to the effective cardiac output, plus the amount of regurgitation. This results in an increase in the ejection fraction. In such cases, both septal and posterior wall excursions are usually increased, with normal or slightly reduced mean posterior wall velocity.[49] The mean velocity of circumferential fiber shortening (V_{CF}) is usually reduced in aortic regurgitation, but determinations of left ventricular performance in patients with dilated chambers must be made with caution (see Chapter 8).

In significant aortic insufficiency, the left atrium is usually dilated. We have found, however, that the left atrial dimensions exceeding 3.0 cm per M^2 are usually associated with simultaneous mitral valve disease. Herbert[50] postulates that dilatation of the left atrium, by increasing the fiber length of the atrial musculature, helps to preserve the normal flow from the atrium to the left ventricle, thus sustaining adequate cardiac output.

Quantification of Regurgitant Volume.   Echocardiographic measure of the aortic regurgitant volume has been approached by various investigators.

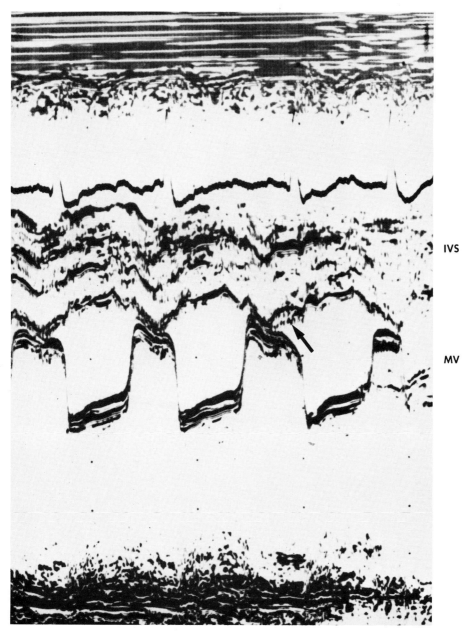

FIGURE 5–26. Aortic stenosis-insufficiency. The mitral EF slope is reduced due to diminished left ventricular compliance, and the mitral valve (MV) is remote from the posterior wall owing to dilatation of the left ventricle. The septum (IVS) is thickened (19 mm) and exhibits a fine diastolic fluttering secondary to the regurgitant flow (arrow).

One method[51] utilizes the difference between the effective cardiac output (which may be determined by the Fick method or by a proposed regression equation using echocardiographic left ventricular volume measurements) and the left ventricular output calculated directly from changes in left ventricular dimensions. The accuracy of this technique diminishes as left ventricular size increases.

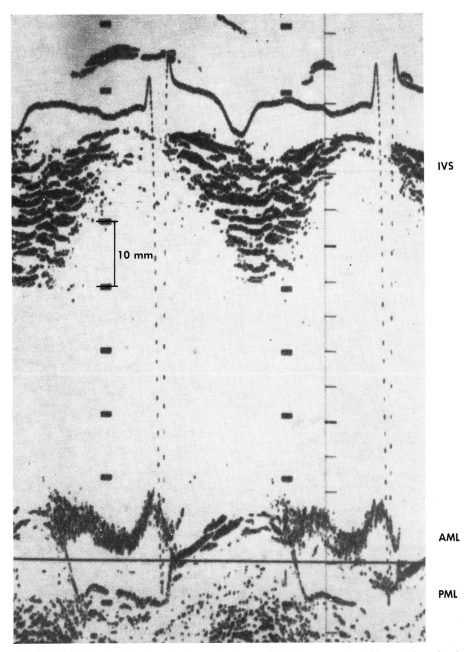

FIGURE 5-27. Aortic regurgitation secondary to dissecting aneurysm. The septal motion is exaggerated with marked fluttering of the anterior mitral leaflet (AML), but the posterior leaflet (PML) shows little fluttering (IVS = interventricular septum).

Another approach utilizes calculation of the difference between the flow across the mitral valve orifice and the flow across the aortic valve orifice, which are normally equal.[49] Again, error in this method results from the overestimation of aortic flow based on the inaccuracies inherent in left ventricular volume estimations taken from the echocardiogram. This method also assumes that the mitral valve is normal and that flow is constant and laminar across that valve; these assumptions will not be valid in every case.

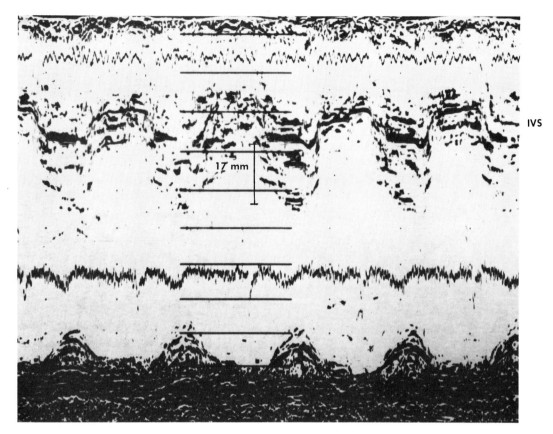

IVS

FIGURE 5-28. Exaggerated septal motion in chronic aortic regurgitation (IVS — interven tricular septum).

Acute Aortic Regurgitation

Acute aortic regurgitation is frequently a genuine medical emergency in which cardiac catheterization is not feasible, and the classic clinical signs of aortic regurgitation are seldom present. Indeed, even the characteristic murmur of aortic insufficiency may be unimpressive. The fact is that acute and chronic forms of aortic insufficiency are two very different pathophysiologic disturbances, the primary distinction being the excellent ability of the left ventricle to accommodate the slowly progressive chronic form and its relative inability to adjust to the acute volume overload.[8, 52, 62]

The most common cause of acute aortic regurgitation is bacterial endocarditis.[8] Of the complications of infective endocarditis involving the aortic valve, acute insufficiency is the most common cause of death. Other causes of acute regurgitation include dissection of the ascending aorta, trauma, and Marfan's disease.[9, 53]

Where there is no prior disease, echocardiographic study of the acutely incompetent aortic valve often does not reveal features to distinguish the abnormal valve from the normal valve. Thickened leaflets due to infective endocarditis[54–56, 67, 68] of a sinus of Valsalva aneurysm into either the right ventricular[57–59] or left ventricular[60] outflow tract, however, should be searched for as causes of acute aortic insufficiency. Aortic dissection may also be detected as a cause.[9-11] When there is pre-existing calcification and fibrosis, the findings sometimes are not distinguishable from those of aortic stenosis. Lee and associates[61] studied four patients with ruptured aortic valve leaflets and found fine linear echoes in the area of the aortic valve leaflets during ventricular systole as well as a band of fine, high-frequency echoes during early- to mid-diastole in the aortic root.

Associated Findings. The mitral valve recording plays an invaluable role in the assessment of acute aortic regurgitation. Normally, mitral closure does not precede the initiation of the QRS complex of the electrocardiogram, as the ventricular pressure does not exceed the atrial pressure until the period of isovolumetric contraction of the left ventricle. (An exception is first-degree heart block, in which early atrial contraction results in atrial emptying early in diastole, with subsequent early mitral valve closure.)

In aortic regurgitation, the left ventricle receives blood from both the atrium and the aorta, with a rapidly expanding volume in early diastole. When the regurgitation is acute, left ventricular compliance is normal, causing the intraventricular pressure to rise rapidly and to exceed left atrial pressure before the initiation of ventricular systole. As a result, the mitral valve closes prematurely (before the beginning of the QRS complex of the electrocardiogram) (Figs. 5–29 and 5–30).[8,43,46,52,53,55,62,63] The premature closure of acute aortic

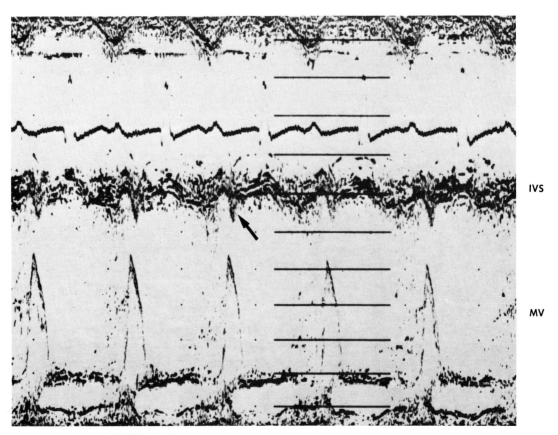

FIGURE 5-29. Acute aortic regurgitation secondary to infective endocarditis. The mitral valve (MV) exhibits a single diastolic opening with marked premature total closure before the onset of the QRS complex of the electrocardiogram. Fine septal (IVS) diastolic oscillations (arrow) are also seen. First-degree heart block is present.

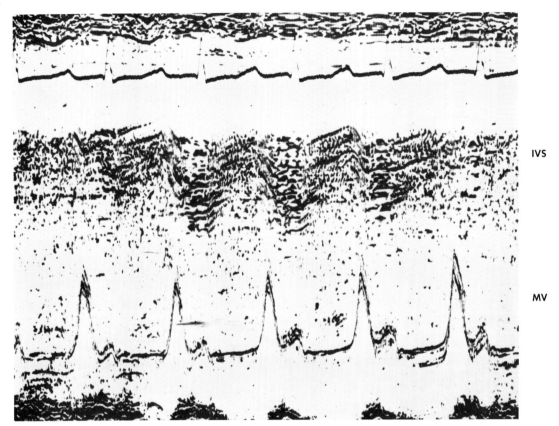

IVS

MV

FIGURE 5–30. Post-valve replacement for acute aortic regurgitation (same patient as Figure 5–29). Despite the persistent first-degree heart block, total mitral closure now occurs at the time of onset of the QRS complex (IVS = interventricular septum; MV = mitral valve).

insufficiency may be absent when there is coexisting mitral stenosis.[46] Amyl nitrite and other vasodilators, by reducing the regurgitant fraction, may also delay the mitral valve closure and have been proposed as a temporary therapeutic intervention in patients with acute aortic insufficiency until surgery can be performed.[46] Clinically, early mitral closure correlates with diminished intensity of the first heart sound.[63] Mann and associates[52] and Wigle and Labrosse[8] found that premature closure of the mitral valve correlated with the degree of elevation of the left ventricular end-diastolic pressure. Contributing further to this early valve closure is the frequent occurrence of first-degree heart block in acute aortic insufficiency. By means of serial recordings, the degree of prematurity of mitral closure may prove to be an objective means of documenting progression of the severity of acute aortic insufficiency.

Early in acute aortic insufficiency, the size of the left ventricle is usually normal or only mildly increased, with progressive dilatation as the disease worsens. It should be emphasized that increasing left ventricular size detected in serial measurements does not necessarily reflect worsening of the disease, but some dilatation should be expected as the ventricle gradually accommodates the extra volume load that is imposed upon it. The amplitudes of septal and posterior wall motions are increased as the stroke volume increases.

Nonobstructive Calcification of the Aortic Root

Degenerative changes accompanied by calcification and fibrosis, progressive with age, are frequent in structures on the left side of the heart, especially the mitral annulus, the mitral valve, and the aortic valve leaflets and annulus.[64] Involvement of the aortic valve usually does not result in significant obstruction of the valve orifice.

This type of calcification is sometimes observed on the echocardiograms of elderly patients in whom systolic murmurs in the area of the aortic outflow tract may be heard (Fig. 5–31). Calcifications in the walls of the ascending aorta and aortic arch are commonly seen on the chest x-rays of these patients. The echoes are more often concentrated near the walls of the aortic root than within the lumen, perhaps as a result of the involvement of the annulus. While discrete leaflet motion may be seen, the mass of echoes sometimes blankets the entire root, obscuring all signs of the leaflets themselves. Often the mitral annulus is thickened, and occasionally the mitral leaflets are similarly affected.

Differentiation of the degenerative type of calcification from calcium deposition secondary to valvular stenosis in some cases may be impossible from echocardiographic features alone. The degenerative type of echoes most often

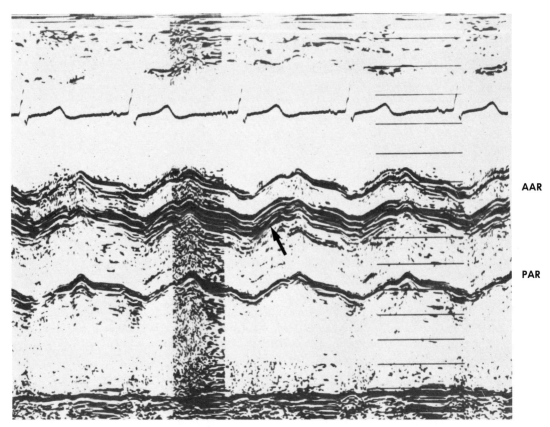

FIGURE 5–31. Nonobstructive aortic root calcification. A heavy mass of echoes (arrow) lies within the aortic root and probably represents calcification and fibrosis of the anterior wall of the ascending aorta (AAR). This appearance may be confused with a dissecting aortic aneurysm except for the fact that the aorta is not dilated (PAR = posterior aortic root wall).

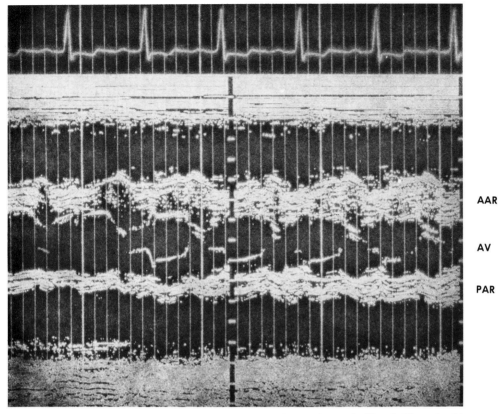

AAR

AV

PAR

FIGURE 5–32. Aneurysm of the ascending aorta. The aortic root is dilated (60 mm), with thickened anterior (20 mm) and posterior (15 mm) walls. (AAR = anterior aortic root wall; PAR = posterior aortic root wall).

cluster near the aortic wall, whereas those of aortic stenosis involve the leaflets themselves.

One note of caution concerning the diagnosis of nonobstructive calcification must be mentioned. If the echo beam is directed to one side of the aortic root, the oblique cut of the beam may produce echoes that suggest an abnormally thick aortic root. This should be considered to be the case when the aortic root dimension appears to be small and especially when the density of the "abnormal" echoes is the same as that of the aortic walls.

Aortic Root Dissection

Acute rupture of the ascending aorta through the intima into the media may occur at any age, but this occurs most often in middle-aged or elderly patients with long-standing hypertension. In these cases the aorta is usually atherosclerotic. Dissection in young persons may occur in the presence of a defective aortic media, such as in Marfan's syndrome and its variants. Brown and associates[65] studied 35 patients with Marfan's syndrome and found 21 to have aortic root dilatation. Acute dissection most often presents as severe chest pain, which may be identical to that experienced in an acute myocardial infarction. The consequences of acute dissection include (1) rupture, usually into the pericardium and resulting in tamponade; (2) obstruction of flow into branches of the aorta, including the coronary arteries and the arch vessels; and (3) acute aortic regurgitation.

Echocardiographic recording of the aortic root in acute dissection is characterized by significant thickening of either or both the anterior and posterior aortic root walls (Fig. 5–32).[9–11,66] A space, either echo-free or containing fine echoes, may be observed within either wall (Fig. 5–33). When the aortic leaflets are recorded, they do not extend beyond the inner wall echo. Another feature is a widening of the dimension of the aortic root, usually exceeding 42 mm[9,10] and in one case, as large as 70 mm.[11] Occasionally, the aortic root of patients without dissection will show a double anterior or posterior wall echo, but the mean aortic root dimension will be normal (Fig. 5–31). Another potential error is the misidentification of the posterior wall of the left atrium as the outer wall of the aortic root. This erroneous finding may be distinguished from a true dissection because the posterior atrial wall does not move in parallel with the aortic wall. When the mitral annulus echo appears within the left atrium, it too must not be mistaken for the posterior aortic wall (Fig. 5–34).

Other echocardiographic abnormalities may occur as a result of the as-

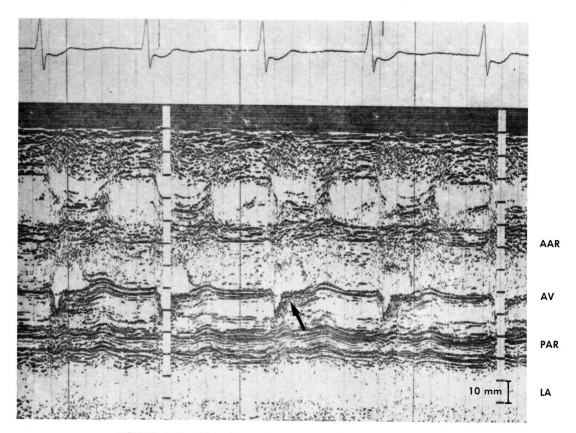

FIGURE 5–33. Dissecting aortic aneurysm. The aortic root is dilated (60 mm) with a double posterior wall (PAR) echo due to the dissection. Note that the aortic valve (AV) noncoronary leaflet (arrow) does not open beyond the inner posterior wall echo and exhibits an abnormal motion of early systolic closure (AAR = anterior aortic root; LA = left atrium).

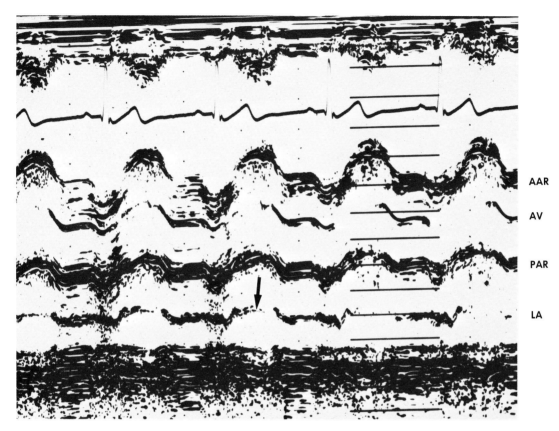

AAR

AV

PAR

LA

FIGURE 5-34. Normal aortic root. The echo (arrow) within the left atrium (LA) is probably the mitral annulus and should not be mistaken for the posterior aortic root wall (PAR), for this would give the appearance of aortic dissection (AAR = anterior aortic root wall; AV = aortic valve).

sociated aortic regurgitation. These include fluttering of the mitral valve and septum, or premature mitral closure in the acute stage. Also, when the dissection ruptures into the pericardium, the echocardiographic features of hemopericardium may be observed (see Chapter 12). A case of rupture of a dissecting aneurysm into the right atrium has been described in which the echocardiogram exhibited the typical features of aortic dissection.[65]

Sinus of Valsalva Aneurysm

Johnson et al.[24] described three cases of rupture of an aneurysm of the right sinus of Valsalva. These were characterized by abnormal early closure of the right coronary cusp, followed by reopening in late systole, with a normal motion of the noncoronary cusp. A single case of sinus of Valsalva aneurysm was reported by Cooperberg and associates[58] in which the right coronary cusp appeared to prolapse through the sinus of Valsalva into the right ventricular outflow tract (Fig. 5-35). An abnormal echo thought to be from the aneurysmal sac was seen in front of the cusp.

A single case of rupture of a right sinus of Valsalva aneurysm into the right atrium was reported by Weyman et al.[57] In this case the aneurysm appeared within the right atrium as a dense mass that prolapsed through the tricuspid orifice during diastole. These authors also noted premature pulmonic valve opening in diastole, a finding regarded as consistent with a communication from the aorta to the right side of the heart. Diastolic fluttering of the anterior mitral valve leaflet also occurred as a consequence of regurgitation.

Whereas most aneurysms of the sinus of Valsalva extend into the right heart, Rothbaum et al.[60] have documented a case in which an aneurysm appeared as an echo mass extending from the aortic root into the left ventricle near the interventricular septum.

Aortic Valve Endocarditis

Dense thickenings of the normally thin aortic cusps are highly suggestive of infective vegetations (Fig. 5–36). [54, 67, 68] This possibility should be particularly

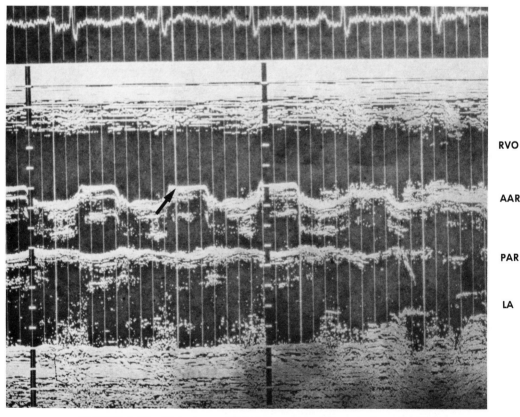

RVO

AAR

PAR

LA

FIGURE 5-35.   Right sinus of Valsalva aneurysm. The anterior wall of the aorta (arrow) exhibits a distinctive motion that resembles valve leaflet motion projecting into the right ventricular outflow tract (RVO) (AAR = anterior aortic wall; PAR = posterior aortic wall; LA = left atrium).

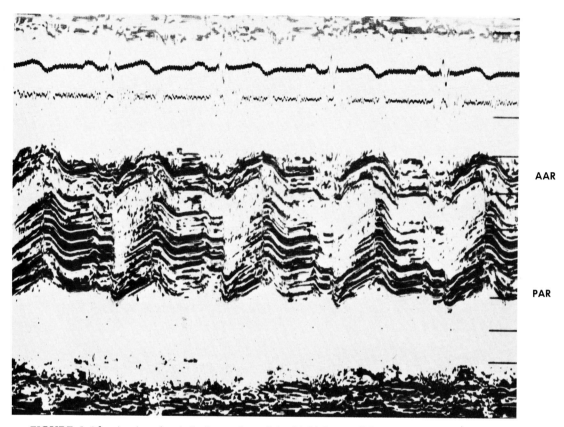

AAR

PAR

FIGURE 5-36. Aortic valve infective endocarditis. Multiple parallel echoes are evident around the valve leaflets, but systolic separation of the valve cusps is normal (AAR = anterior aortic root wall; PAR = posterior aortic wall).

suspected when valve pliability appears normal in spite of very thick leaflet echoes. Gottlieb et al.[54] found that two patients with proven infective endocarditis had dense, highly mobile echo masses within the aortic root in diastole. In four patients in their study, premature mitral valve closure suggested acute aortic regurgitation as well. Hirschfeld and Schiller[56] found that echocardiographic evidence of leaflet thickening in aortic valve endocarditis correlated with the presence of anatomically proven vegetations exceeding 5 mm in diameter. Wray[69] reported a case of bacterial endocarditis in which flail aortic valve leaflets appeared as a disorganized echo mass in the left ventricular outflow tract during ventricular systole.

References

1. Loew DE, Harken DE, and Ellis LB: Valvular heart disease: Undiagnosed valvular involvement, concomitant coronary artery disease and systemic embolization. Am J Cardiol *30*:222–228, 1972.
2. Zitnick RS, Piemme TE, Messer RJ, et al.: The masking of aortic stenosis by mitral stenosis. Am Heart J *69*:22–30, 1965.

3. Segal BL, Likoff W, and Kaspar AJ: "Silent" rheumatic aortic regurgitation. Am J Cardiol 14:628–632, 1964.

4. Gramiak R, and Shah PM: Echocardiography of the aortic root. Invest Radiol 3:356–366, 1968.

5. Goldberg BB: Suprasternal ultrasonography. JAMA 215:245–250, 1971.

6. Chang S, and Feigenbaum H: Subxiphoid echocardiography. J Clin Ultrasound 1:14–20, 1973.

7. Hernberg J, Weiss B, and Keegan A: The ultrasonic recording of aortic valve motion. Radiology 94:361–368, 1970.

8. Wigle ED, and Labrosse CJ: Sudden, severe aortic insufficiency. Circulation 32:708–720, 1965.

9. Nanda NC, Gramiak R, and Shah PM: Diagnosis of aortic root dissection by echocardiography. Circulation 48:506–513, 1973.

10. Moothart RW, Spangler RD, and Blount SG, Jr.: Echocardiography in aortic root dissection and dilatation. Am J Cardiol 36:11–16, 1975.

11. Brown OR, Popp RL, and Kloster FE: Echocardiographic criteria for aortic root dissection. Am J Cardiol 36:17–20, 1975.

12. Gramiak R, and Shah PM: Echocardiography of the normal and diseased aortic valve. Radiology 96:1–8, 1970.

13. Vredevoe LA, Creekmore SP, and Schiller NB: The measurement of systolic time intervals by echocardiography. J Clin Ultrasound 2:99–104, 1974.

14. Anastassiades PC, Quinones MA, Gaasch WH, et al.: Relation of aortic valve closure to the second heart sound: Echocardiographic and phonocardiographic assessment (Abstr). Circulation (Suppl III) 49,50:85, 1974.

15. Chandraratna PAN, Lopez JM, and Cohen LS: Echocardiographic observations on the mechanism of production of the second heart sound. Circulation 51:292–296, 1975.

16. Paraskos JA, and Montesclaros LA: Relation of the second heart sound to aortic valve closure as assessed by echocardiography (Abstr). Circulation (Suppl III) 49,50:239, 1974.

17. Edwards JE: Pathology of left ventricular outflow tract obstruction. Circulation 31:586–599, 1965.

18. Bristow JD: Recognition of left ventricular outflow obstruction. Circulation 31:600–611, 1965.

19. Popp RL, Silverman JF, French JW, et al.: Echocardiographic findings in discrete subvalvular aortic stenosis. Circulation 49:226–231, 1974.

20. Ultan LB, Segal BL, and Likoff W: Echocardiography in congenital heart disease: Preliminary observations. Am J Cardiol 19:74–83, 1967.

21. Laurenceau J-L, Guay JM, and Gagné S: Echocardiography in the diagnosis of subaortic membranous stenosis (Abstr). Circulation (Suppl IV) 48:46, 1973.

22. Davis RH, Feigenbaum H, Chang S, et al.: Echocardiographic manifestations of discrete subaortic stenosis. Am J Cardiol 33:277–280, 1974.

23. Lundström N, and Edler I: Ultrasound cardiology in infants and children. Acta Paediatr Scand 60:117, 1971.

24. Johnson ML, Warren SG, Waugh RA, et al.: Echocardiography of the aortic valve in non-rheumatic left ventricular outflow tract lesions. Radiology 112:677–684, 1974.

25. McIntosh HD, Sealy WC, Whalen RE, et al.: Obstruction to outflow tract of left ventricle. Arch Intern Med 110:84–94, 1962.

26. Perloff JK: The Clinical Recognition of Congenital Heart Disease. Philadelphia, W. B. Saunders Company, 1970.

27. Roberts WC: The structure of the aortic valve in clinically isolated aortic stenosis: An autopsy study of 162 patients over 15 years of age. Circulation 42:91–97, 1970.

28. Hancock EW: Differentiation of valvular, subvalvular and supravalvular aortic stenosis. Guy's Hosp Rep 110:1, 1961.

29. Yeh H-C, Winsberg F, and Mercer EN: Echographic aortic valve oriface [sic] dimension: Its use in evaluating aortic stenosis and cardiac output. J Clin Ultrasound 1:182–189, 1973.

30. Nanda NC, Gramiak R, Manning J, et al.: Echocardiographic recognition of the congenital bicuspid aortic valve. Circulation 49:870–875, 1974.

31. Rotman M, Morris JJ, Jr., Behar VS, et al.: Aortic valvular disease: Comparison of types and their medical and surgical management. Am J Med 51:241–257, 1971.

32. Bloom KR, Meyer RA, Bove KE, and Kaplan S: The association of fixed and dynamic left ventricular outflow obstruction. Am Heart J 89:586–590, 1975.

33. Hirata T, Wolfe SB, Popp RL, et al.: Estimation of left atrial size using ultrasound. Am Heart J 78:43–52, 1969.

34. Brown OR, Harrison DC, and Popp RL: An improved method for echographic detection of left atrial enlargement. Circulation 50:58–64, 1974.

35. Meyers AR, and Willis PW, III: Clinical spectrum of supravalvular aortic stenosis. Arch Intern Med 118:553–561, 1966.

36. Meyer RA, Schwartz DC, and Kaplan S: The diagnosis of aortic atresia by echocardiography (Abstr). Am J Cardiol 29:280, 1972.

37. Usher BW, Goulden D, and Murgo JP: Echocardiographic detection of supravalvular aortic stenosis. Circulation *49*:1257–1259, 1974.

38. Becker AE, Becker MJ, and Edwards JE: Mitral valvular abnormalities associated with supravalvular aortic stenosis: Observations in 3 cases. Am J Cardiol *29*:90–94, 1972.

39. Eliot RS, Woodburn RL, and Edwards JE: Conditions of the ascending aorta simulating aortic valvular incompetence. Am J Cardiol *14*:679–694, 1964.

40. Carter JB, Sethi S, Lee GB, and Edwards JE: Prolapse of semilunar cusps as causes of aortic insufficiency. Circulation *43*:922–932, 1971.

41. Glancy DL, Freed TA, O'Brien KP, and Epstein SE: Calcium in the aortic valve: Roentgenologic and hemodynamic correlations in 148 patients. Ann Intern Med *71*:245–250, 1969.

42. Edwards JE, and Burchell HB: Endocardial and intimal lesions (jet impact) as possible sites of origin of murmurs. Circulation *18*:946–960, 1958.

43. Pridie RB, Benham R, and Oakley CM: Echocardiography of the mitral valve in aortic valve disease. Br Heart J *33*:296–304, 1971.

44. Joyner CR, Jr., Dyrda I, and Reid JM: Behavior of the anterior leaflet of the mitral valve in patients with the Austin Flint murmur (Abstr). Clin Res *14*:251, 1966.

45. Winsberg F, Gabor GE, Hernberg JG, and Weiss B: Fluttering of the mitral valve in aortic insufficiency. Circulation *41*:225–229, 1970.

46. Botvinick EH, Schiller NB, Wickramasekaran R, Klausner SC, and Gertz E: Echocardiographic demonstration of early mitral valve closure in severe aortic insufficiency: Its clinical implications. Circulation *51*:836–847, 1975.

47. Friedewald VE, Futral JE, Kinard SA, and Phillips B: Oscillations of the interventricular septum in aortic insufficiency (Abstr). In White D (Ed.): Ultrasound in Medicine, New York, Plenum Press, 1975, p. 88.

48. Cope GD, Kisslo JA, Johnson ML, and Myers S: Diastolic vibration of the interventricular septum in aortic insufficiency. Circulation *51*:589–593, 1975.

49. Danford HG, Danford DA, Mielke JE, and Peterson LF: Echocardiographic evaluation of the hemodynamic effects of chronic aortic insufficiency with observations on left ventricular performance. Circulation *48*:253–262, 1973.

50. Herbert WH: Atrial transport and aortic insufficiency. Br Heart J *29*:559–562, 1967.

51. Popp RL, and Harrison DC: Ultrasonic cardiac echography for determining stroke volume and valvular regurgitation. Circulation *41*:493–502, 1970.

52. Mann T, McLaurin L, Grossman W, and Craige E: Assessing the hemodynamic severity of acute aortic regurgitation due to infective endocarditis. N Engl J Med *293*:108–113, 1975.

53. Pridie RB, Benham R, and Oakley CM: Recognition of aortic regurgitation of recent onset by ultrasound technique (Abstr). Am J Cardiol *26*:654–655, 1970.

54. Gottlieb S, Khuddus SA, Bolooki H, et al.: Echocardiographic diagnosis of aortic valve vegetations in Candida endocarditis. Circulation *50*:826–830, 1974.

55. Gottlieb S, Khuddus SA, Bolooki H, and Myerburg RJ: Echocardiographic diagnosis of endocarditis (Abstr). Circulation (Suppl III) *49,50*:76, 1974.

56. Hirschfeld D, and Schiller NB: Echocardiographic localization of aortic valve vegetations (Abstr). Circulation (Suppl III) *49,50*:143, 1974.

57. Weyman AE, Dillon JC, Feigenbaum H, and Chang S: Premature pulmonic valve opening following sinus of Valsalva aneurysm rupture into the right atrium. Circulation *51*:556–560, 1975.

58. Cooperberg P, Mercer EN, Mulder DS, and Winsberg F: Rupture of a sinus of Valsalva aneurysm. Radiology *113*:171–172, 1974.

59. Warren SG, Waugh RA, Kisslo J, and Johnson ML: Echocardiographic abnormalities in ruptured right coronary sinus of Valsalva aneurysm (Abstr). Circulation (Suppl III) *49,50*:249, 1974.

60. Rothbaum DA, Dillon JC, Chang S, and Feigenbaum H: Echocardiographic manifestation of right sinus of Valsalva aneurysm. Circulation *49*:768–771, 1974.

61. Lee C-C, Das G, and Weissler AM: Characteristic echocardiographic manifestations in ruptured aortic valve leaflet (Abstr). Circulation (Suppl III) *49,50*:144, 1974.

62. Rees JR, Epstein EJ, Criley JM, and Ross RS: Haemodynamic effects of severe aortic regurgitation. Br Heart J *26*:412–421, 1964.

63. Meadows WR, Van Praagh S, Indreika M, and Sharp JT: Premature mitral valve closure: A hemodynamic explanation for absence of the first sound in aortic insufficiency. Circulation *28*:251–258, 1963.

64. Pomerance A: Ageing changes in human heart valves. Br Heart J *29*:222–230, 1967.

65. Brown OR, DeMots H, Kloster F, Roberts A, Menashe VD, and Beals RK: Aortic root dilatation and mitral valve prolapse in Marfan's syndrome: An echocardiographic study. Circulation *52*:651–657, 1975.

66. Millward DK, Robinson NJ, and Craige E: Dissecting aortic aneurysm diagnosed by echocardiography in a patient with rupture of the aneurysm into the right atrium: Rare cause for continuous murmur. Am J Cardiol *30*:427–431, 1972.

67. DeMaria AN, King JF, Salel AF, et al.: Echography and phonography of acute aortic regurgitation in bacterial endocarditis. Ann Intern Med *82*:329–335, 1975.

68. Wray TM: The variable echocardiographic features in aortic valve endocarditis. Circulation *52*:658–663, 1975.

69. Wray TM: Echocardiographic manifestations of flail aortic valve leaflets in bacterial endocarditis. Circulation *51*:832–835, 1975.

70. Bolen JL, Popp RL, and French JW: Echocardiographic features of supravalvular aortic stenosis Circulation *52*:817–822, 1975.

71. Chandraratna PAN, Samet P, and Robinson MJ: Echocardiography of the "floppy" aortic valve. Circulation *52*:959–962, 1975.

6
The Left Atrium

Echocardiographic study of the left atrium is of particular importance because the posterior location of the atrium within the heart makes this chamber especially difficult to assess on physical examination and with routine chest x-rays. Furthermore, it is the most difficult of the four cardiac chambers to study by angiography. Because the determination of the left atrial size is very important in the assessment of many congenital and acquired cardiac diseases,[1] it is fortunate that measurement of left atrial dimensions is easily accomplished by echocardiography. Detection of intra-atrial masses is also possible with the echocardiogram.

ANATOMY AND PHYSIOLOGY

The left atrium is bordered anteriorly by the aortic root, which is its most important echocardiographic relationship. Posterior to the left atrium are the descending thoracic aorta and the esophagus. The right atrium is located to the right of and anterior to the left atrium; the left ventricle is located anteriorly, inferiorly, and to the left. The pulmonary veins enter the left atrium posteriorly and may be surrounded by thickenings of the atrial musculature extending 1 to 2 cm into the chamber.[2]

The left atrium functions principally (1) as a reservoir for blood returning from the lungs and (2) as a muscular structure that actively augments ventricular filling,[3-5] especially in the presence of reduced left ventricular compliance[6] and possibly in mitral stenosis.[7] In addition, the posterior wall of the left atrium adjoins the posterior mitral leaflet and therefore plays a part in maintaining the integrity of the mitral valve.

The left atrium is a low-pressure chamber with a mean pressure of 7 mm Hg and a pressure range of 3 to 13 mm Hg.[8] Left atrial pressure may be assessed directly or, more commonly, indirectly by measurement of the pulmonary capillary wedge pressure. Three pressure waves occur in each cardiac cycle. The first, the "a" wave, occurs with atrial contraction; the second, the "c" wave, at the onset of ventricular systole; and the third, the "v" wave, at the end of ventricular systole as the atrium becomes filled. The pressure differential between the left atrium and left ventricle at the end of ventricular systole and diastole determines the timing of the opening and closing of the mitral valve.

The left atrial myocardium possesses the same contractile properties as other cardiac musculature. It must first be electrically depolarized before contraction occurs. Because cardiac depolarization normally begins in the sinus node, which is located in the right atrium, left atrial contraction begins after that of the right atrium. Depolarization of the left atrial structure is represented by the terminal portion of the P wave on the surface electrocardiogram.

NORMAL ECHOCARDIOGRAPHIC FEATURES

The left atrium is best studied from the third or fourth intercostal space, as it is recorded simultaneously with the aortic root (see Fig. 5–1).

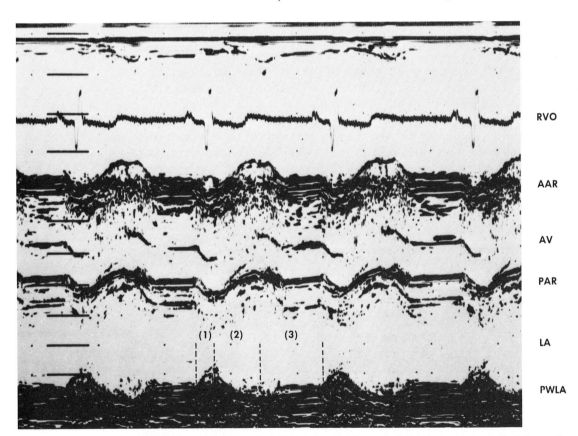

FIGURE 6–1.   The left atrium (LA) is bordered anteriorly by the posterior wall of the aortic root (PAR). The posterior wall of the left atrium (PWLA) exhibits three phases of motion: (1) anterior movement during atrial systole, (2) posterior movement during ventricular systole, and (3) anterior movement during early ventricular diastole followed by flattening until the next atrial contraction. (RVO = right ventricular outflow tract; AAR = anterior aortic root wall; AV = aortic valve.)

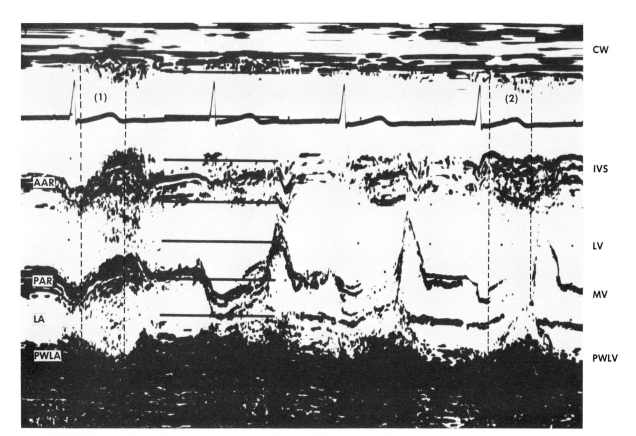

CW

IVS

LV

MV

PWLV

FIGURE 6-2. A scan from the left atrium (LA) to the left ventricle (LV) demonstrates posterior motion of the posterior wall of the left atrium (PWLA) during ventricular systole (1). In contrast, the posterior wall of the left ventricle (PWLV) moves anteriorly during systole (2). Note also that the left atrial wall and the left ventricular wall lie approximately at the same distance from the anterior chest wall (CW) (AAR = anterior aortic root; PAR = posterior aortic root; IVS = interventricular septum; MV = mitral valve).

Wall Motion

The anterior left atrial wall is ultrasonically inseparable from the posterior wall of the aortic root. Thus, its motion is the same as that of the cardiac skeleton, as described in Chapter 4. In the early literature, the left atrial wall motion was confused with that of the anterior mitral leaflet.[9] The posterior atrial wall has a distinctive motion that occurs in three phases (Figs. 6-1 to 6-3).

In phase 1, following the onset of the electrocardiographic P wave, wall motion is anterior in direction. On the echocardiogram, this contraction of the atrial wall may appear rounded (Fig. 6-1) or infrequently may exhibit a sharp, peaked appearance (Fig. 6-3).

In phase 2, following the QRS complex of the electrocardiogram, left atrial wall motion is posterior in direction. This posterior expansion may be accounted for by the combination of atrial filling from the pulmonary veins and an effective reduction in the chamber size of the left atrium as the mitral leaflets have closed.

Phase 3 is characterized by a short, abrupt anterior displacement of the atrial

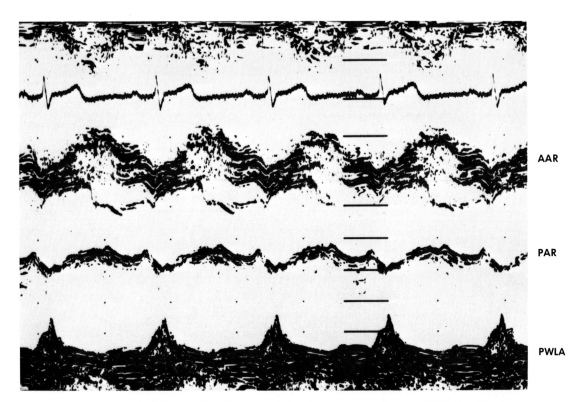

FIGURE 6-3. In this normal left atrium, the posterior wall (PWLA) exhibits a very sharp anterior motion during atrial systole (AAR = anterior aortic root wall; PAR = posterior aortic root wall).

wall and a neutral position until the commencement of the next atrial contraction.

Because the amplitude of the posterior wall motion in each of the three phases is small, the echo beam must approach 90 degrees to the posterior wall, or all motion will go undetected. Furthermore, movements of the posterior wall may be obscured by other echoes originating in the atrium. Flattened posterior wall motion is usually present when the left atrium is dilated (Fig. 6–4). Failure of synchronous atrial contraction, such as atrial fibrillation, will also result in an absence of the anterior (phase 1) displacement prior to ventricular systole. Patients in atrial flutter may be observed to have regular posterior atrial wall undulations that coincide with the flutter waves on the electrocardiogram.[10]

Dimension

Measurement of the single anterior–posterior dimension of the left atrium by echocardiography is particularly useful because atrial enlargement occurs concentrically. In children this dimension has been correlated with left atrial volumes determined by cineangiography in normals and in patients with atrial dilatation.[11] Various ways of measuring this dimension are utilized in different laboratories, and each method has its own value and limitations. Normal values are obviously dependent on the technique adopted.

The most widely used method is that described by Hirata et al.[12] and Brown et al.[13] The anterior–posterior dimension of the left atrium is measured from the anterior border of the posterior aortic wall at its peak systolic position to the posterior left atrial wall (Fig. 6–4). In adults, this dimension normally does not exceed 4.0 cm. Corrected for body surface area, the normal anterior-posterior left atrial dimension is 1.0 to 2.0 cm per M².[12] In the application of this method, several technical errors must be guarded against.

1. This dimension is not valid in the subxiphoid examination.

2. The true posterior wall echo must be used and not those fainter echoes sometimes observable in front of the posterior wall (Fig. 6–5).

3. The calcified or sclerotic aortic annulus sometimes seen in elderly persons or in patients with aortic valvular disease may cause the aortic wall to be unusually thick and cause a spurious increase of the atrial measurement.

Francis and Hagan studied 100 normal males and females for atrial size.[14] They measured the left atrial dimension from the posterior edge of the aortic wall echo at end-diastole. With this method the mean left atrial dimension was 20.7 mm ± 4.8 S.D. in males and 18.3 mm ± 4.4 S.D. in females, a significant difference between the sexes. The range was 16 mm to 40 mm. In contrast to other studies, there was no apparent correlation with the body surface area.

The left atrial maximal dimension (at the time of left ventricular end-systole) can also be compared to the left ventricular end-diastolic aortic root dimension (LA–AO ratio) as an index for enlargement.[13, 15] With this method, the ratio of the dimension of the left atrium to that of the aortic root ranges from

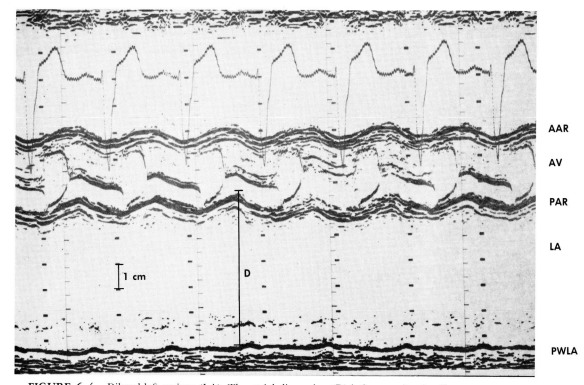

FIGURE 6–4. Dilated left atrium (LA). The atrial dimension (D) is 6 cm, twice the dimension of the aortic root. Posterior left atrial wall (PWLA) motion is flat (AAR = anterior aortic root; PAR = posterior aortic root; AV = aortic valve).

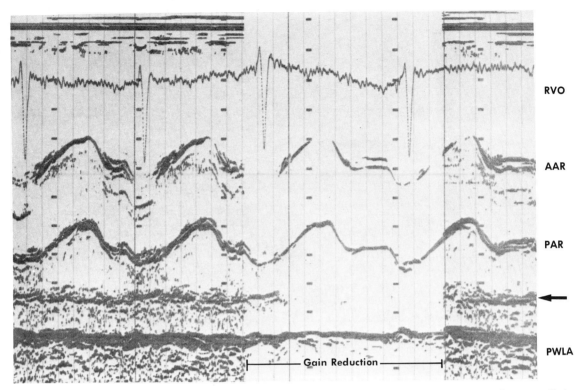

RVO

AAR

PAR

PWLA

Gain Reduction

FIGURE 6-5. Intracavity echoes within the left atrium (arrow). These echoes are distinguishable from those reflected by the posterior left atrial wall (PWLA) by their lower intensity. Such low-intensity echoes can be eliminated by a reduction in gain without eliminating the echoes from the posterior wall and the aortic root. (RVO = right ventricular outflow tract; AAR = anterior aortic root; PAR = posterior aortic root).

0.87 to 1.11. This ratio should not be used, however, when the aortic root is dilated, as in aneurysmal disease of the ascending aorta. The aortic root dimension may also be increased in aortic stenosis if the echo beam transects the aorta above its stenotic portion, thereby "normalizing" the ratio when the left atrium is also dilated. (An aortic root dimension exceeding 4.2 cm may be assumed to be enlarged.) In the case of low cardiac output states, the aortic root may be abnormally small. In these cases the LA–AO ratio can increase irrespective of the true left atrial size.

Wall Thickness

The posterior left atrial wall is normally approximately 3 mm thick.[16] With the newer recorders, and especially those with gray scale, the outer boundary of this thin echo can be discriminated from the echoes reflected from adjacent tissue (Fig. 6–5). When the full thickness of the wall can be delineated, it demonstrates slight thickening during atrial systole.

The echo of the anterior portion of the left atrial myocardium is contiguous with that of the aortic wall and cannot be measured because its left atrial edge is indistinct.

Intracavitary Echoes

Very often a band of echoes is recorded within the left atrial chamber (Fig. 6–5). These echoes may be differentiated from the true posterior atrial wall echo in that they are somewhat fainter and are discontinuous. If they are mistaken for the posterior wall, the left atrial measurement will be erroneously reduced.

The origins of these echoes are in doubt, but they probably reflect at least two structures, and possibly three, depending on transducer angle:

1. The mitral annulus. The intracavitary echo band is especially common among persons having a thick annulus, which in some cases may actually project into the left atrium (see Chapter 4).

2. Thickened atrial muscle around the orifices of the pulmonary veins.[2]

3. Transverse sinus of the pericardium in the presence of pericardial effusion.[17]

LEFT ATRIAL DILATATION

Echocardiographic measurement of the left atrial dimension has been shown to be a very sensitive index for dilatation of this chamber, especially when compared to the aortic root dimension.[13, 15] Hirata et al.[12] have classified left atrial enlargement, corrected for body surface area, as mild (2.0 to 3.0 cm per M^2), moderate (3.0 to 4.0 cm per M^2) or marked (over 4.0 cm per M^2). Brown et al.[13] found that a left atrial–aortic root ratio of 1.17 or greater was always associated with left atrial dilatation. The specificity of an increased left atrial dimension for true dilatation has been documented by ten Cate,[15] who found that only 2 of 25 normal patients exhibited an LA–AO ratio exceeding 1.0.

Another feature of left atrial dilatation is the displacement of the posterior atrial wall behind the position of the posterior left ventricular wall, provided the left ventricle is not enlarged. This is evident on the scan from the left atrium to the left ventricle (Fig. 6–6).

Waggoner[18] compared the relative ability of the echocardiogram and the electrocardiogram to detect left atrial enlargement in 302 patients in sinus rhythm. Electrocardiographic criteria were highly specific (81 percent) but much less sensitive (64 percent) than the echocardiogram.

Chronic mitral regurgitation causes marked left atrial dilatation, which may exceed 2 liters.[19] Among patients with mitral regurgitation, the degree of atrial dilatation shows considerable variation. It may become extensive with maintenance of normal atrial and pulmonary artery pressures.[20] In some cases, however, there is much less accommodation of the regurgitant flow by means of left atrial dilatation, and pulmonary hypertension develops and may become extreme. Consequently, neither the severity of mitral regurgitation nor the atrial pressure can be predicted on the basis of the echocardiographic left atrial dimension. Nevertheless, the atrial dimension is very sensitive to the presence of even minimal mitral insufficiency.[13] Mitral stenosis also causes enlargement of the left atrium, although generally not to the same degree observed in severe mitral insufficiency.[21]

Reduction of left ventricular compliance and left ventricular failure are sometimes associated with left atrial enlargement. Left atrial volume has been shown to correlate with atrial pressure in these patients.[21] Brown et al.[13] found that seven of 40 patients with aortic valve disease had left atrial enlargement exceeding 2.0 cm per M^2. In twelve of the 40, the left atrial dimension was at least 17 percent greater than the aortic root dimension.

One of the most useful applications of left atrial dimension is in the assessment for patent ductus arteriosus (PDA) in premature newborn infants in respiratory distress (Fig. 6-7). Differentiation of this entity from idiopathic respiratory distress syndrome is important because ligation of a significant patent ductus results in rapid improvement. Circumvention of catheterization by noninvasive echocardiographic diagnosis in neonates with the respiratory distress syndrome is obviously invaluable. Baylen et al.[22] found both the left atrial and left ventricular dimensions to be increased in infants with PDA's, and in most cases, following ductal ligation, chamber sizes returned to normal. Silverman et al.[23] found that the LA-AO ratio was 1.28 ± 0.23 in premature infants with PDA's, compared to 0.86 ± 0.10 among controls. Furthermore, in only one infant with an LA–AO ratio over 1.15 did the PDA close spontaneously. Surgical intervention was required in all other infants in whom the ratio exceeded 1.15. Following ligation of the ductus arteriosus, the LA–AO ratio fell below 1.0 within 24 hours. In contrast, the LA–AO ratio was normal in those infants with severe respiratory distress without a left-to-right shunt caused by a PDA. It must be re-emphasized that caution be used in interpreting

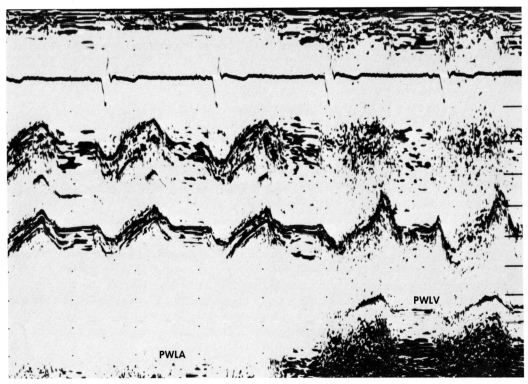

FIGURE 6-6.   Dilated left atrium on scan to the mitral valve. The posterior left atrial wall (PWLA) is displaced posteriorly relative to the posterior wall of the left ventricle (PWLV) (see also Figure 6-2).

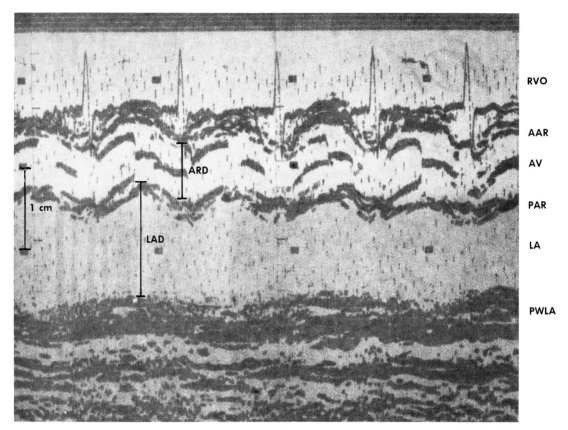

FIGURE 6-7. Patent ductus arteriosus in a 3-week-old premature infant. The left atrial dimension (LAD) is 1.3 cm, and the aortic root (ARD) measures 0.7 cm (LA–AO ratio = 1.9:1) (RVO = right ventricular outflow tract; AAR = anterior aortic root wall; AV = aortic valve; PAR = posterior aortic root wall; LA = left atrium; PWLA = posterior wall of the left atrium).

an altered LA–AO ratio in distressed infants, because any cause of left ventricular failure can enlarge the left atrium in proportion to the aortic root.

The LA–AO ratio is also altered in isolated ventricular septal defect,[24, 25] and it may be used as an index for the degree of shunting in such patients. (For further discussion, see Chapter 7.)

ATRIAL SEPTAL (SECUNDUM) DEFECT

The most commonly recognized echocardiographic feature of secundum septal defects is altered motion of the interventricular septum, a characteristic of all right ventricular diastolic volume overload states (Table 6–1, Fig. 6–8). The left atrium itself is normal or shows a borderline increase in size.[12] Marked enlargement of the left atrium in any patient with an atrial septal defect should raise the possibility of associated mitral valve disease.

Several recent studies[27-29] have documented the frequent association of cineangiographic evidence of mitral valve prolapse and secundum atrial septal defect. Overt mitral insufficiency occurs in some patients. Echocardiographic evidence of mitral prolapse has been reported in 30 percent of patients with

TABLE 6-1   ECHOCARDIOGRAPHIC FEATURES OF ATRIAL SEPTAL DEFECT

Normal or slightly enlarged left atrium
Abnormal septal motion
Dilated right ventricle
Tricuspid valve visible and sometimes showing fluttering
Mitral valve thickening and prolapse

atrial septal defect.[30] The mechanism of mitral prolapse is unclear, but there has been speculation that it is a result of chordal deformity,[27] valve trauma secondary to altered blood flow,[30, 31] or a congenital biochemical abnormality.[30] The mitral valve leaflets may also appear thickened on the echocardiogram, a change that has been demonstrated pathologically in most cases of septum secundum defects.[31, 32]

The tricuspid valve is often recorded in the presence of a large atrial septal defect, probably as a result of the volume overload of the right ventricle that has rotated anteriorly. A fluttering motion of the tricuspid leaflets has been described by Nanda et al.,[33] who attributed this abnormality to increased flow across the valve. The internal dimension of the right ventricle is increased.[26, 34]

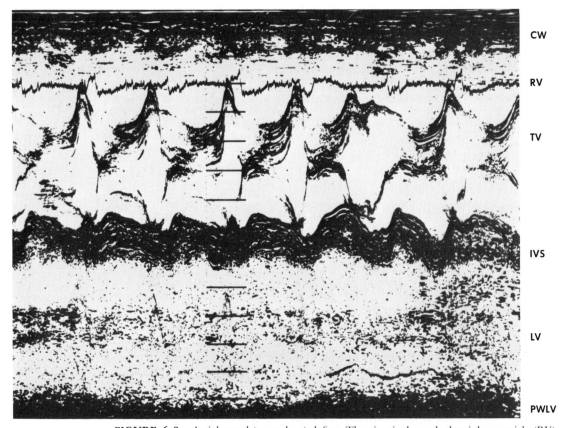

FIGURE 6-8. Atrial septal (secundum) defect. The view is through the right ventricle (RV) and left ventricle (LV). Two of the tricuspid valve (TV) leaflets are prominent and the right ventricular internal dimension is increased to 5 cm. The motion of the septum (IVS) is anterior in ventricular systole (CW = chest wall; PWLV = posterior wall of the left ventricle).

Further discussion of the right ventricular volume overload states is included in Chapter 7.

ATRIAL SEPTAL PRIMUM DEFECT

Atrial septal primum defect involves the lowermost portion of the atrial septum and is one type of a group of congenital abnormalities termed endocardial cushion defects. These include maldevelopment of the atrial septum, the ventricular septum, the mitral valve, and the tricuspid valve. All these structures (complete endocardial cushion defect) or various combinations (incomplete endocardial cushion defect) may be involved.

Ostium primum defect is usually associated with a cleft mitral valve in which the anterior mitral leaflet is divided into two parts,[35] causing mitral insufficiency. When this is the case, the interventricular septum usually moves paradoxically, and the right ventricle is dilated, as in secundum defects.[26] The left atrium is dilated when mitral insufficiency is present, and the left ventricle may also become enlarged as insufficiency increases. When this occurs, septal motion may become normal. Diamond et al.[26] found, however, that paradoxical septal motion persisted in patients with moderate mitral insufficiency and septum primum defects.

In the presence of cushion defects, the mitral valve echo is abnormal in that it appears somewhat superiorly and medially in the left ventricular outflow tract and is continuous with the anterior wall of the aortic root (owing to its attachment to the crest of the interventricular septum.)[36] Nanda et al.[37,38] have identified the echo from the interatrial septum behind the tricuspid valve. Normally this echo is continuous with the mitral valve leaflet. Whereas this continuity is preserved in patients with septum secundum defects, it may appear discontinuous with the mitral valve in septum primum defects. In some cases, the mitral valve echo actually appears to traverse the septum.[36,39]

LEFT ATRIAL MYXOMA

Diagnosis of the left atrial myxoma was one of the first clinical applications of cardiac ultrasound, which has subsequently become the best means for detection of this rare cardiac tumor.

The left atrial myxoma is the most common primary tumor of the heart. Three fourths of cardiac myxomas occur in the left atrium, and most of the remainder are found in the right atrium.[40-42] Very rarely do such tumors occur in the ventricles or on the mitral valve. In the atria they usually arise near the fossa ovalis and are attached to pedicles of variable length. When the pedicles are sufficiently long, myxomas may be quite mobile, intermittently moving across the mitral orifice into the left ventricle.

The clinical manifestations of myxomas simulate a variety of cardiac diseases.[43-45] Goodwin[46] classifies the features of the left atrial myxoma as obstructive, embolic, and constitutional. Intermittent obstruction of the mitral orifice causes dyspnea and pulmonary hypertension. When the tumor traumatizes the mitral leaflets, mitral insufficiency may occur. Mitral insufficiency may also result from failure of the tumor to retract totally during ventricular systole, interfering with mitral leaflet closure.[47] A diastolic murmur simulating the murmur of mitral stenosis is sometimes present as well. Acute obstruction at the mitral orifice may cause a sudden reduction in cardiac output with syncope and, occasionally, sudden death.

Peripheral embolism either of a portion of the atrial tumor itself or of thrombus formed on the surface may occur. For this reason, any patient with evidence of a systemic embolus should be evaluated for atrial myxoma.[48] Pulmonary embolism is also a common occurrence in patients with left atrial myxomas.

The constitutional effects of an atrial myxoma include weight loss, fever, anemia, increased sedimentation rate, and increased serum gamma globulin.

Diagnosis of a left atrial myxoma in a patient who has no obvious reason for the clinical features described may be accomplished with the echocardiogram. Echocardiography should always be employed in patients who appear to have mitral stenosis as well, because an obstructing myoxma and mitral stenosis are clinically similar. Because the treatments are totally different for the two entities, the differential diagnosis is essential. Also, an echocardiogram should serve as an essential prelude to cardiac catheterization for any patient with possible atrial myxoma for at least two reasons. First, the hazard of traumatic catheter-

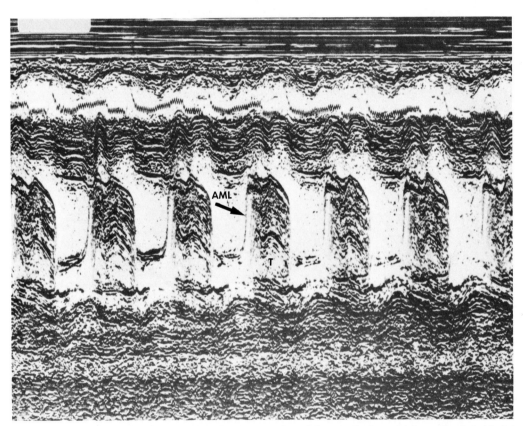

FIGURE 6–9. Left atrial myxoma. The solid mass of echoes (T) immediately behind the anterior mitral leaflet (AML) is the tumor protruding through the mitral orifice during valve opening. Note that there is a slight delay from the time of valve opening until the tumor echoes appear (IVS = interventricular septum). (Recording courtesy of M. Johnson, M.D., Duke University Medical Center, Durham, North Carolina.)

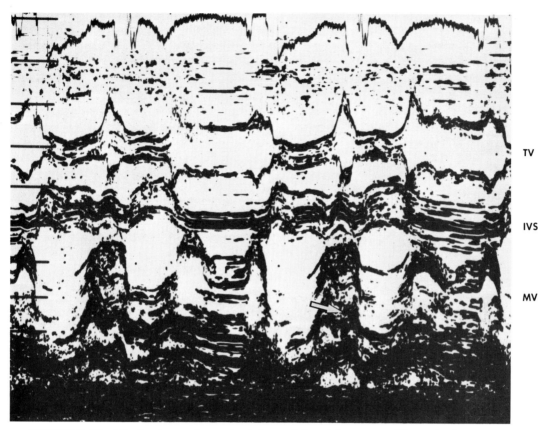

FIGURE 6-10. Mitral valve prolapse simulating a left atrial myxoma. The redundant valvular tissue appears as a mass resembling a protruding myxoma (arrow). The tricuspid valve is prominent as pulmonary hypertension is present (TV = tricuspid valve; IVS = intervntricular septum; MV = mitral valve).

TV

IVS

MV

induced tumor embolism is reduced if a myxoma is detected prior to this invasive procedure, especially if transseptal puncture is contemplated.[49, 51] Second, a myxoma may be missed by "routine" catheterization unless prior evidence suggests its presence.[52, 53] Because these tumors appear to be familial in some instances, routine screening of relatives of patients with myxomas has been advocated.[54, 55]

Echocardiographic detection of the left atrial myxoma is principally contingent upon the tumor's extending through the mitral orifice during mitral valve opening. Such protrusion probably occurs in the majority of cases. In Goodwin's collection of 45 cases,[46] 90 percent had some evidence of mitral orifice obstruction. This gives the appearance of a mass of echoes filling in immediately behind the anterior valve leaflet (Fig. 6-9).[50, 51, 56-60] The technologist who is not informed of the possibility of a myxoma or who is unfamiliar with its echocardiographic appearance may make an effort to "clean up" these echoes by reducing echo intensity to the point that the tumor echoes are poorly recorded. The diagnosis will also be missed if the tumor is not traversing the orifice at the time of the examination. When the diagnosis is suspected, therefore, long, uninterrupted recordings of the mitral valve with the patient in various positions may be necessary to confirm or deny the presence of a myxoma. When the index of suspicion is high and echocardiographic results are negative, repeat examinations may be warranted.

A mass of echoes appearing posterior to the anterior mitral leaflet during its diastolic opening cannot be considered absolutely diagnostic of a myxoma. The markedly redundant mitral leaflets of valvular myxomatous degeneration associated with mitral prolapse give a similar appearance[76] (Fig. 6–10). This may be especially misleading in some cases of mitral valve prolapse associated with pulmonary hypertension (personal communication, R. L. Popp).[61] Marked thickening of the mitral leaflets in some cases of mitral stenosis can also result in dense echoes which resemble a protruding tumor (Fig. 6–11). Thickened leaflet echoes, however, are present from the onset of valve opening, whereas there is usually a slight delay following mitral opening before the tumor echoes appear.[47]

The flail posterior mitral leaflet in cases of ruptured chordae tendineae or transected papillary muscle may also cause a diastolic echo to appear posterior to the anterior leaflet (Fig. 6–12). Clinically, a ruptured chorda should pose little difficulty in differentiation from a myxoma. (It should be recalled, however, that on occasion chordal rupture secondary to a "wrecking ball" myxoma may occur.[62]) Massive calcification of the mitral annulus presents a heavy echo behind the mitral leaflets but is differentiated by its systolic anterior and diastolic posterior motion, opposite to that of the myxoma. Finally, it is possible that an atrial thrombus could also appear as a myxoma through the mitral orifice, although this is probably quite rare.

While the atrial myxoma is usually detected only as it protrudes through the mitral orifice, it occasionally is visualized as an echo mass within the left

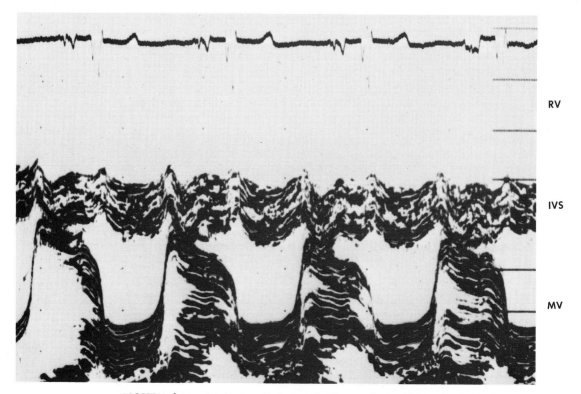

RV

IVS

MV

FIGURE 6-11. Moderate mitral stenosis. The markedly thickened valve leaflets resemble a protruding atrial tumor (RV = right ventricle; IVS = interventricular septum; MV = mitral valve).

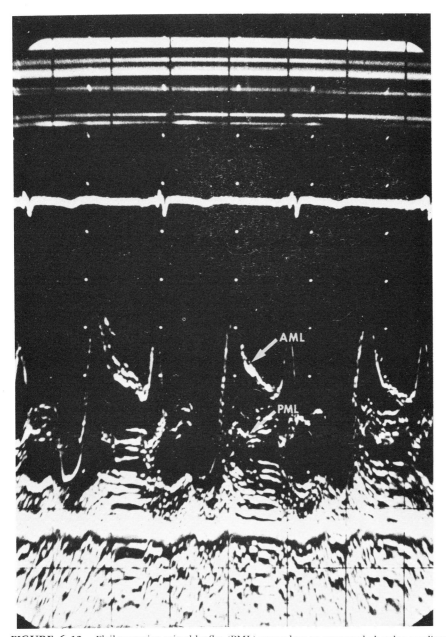

FIGURE 6–12. Flail posterior mitral leaflet (PML) secondary to ruptured chordae tendinae. During diastolic opening the posterior leaflet appears as an echo mass behind the anterior leaflet (AML) and resembles a myxoma.

atrium either during ventricular systole only[53] or throughout the cardiac cycle (Fig. 6–13).[63, 77] The left atrium itself may be dilated.

In the presence of an atrial myxoma, the motion of the mitral valve is altered principally in that the EF slope is reduced as a result of decreased flow across the obstructed mitral orifice and because the tumor physically prevents normal partial closure of the valve in mid-diastole.[64] Distinct leaflet echoes, especially those of the posterior leaflet, may be difficult or impossible to record in some patients as they become obscured by the dense tumor echoes.

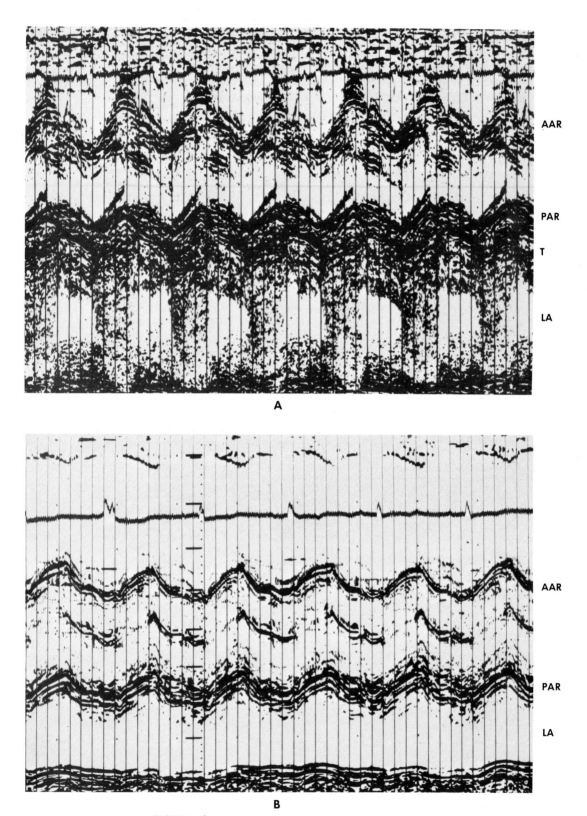

AAR

PAR

T

LA

A

AAR

PAR

LA

B

FIGURE 6-13. Left atrial myxoma. *A*. Preoperative recording through the aortic root and left atrium (LA). The tumor (T) appears as a mass of echoes adjacent to the posterior aortic root wall (PAR). The tumor fills the entire atrium during ventricular systole when the pedunculated portion recedes through the mitral orifice. *B*. Postoperative recording. Following resection, tumor echoes are no longer seen in the left atrium. (AAR = anterior aortic root wall.)

Also, the right ventricle may be dilated, and when pulmonary hypertension occurs the septum may be asymmetrically thickened. Because on rare occasions myxomas are bilateral,[65] the tricuspid valve area should be routinely scanned for evidence of a tumor prolapsing from the right atrium through the tricuspid orifice.[51, 54, 59]

Surgical excision of an atrial myxoma is usually curative.[66] Following operation, the echocardiogram can be expected to be normal.[52, 56] Also, the mitral EF slope will return to normal.[51, 53, 54, 58, 66-68] However, because atrial myxomas may recur,[69] regular long-term follow-up echocardiography is indicated.[53]

COR TRIATRIATUM

Cor triatriatum is a rare congenital anomaly in which an accessory chamber receives blood from the pulmonary veins and communicates with the left atrium through openings of varying numbers and sizes. Clinically this condition resembles mitral stenosis. Associated cardiac anomalies are common and often determine the prognosis as the intra-atrial partition itself is resectable.[70]

The characteristic echocardiographic feature of cor triatriatum is the presence of a continuous band of echoes within the left atrial chamber.[71, 72] Such intra-atrial echoes must be interpreted most cautiously in view of the frequent occurrence of similar echoes described previously. In two reports of cor triatriatum,[73, 74] echoes presumed to be produced by the atrial partition were seen posterior to the mitral valve. A thin echo of this type behind the anterior mitral leaflet could be confused with the mitral annulus and the posterior mitral leaflet as well as a non-prolapsing atrial myxoma or thrombus. Therefore, the diagnosis of cor triatriatum should not be made unless the partition is seen within the atrial chamber itself.

INTRA-ATRIAL ECHO FROM RUPTURED CHORDAE TENDINEAE

The appearance of a fine echo within the atrial chamber during each ventricular systole is suggestive of a ruptured chorda tendineae with prolapse of a mitral leaflet into the atrium. (See Chapter 4 for further discussion.)

LEFT ATRIAL THROMBUS

The ultrasonic diagnosis of thrombus formation within the left atrium is unreliable.[75] Failure to detect atrial thrombi is due principally to the fact that, unless they are calcified, they seldom reflect echoes of sufficient intensity to be distinguished from blood.

References

1. Castellanos A, and Hernandez F: Angiocardiographic determination of size of left atrium in congenital heart disease. Acta Radiol 6:433–452, 1967.

2. Nathan H, and Eliakim M: The junction between the left atrium and the pulmonary veins. Circulation *34*:412–422, 1966.

3. Nolan SP, Dixon SH, Jr., Fisher RD, and Morrow AG: The influence of atrial contraction and mitral valve mechanics on ventricular filling. Am Heart J *77*:784–791, 1969.

4. Thompson ME, Metzger CC, Shaver JA, et al.: Assessment of left atrial transport function immediately after cardioversion. Am J Cardiol *29*:481–489, 1972.

5. DeMaria AN, Lies JE, King JF, et al.: Echographic assessment of atrial transport, mitral movement, and ventricular performance following electroversion of supraventricular arrhythmias. Circulation *51*:273–282, 1975.

6. Stott DK, Marpole DGF, Bristow JD, et al.: The role of left atrial transport in aortic and mitral stenosis. Circulation *41*:1031–1041, 1970.

7. Heidenreich FP, Thompson ME, Shaver JA, and Leonard JJ: Left atrial transport in mitral stenosis. Circulation *40*:545–554, 1969.

8. Schlant RC: Normal physiology of the cardiovascular system. *In* Hurst JW, and Logue RB (Eds.): The Heart. New York, McGraw-Hill Book Company, 1970, p. 90.

9. Edler I, and Gustafson A: Ultrasonic cardiogram in mitral stenosis. Acta Med Scand *159*:85–90, 1957.

10. Zoneraich S, Zoneraich O, and Rhee JJ: Echocardiographic findings in atrial flutter. Circulation *52*:455–459, 1975.

11. Yabek SM, Isabel-Jones J, Bhatt D, Villoria G, and Jarmakani JM: Echocardiographic determination of left atrial volumes in children (Abstr). Circulation (Suppl II) *52*:259, 1975.

12. Hirata T, Wolfe SB, Popp RL, et al.: Experimental and laboratory reports: Estimation of left atrial size using ultrasound. Am Heart J *78*:43–52, 1969.

13. Brown OR, Harrison DC, and Popp RL: An improved method for echographic detection of left atrial enlargement. Circulation *50*:58–64, 1974.

14. Francis GS, and Hagan AD: Echocardiographic criteria of normal left atrial size in adults (Abstr). Circulation (Suppl III) *49,50*:76, 1974.

15. ten Cate FJ, Kloster FE, van Dorp WG, et al.: Dimensions and volumes of left atrium and ventricle determined by single beam echocardiography. Br Heart J *36*:737–746, 1974.

16. Gray H: Anatomy of the Human Body, 27th ed. Philadelphia, Lea & Febiger, 1973.

17. King D: Fundamentals of Abdominal Pelvic Ultrasonography. Philadelphia, W. B. Saunders Company, 1975.

18. Waggoner AD, Adyanthaya AV, Quenonis MA, and Alexander JK: Left atrial enlargement: Echocardiographic validation of electrocardiographic criteria (Abstr). Am J Cardiol *35*:175, 1975.

19. DeSanctis RW, Dean DC, and Bland EF: Extreme left atrial enlargement: Some characteristic features. Circulation *29*:14–23, 1964.

20. Braunwald E, and Awe WC: The syndrome of severe mitral regurgitation with normal left atrial pressure. Circulation *27*:29–35, 1963.

21. Sauter HJ, Dodge HT, Johnston RR, and Graham TP: The relationship of left atrial pressure and volume in patients with heart disease. Am Heart J *67*:635–642, 1964.

22. Baylen B, Meyers A, and Kaplan S: Echocardiographic assessment of patent ductus arteriosus in prematures with respiratory distress (Abstr). Circulation (Suppl III) *49,50*:16, 1974.

23. Silverman NH, Lewis AB, Heymann MA, and Rudolph AM: Echocardiographic assessment of ductus arteriosus shunt in premature infants. Circulation *50*:821–825, 1974.

24. Carter WH, and Bowman CR: Estimation of shunt flow in isolated ventricular septal defect by echocardiogram (Abstr). Circulation (Suppl IV) *48*:64, 1973.

25. Yoshikawa J, Owaki T, Kato H, and Tanaka K: Abnormal motion of interventricular septum of patients with prosthetic valve (Abstr). *In* White D (Ed.): Ultrasound in Medicine. New York, Plenum Press, 1974, p. 1.

26. Diamond MA, Dillon JC, Haine CL, Chang S, and Feigenbaum H: Echocardiographic features of atrial septal defect. Circulation *43*:129–135, 1971.

27. McDonald A, Harris A, Jefferson K, et al.: Association of prolapse of posterior cusp of mitral valve and atrial septal defect. Br Heart J *33*:383–387, 1971.

28. Hynes KM, Frye R., Brandenburg RO, et al.: Atrial septal defect (secundum) associated with mitral regurgitation. Am J Cardiol *34*:333–337, 1974.

29. Betriu A, Wigle ED, Felderhof CH, and McLoughlin MJ: Prolapse of the posterior leaflet of the mitral valve associated with secundum atrial septal defect. Am J Cardiol *35*:363–369, 1975.

30. Owens JP, Williams RG, and Fellows KE: Prolapsing mitral leaflet associated with secundum atrial septal defect (Abstr). Circulation (Suppl III) *49,50*:239, 1974.

31. Okada R, Glagov S, and Lev M: Relation of shunt flow and right ventricular pressure to heart valve structure in atrial septal defect. Am Heart J *78*:781–795, 1969.

32. Kamigaki M, and Goldschlager N: Echocardiographic analysis of mitral valve motion in atrial septal defect. Am J Cardiol *30*:343–348, 1972.

33. Nanda NC, Gramiak R, and Manning JA: Echocardiographic studies of the tricuspid valve in atrial septal defect. In White D (Ed.): Ultrasound in Medicine. New York, Plenum Press, 1975, pp. 11–17.

34. Tajik J, Gau GT, and Schattenberg TT: Echocardiogram in atrial septal defect. Chest 62:213–214, 1972.
35. Perloff JK: The Clinical Recognition of Congenital Heart Disease. Philadelphia, W. B. Saunders Company, 1970.
36. Williams RG, and Rudd M: Echocardiographic features of endocardial cushion defects. Circulation 49:418–422, 1974.
37. Nanda NC, Gramiak R, Manning J, and Gross CM: Echocardiographic identification of the inter-atrial septum: Clinical usefulness (Abstr). Circulation (Suppl II) 51,52:221, 1975.
38. Nanda NC, Gramiak R, Viles P, Manning J, and Gross C: Echocardiographic identification of the inter-atrial septum behind the tricuspid valve (Abstr). Circulation (Suppl II) 51,52:221, 1975.
39. Pieroni DR, Homcy E, and Freedom RM: Echocardiography in atrioventricular canal defect: A clinical spectrum. Am J Cardiol 35:54–58, 1975.
40. Greenwood WF: Profile of atrial myxoma. Am J Cardiol 21:367–375, 1968.
41. Heath D: Pathology of cardiac tumors. Am J Cardiol 21:315–327, 1968.
42. Waxler EB, Kawai N, and Kasparian H: Right atrial myxoma: Echocardiographic, phonocardiographic, and hemodynamic signs. Am Heart J 83:251–257, 1972.
43. Selzer A, Sakai FJ, and Popper RW: Protean clinical manifestations of primary tumors of the heart. Am J Med 52:9–17, 1972.
44. Zitnik RS, and Giuliani ER: Clinical recognition of atrial myxoma. Am Heart J 80:689–700, 1970.
45. Goodwin JF: Symposium on cardiac tumors. Introduction: The spectrum of cardiac tumors. Am J Cardiol 21:307–314, 1968.
46. Goodwin JF: Diagnosis of left atrial myxoma. Lancet 1:464–467, 1963.
47. Moscovitz HL, Pantazopoulos J, Bodenheimer M, et al.: Simulated left atrial tumor: A hemodynamic, echocardiographic and cineangiographic study. Am J Cardiol 34:63–71, 1974.
48. Spencer WH, III, Peter RH, and Orgain ES: Detection of a left atrial myxoma by echocardiography. Arch Intern Med 128:787–789, 1971.
49. Pindyck F, Peirce EC, II, Baron MG, and Lukban SB: Embolization of left atrial myxoma after transseptal cardiac catheterization. Am J Cardiol 30:569–571, 1972.
50. Schattenberg TT: Echocardiographic diagnosis of left atrial myxoma. Mayo Clinic Proc 43:620–627, 1968.
51. Wolfe SB, Popp RL, and Feigenbaum H: Diagnosis of atrial tumors by ultrasound. Circulation 39:615–622, 1969.
52. Popp RL, and Harrison DC: Ultrasound for the diagnosis of atrial tumor. Ann Intern Med 71:785–787, 1969.
53. Martinez EC, Giles TD, and Burch GE: Echocardiographic diagnosis of left atrial myxoma. Am J Cardiol 33:281–285, 1974.
54. Kleid JJ, Klugman J, Haas J, and Battock D: Familial atrial myxoma. Am J Cardiol 32:361–364, 1973.
55. Farah MG: Familial atrial myxoma. Ann Intern Med 83:358–360, 1975.
56. Glasser SP, Bedynek JL, Hall RJ, Hopeman AR, et al.: Left atrial myxoma: Report of a case including hemodynamic, surgical, histologic and histochemical characteristics. Am J Med 50:113–121, 1971.
57. Kostis JB, and Moghadam AN: Echocardiographic diagnosis of left atrial myxoma. Chest 58:550–552, 1970.
58. Trinkle JK, Edelstein SG, and Yoshonis KF: Left atrial myxoma: Diagnosis and excision. J Thorac Cardiovasc Surg 61:765–767, 1971.
59. Dadd MJ, and Wilcken DEL: Echocardiography in left atrial myxoma: Relation to the findings in mitral stenosis. Aust NZ J Med 2:124–127, 1972.
60. Nasser WK, Davis RH, Dillon JC, et al.: Atrial myxoma: II. Phonocardiographic, echocardiographic, hemodynamic, and angiographic features in nine cases. Am Heart J 83:810–824, 1972.
61. Phillips B, Diethrich EB, Friedewald VE, Jr., and Ellis J: Calcified intra-atrial mass detected by M-mode echocardiography and multi-head transducer scanning: A case report. In White D (Ed.): Ultrasound in Medicine, New York, Plenum Press, 1975, pp. 49–53.
62. Castleman B, Scully RE, and McNeely BU: Case records of the Massachusetts General Hospital, Case 42–1793. N Engl J Med 289:853–859, 1973.
63. Johnson ML, Sieker HO, Behar VS, and Whalen RE: Echocardiographic diagnosis of a left atrial myxoma found attached to the free left atrial wall. J Clin Ultrasound 1:75–81, 1973.
64. Bodenheimer MM, Moscovitz HL, Pantazopoulous J, and Donoso E: Echocardiographic features of experimental left atrial tumor. Am Heart J 88:615–620, 1974.
65. Harvey WP: Clinical aspects of cardiac tumors. Am J Cardiol 21:328–343, 1968.
66. Croxson RS, Jewitt D, Bentall HH, Cleland WP, et al.: Long-term follow-up of atrial myxoma. Br Heart J 34:1018–1023, 1972.
67. Srivastava TN, and Fletcher E: The echocardiogram in left atrial myxoma. Am J Med 54:136–139, 1973.

68. Finegan RE, and Harrison DC: Diagnosis of left atrial myxoma by echocardiography. N Engl J Med *282:*1022–1023, 1970.

69. Walton JA, Jr, Kahn DR, and Willis PW, III: Recurrence of a left atrial myxoma. Am J Cardiol *29:*872–876, 1972.

70. Martin-Gardía J, Tandon R, Lucas RV, Jr., and Edwards JE: Cor triatriatum: Study of 20 cases. Am J Cardiol *35:*59–66, 1975.

71. Nimura Y, Matsumoto M, Beppu S, et al.: Noninvasive preoperative diagnosis of cor triatriatum with ultrasonocardiotomogram and conventional echocardiogram. Am Heart J *88:*240–250, 1974.

72. Troy BL, Panepinto M, Harp R, et al.: Diagnosis of cor triatriatum by echocardiography (Abstr). J Clin Ultrasound *1:*257, 1973.

73. Gibson DG, Honey M, and Lennox SC: Cor triatriatum: Diagnosis by echocardiography. Br Heart J *36:*835–838, 1974.

74. Lundström N-R: Ultrasoundcardiographic studies of the mitral valve region in young infants with mitral atresia, mitral stenosis, hypoplasia of the left ventricle, and cor triatriatum. Circulation *45:*324–334, 1972.

75. Tallury VK, and DePasquale NP: Ultrasound cardiography in the diagnosis of left atrial thrombus. Chest *59:*501–503, 1971.

76. Watts LE, Nomeir AM, and DeMelo RA: Echocardiographic findings in patients with mitral valve prolapse mimicking left atrial tumor (Abstr). *In* White D (Ed.): Ultrasound in Medicine, New York, Plenum Press, 1975, p. 100.

77. Coltart DJ, Billingham ME, Popp RL, et al.: Left atrial myxoma. JAMA *234:*950–953, 1975.

7

The Interventricular Septum

An abundance of new information concerning the interventricular septum has been made available by echocardiography. Specifically, the complex motion of the normal septum, heretofore not fully appreciated, has been recorded echocardiographically. Furthermore, recognition that the motion of the septum becomes altered in a variety of pathophysiological states has been of paramount importance. In no instance, however, has the ultrasonic assessment of cardiac structures been more rewarding than in studies of septal thickness in cases of asymmetric septal hypertrophy.

NORMAL ANATOMY

The septum dividing the ventricles is composed of two distinct portions, the membranous septum and the muscular septum. The *membranous septum* is contiguous with the interatrial septum, the atrioventricular (A-V) valve rings, and the aortic and pulmonary trunks, and is part of the fibrous skeleton of the heart.[1] The membranous septum is the last portion of the septum to close during embryonic development. The *muscular septum* comprises the remainder and the bulk of the interventricular septum, and it separates the main chambers of the left and right ventricles.

The anterior portion of the septum derives its blood supply from perforating branches of the anterior descending coronary artery. The posterior part of the septum is supplied by the posterior descending artery, which is a branch of the right coronary vessel in most instances; in some cases, however, the posterior septum is supplied by both the circumflex and right coronary arteries or by the circumflex coronary artery alone.

The septum houses portions of the cardiac conduction system. The lower A-V node and bundle of His are in the membranous septum at its posterior margin, extending into the upper part of the muscular septum. The common bundle divides into the right and left bundle branches, which course along the subendocardial surfaces of each side of the septum.

Normal electrical depolarization of the septum is initiated from the left bundle branch system, with the wave of depolarization extending from left to right across the septum. The septum is the first portion of the ventricles to contract in ventricular systole.

ECHOCARDIOGRAPHIC FEATURES

The upper portion, or membranous septum, forms part of the anteromedial border of the left ventricular outflow tract, opposite the ventricular surface of the anterior mitral leaflet in diastole. It is continuous with the anterior wall of the aortic root (Fig. 7–1). Because the membranous septum is actually part

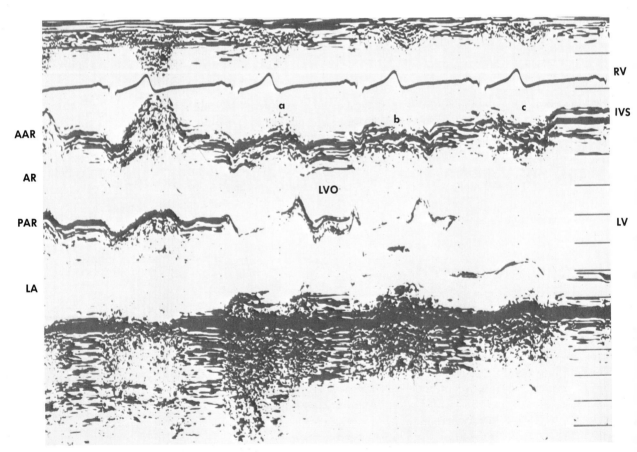

FIGURE 7–1. Scan from the aortic root (AR) to the left ventricle (LV). The septum (IVS) bordering the left ventricular outflow tract (LVO) is contiguous with the anterior wall of the aortic root (AAR) and moves anteriorly during ventricular systole (a,b). Within the body of the left ventricular chamber, it moves posteriorly during systole (c) (PAR = posterior aortic root wall; LA = left atrium; RV = right ventricle).

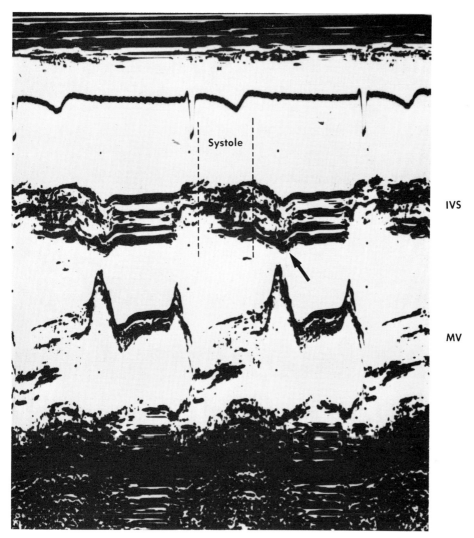

FIGURE 7–2. The upper septum (IVS). During ventricular systole the septal motion is often flat or anterior in direction when the mitral valve (MV) is well recorded. Note the small notch (arrow) immediately after the E point of the mitral valve motion.

of the cardiac skeleton and does not itself have muscular contractility, its motion is entirely passive. For this reason, normal membranous septal motion is similar to that of the aortic root walls, i.e., anterior in systole and posterior in early diastole. This motion is opposite that of the muscular septum, and this becomes apparent in a continuous echocardiographic scan of the septum from the membranous to the muscular portion (Fig. 7–1). Consequently, an erroneous diagnosis of "paradoxical" septal motion may be made if the echo beam intersects the septum at such a high point on that structure that the mitral motion is seen in its entirety (Fig. 7–2). Following the anterior motion of the membranous septum during systole, a small "notch" of low-amplitude, short-duration posterior displacement occurs immediately after the E point of the mitral valve (Fig. 7–2). This notch is exaggerated in patients with mitral stenosis (Fig. 7–3).

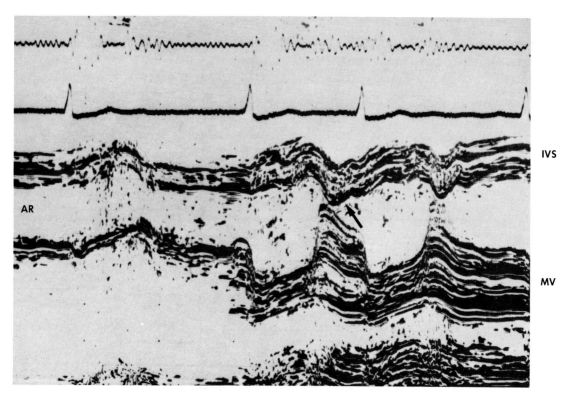

FIGURE 7–3.   Septal motion in mitral stenosis. The exaggerated notch (arrow) following the E point of the mitral valve (MV) motion is frequently seen in mitral stenosis (AR = aortic root; IVS = interventricular septum).

The upper portion of the muscular septum also forms part of the left ventricular outflow tract and it may exhibit a small degree of anterior motion during ventricular systole. The midportion of the muscular septum, however, normally thickens by about one third during ventricular systolic contraction, and this thickening is predominantly posterior into the left ventricle (Fig. 7–4). The left ventricular aspect of the septal wall moves more posteriorly than its right ventricular side. Thus, the septum appears to function primarily as part of the left ventricle. The amplitude of its posterior motion is lessened by the simultaneous anterior excursion of the entire heart during ventricular systole. Maximal posterior systolic movement occurs slightly before the peak posterior wall systolic excursion. After ventricular systole the septum moves anteriorly to its diastolic position, a motion sometimes interrupted by a short posterior notch in early diastole.[2] It reaches its smallest width in late diastole. Septal thickness should therefore be measured at the time immediately preceding the P wave or at the beginning of the QRS complex of the electrocardiogram. Sometimes a low-amplitude anterior motion of the septum may be recorded just after the P wave. This may be a result of atrial filling of the left ventricle.[3]

When the septum is recorded near the cardiac apex, its motion may appear anterior in direction during systole. At that level, this is probably a result of the predominant motion of the whole apical region of the heart as it moves anteriorly and superiorly. Thus, it should be reiterated that an erroneous impression of paradoxical septal motion may be given if the ultrasound beam is

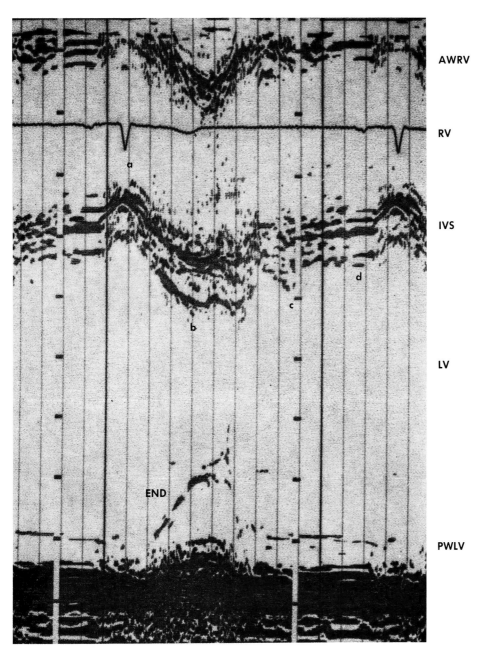

AWRV

RV

IVS

LV

PWLV

FIGURE 7-4. The muscular septum (IVS). A small-amplitude anterior motion (a) normally occurs immediately following the P wave of the ECG. Ventricular systolic motion is posterior in direction (b) after the QRS complex of the ECG, opposing the motion of the left ventricular posterior wall (PWLV). Anterior motion characterizes septal relaxation and is sometimes interrupted by a small notch (c). During late diastole the septum is motionless, and at this time (d) septal width should be measured (AWRV = anterior wall of right ventricle; RV = right ventricle; LV = left ventricle; END = endocardium).

angled too superiorly into the membranous and muscular portions bordering the left ventricular outflow tract, or too inferiorly into the cardiac apex.

ABNORMAL SEPTAL MOTION

Analysis of septal motion can be enormously informative because this motion may be affected by hemodynamic changes on both the left and right sides of the heart, as well as by abnormalities of the septum itself. Alterations in electrical depolarization may also alter septal motion.

Jacobs et al.[4] have categorized changes in systolic septal motion in adults as (1) diminished, or less than 3 mm posterior systolic motion; (2) flat, or absent systolic motion (Fig. 7–5); and (3) paradoxical, or anterior motion during systole (Fig. 7–6). The abnormal anterior systolic septal motion has been designated "type A" motion and the flattened septal motion, "Type B."[5] Any of several different mechanisms of altered septal motion may occur, depending on the underlying pathophysiology.

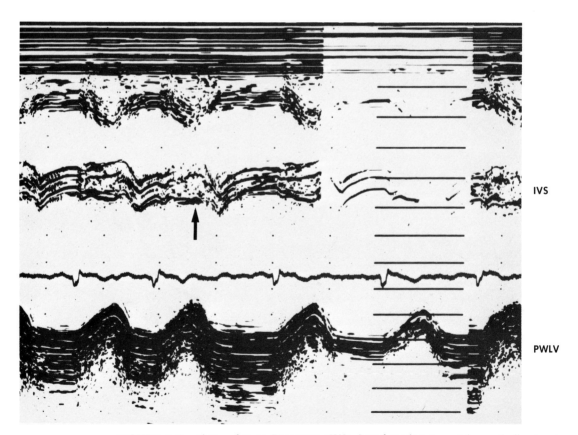

IVS

PWLV

FIGURE 7–5. Flattened (type B) septum (IVS). Septal motion (arrow) is practically absent during ventricular systole (PWLV = posterior left ventricular wall).

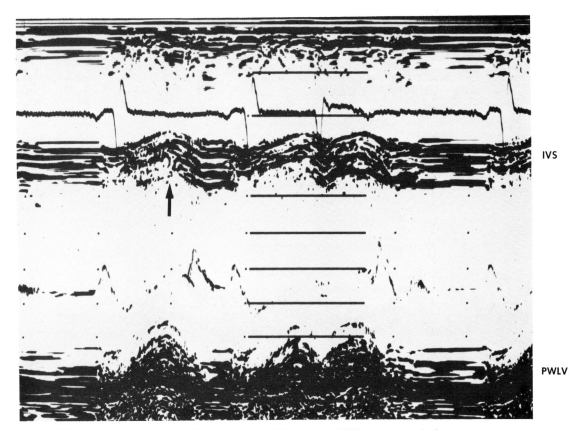

IVS

PWLV

FIGURE 7–6. Reversed (type A) septal motion. The septum (IVS) moves anteriorly (arrow) during ventricular systole (PWLV = posterior wall of left ventricle).

Right Ventricular Volume Excess

The classic example of right ventricular volume overload is the case of atrial septal defect. Meyer et al. have speculated that the paradoxical septal motion in patients with increased right ventricular volume is due to the more anterior position of the right ventricle when it is dilated, with rotation of the left ventricle posteriorly.[6] As the excessive volume of blood is ejected from the right ventricle, the anterior movement of the entire heart has an amplitude that exceeds the posterior motion of the septum. Thus, the net septal motion becomes anterior during systole (Fig. 7–7). Pearlman has stated that the position of the septum relative to the dimension between the right ventricular and left ventricular epicardial echoes is the determinant of flat or paradoxical septal motion.[7] He and his associates found that as the septum is shifted farther posteriorly in relation to the anterior and posterior wall echoes, regardless of cause, the degree of paradoxical septal motion increases.

The causes of right ventricular volume excess are summarized in Table 7–1. Most commonly these result from left-to-right shunting occurring at a level proximal to the mitral valve.[8] The septal motion may be used in a gross assessment of the volume of shunt flow. Kerber and associates found that as the shunt flow was increased in experimental animals, a flattening of septal systolic

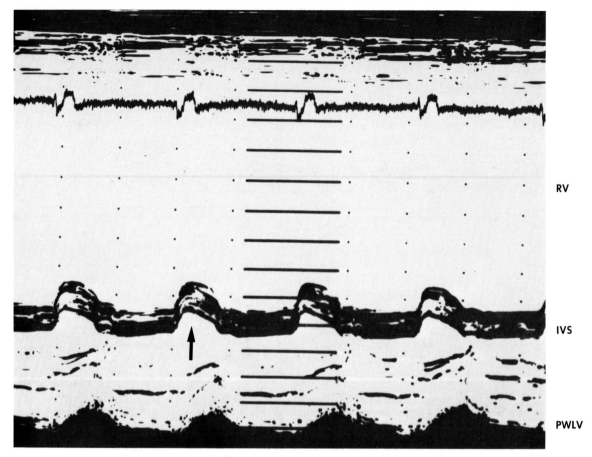

RV

IVS

PWLV

FIGURE 7–7.   Paradoxical septal motion in right ventricular volume overload. In this case of atrial septal secundum defect, the right ventricle (RV) is markedly dilated. The interventricular septum (IVS) moves anteriorly (arrow) during ventricular systole, paralleling the motion of the posterior left ventricular wall (PWLV).

motion (type B) preceded actual reversal to anterior direction (type A).[9] In their series of patients with left-to-right shunts, the mean ratio of pulmonic to systemic blood flow was 1.9 in those with normal septal motion, compared to 2.4 in cases of abnormal septal motion. Abnormal septal motion has been

TABLE 7–1   CAUSES OF RIGHT VENTRICULAR VOLUME EXCESS ASSOCIATED WITH ABNORMAL SEPTAL MOTION

Left-to-right shunts
    Atrial septal defect (ostium secundum defect)
    Anomalous pulmonary drainage
    Common A-V canal (ostium primum defect)
    Sinus venosus defect
    Peripheral arteriovenous shunt

Tricuspid valve lesions
    Tricuspid regurgitation
    Ebstein's anomaly

Pulmonic valve lesion
    Pulmonic regurgitation

reported in over 75 percent of cases of right ventricular hypervolemia,[5, 6, 9-12] although in one series, the septum was definitely abnormal in as few as 60 percent of the patients studied.[13] The septal motion is usually normal when the shunting is associated with pulmonary hypertension.[5, 6] With complete correction of the shunt defect, normal septal motion returns in some cases, but the frequency of this occurrence among reported series is extremely variable.[6, 9] In some cases, normal septal motion does not return until more than one year following surgery. Furthermore, the septal motion may flatten (type B) without completely returning to normal following operative intervention.[6, 9]

In addition to intracardiac left-to-right shunting as a cause of paradoxical septal motion, one case of peripheral arteriovenous shunting has been reported.[14] In this patient, septal motion remained abnormal 4 months after surgical correction, although the right ventricular dimension had returned to normal almost immediately after operation.

Abnormalities of the tricuspid valve that result in right ventricular hypervolemia include tricuspid regurgitation[5] and Ebstein's anomaly.[37] Severe pulmonic insufficiency also causes abnormal motion of the septum.

Dysfunction of the Septal Myocardium

In diseases that cause dysfunction of the septal myocardium, the contractile elements comprising the septum have decreased or absent activity. In the ischemic and hypertrophic cardiomyopathies, septal motion is usually normal in direction but low in amplitude or, in some cases, does not occur at all.[4, 16-18] Obstruction of the left anterior descending coronary artery frequently causes abnormal septal motion because the echo beam traverses the anterior portion of the septum. The motion is usually abnormal when anteroseptal infarction has occurred.[4] It has also been suggested that ischemia alone can produce this change.[4] (For a further explanation of the effects of ischemia, see Chapter 14; and for cardiomyopathy, see Chapter 8.)

Altered Sequence of Depolarization

Contraction of the myocardial elements of the septum is preceded by electrical depolarization, which normally progresses from left to right, superior to inferior. Alteration of electrical conduction, as in left bundle branch block and pre-excitation syndromes, causes changes in the timing of septal contraction in relation to contraction of the remainder of the left ventricular myocardium. This can result in septal motion that appears distinctly abnormal and frankly paradoxical in many cases.

In left bundle branch block, the septum typically exhibits a low-amplitude posterior displacement within 0.04 sec after the onset of the QRS complex of the electrocardiogram, corresponding to the pre-ejection period of left ventricular systole (Fig. 7–8).[3, 19, 20] This is followed by a slow anterior motion during left ventricular ejection. Sometimes the systolic motion is flat (Fig. 7–9), but only rarely is it posterior in direction. The notch often present at the beginning of diastole is frequently absent, but the low-amplitude anterior septal excursion after the P wave of the electrocardiogram remains preserved.

The same motion of the septum occurs in cases of beats originating in the right ventricle (see Fig. 3–2).[21] In these instances the septum is depolarized from right to left, as in left bundle branch block. The same mechanism accounts for paradoxical septal motion in patients who have right ventricular implanted pacemakers (Fig. 7–10), although septal motion is often normal in these patients.[3] When the left ventricle is the origin of an extra-systole, however, the normal sequence of septal depolarization from left to right is preserved, and septal motion is normal. Right bundle branch block is also associated with normal motion of the septum.

In the pre-excitation syndromes, part or all of the septal conduction tissue is bypassed, and ventricular depolarization begins in either the left or the right ventricle, in locations often remote from the septum. In some such cases, the septal motion is abnormal. In five of seven patients with type A Wolff-Parkinson-White syndrome, DeMaria et al. found that initial and maximal posterior septal systolic motion occurred later than in normals.[22] Theroux and associates have found a characteristic pattern of early septal posterior motion among type B Wolff-Parkinson-White patients but normal motion during ventricular ejection and relaxation.[23] These authors found normal septal motion in those persons with type A Wolff-Parkinson-White syndrome. Kanakis et al.

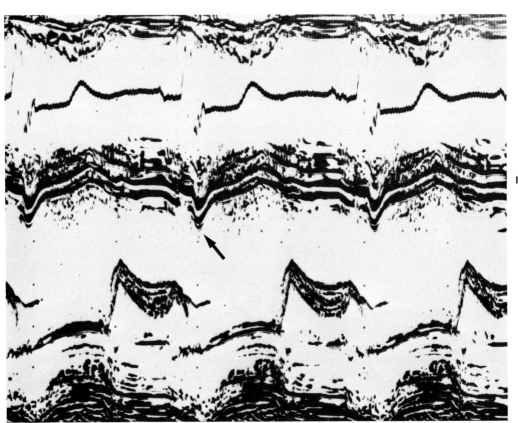

IVS

FIGURE 7–8. Left bundle branch block. The septum (IVS) exhibits an abrupt, low-amplitude posterior motion (arrow) immediately following onset of the QRS complex of the electrocardiogram. The septum then moves anteriorly during systolic ejection. Note also that the early diastolic notch is absent.

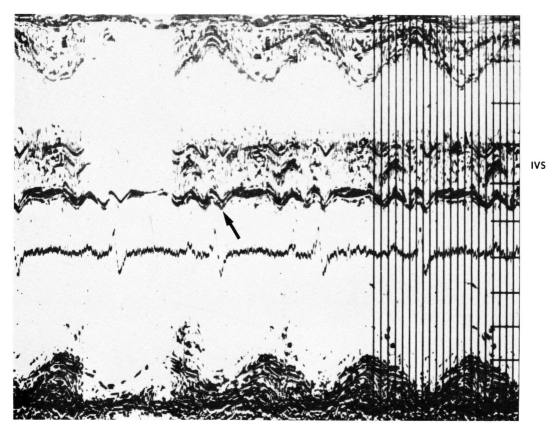

IVS

FIGURE 7-9. Left bundle branch block. The posterior notch (arrow) during the QRS complex of the ECG is followed by flattened septal motion (IVS) during the left ventricular ejection period.

found paradoxical septal motion to be present in six of seven patients with right anterior pre-excitation.[24] Chandra and associates also related abnormal septal motion, principally among patients with right ventricular (type I) Wolff-Parkinson-White syndrome.[36] The apparent disparities among different studies of septal motion in patients with pre-excitation syndromes may be due to the complexities of the syndromes themselves, and to the lack of precision in clinically determining the exact alteration in the depolarization sequence in individual patients.

Pericardial Effusion

In the presence of large pericardial effusions, the anterior–posterior motion of the entire heart becomes exaggerated. When this occurs, the composite direction of systolic motion of the septum may become anterior. In these cases, the anterior myocardium also moves anteriorly during systole. The resultant parallel motion of the septum and anterior and posterior cardiac walls has been termed "the swinging heart"[25] (see Chapter 12).

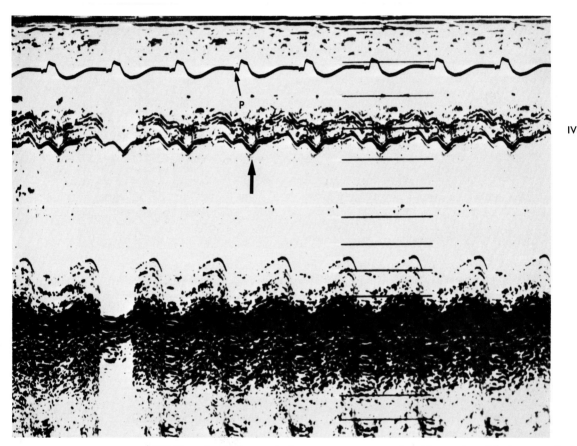

IVS

FIGURE 7–10. Right ventricular transvenous pacemaker. The motion of the interventricular septum (IVS) resembles the pattern of left bundle branch block, with a posterior notch (arrow) during the QRS complex and anterior movement in ventricular systole (P = pacemaker artifact).

Cardiac Surgery

The interventricular septum is frequently seen to exhibit altered motion following cardiac surgery.[19, 26-28] This may occur in the absence of any evidence of infarction or abnormal ventricular depolarization.

Yoshikawa found that 80 percent of patients undergoing aortic or mitral prosthetic valve replacement exhibited paradoxical or flat septal motion after operation.[27] Among 45 patients undergoing coronary artery bypass in another series, 12 developed anterior systolic septal motion postoperatively.[28]

The mechanism of postoperative paradoxical septal motion is controversial. Some cases, especially those in the coronary disease group, may have sustained intraoperative infarction, but this probably represents only a minority. Other possible explanations include cardiac rotation as a result of operation and unexplained alterations in the sequence of septal depolarization.

Constrictive Pericarditis

Gibson et al. found that 19 of 20 patients with constrictive pericarditis had paradoxical septal motion.[29] This motion persisted in all of the five patients studied after pericardial stripping. In a separate study, one of two patients with constrictive pericarditis showed a return to normal septal motion following operation.[30] The mechanism of abnormal septal motion in association with constrictive pericarditis is probably related to an abnormal pressure relationship between the two ventricles.

EXAGGERATED SEPTAL MOTION

The septum may exhibit increased posterior systolic motion either as a result of increased volume demand imposed upon the left ventricle or as an apparent compensatory mechanism in segmental nonseptal myocardial dysfunction as a result of coronary artery disease. (For further discussion, see Chapter 5, Mitral Regurgitation; Chapter 6, Aortic Regurgitation; and Chapter 14, Coronary Artery Disease.)

THE THICKENED SEPTUM

The septum becomes thickened as a result of right or left ventricular hypertrophy (concentric chamber hypertrophy) and infiltrative myocardial diseases (see Chapter 8). It may also thicken by the primary pathologic process known as asymmetric septal hypertrophy (ASH). Because of the unique importance of ASH to the echocardiographer, a separate chapter is devoted to its discussion (see Chapter 13).

VENTRICULAR SEPTAL DEFECT

A ventricular septal defect can be identified by means of the B-scan technique,[31] but in M-mode recordings the septum appears intact, except when the defect is very large and fortuitously located in the path of the single echo beam. The echocardiogram has, however, been useful in estimating the volume of shunt flow. Such calculations are based on the fact that the left atrium dilates in order to accommodate the increased flow from the right side of the heart. Carter and Bowman found the left atrial dimension (corrected for body surface area) to be 2.5 cm or smaller in the presence of shunts of less than 1.5:1.0 (pulmonic-to-systemic flow).[32] When the shunt exceeded 2.0:1.0, the corrected left atrial dimension was 3.0 cm or greater. In a study by Laird and Fixler, the mean corrected left atrial dimension was 2.42 ± 0.40 cm when the shunt was 1.5:1.0 or less, whereas among patients with shunts exceeding 1.5:1.0, they found that the mean left atrial dimension was 6.3 ± 0.57 cm.[33] In this series all patients with a shunt exceeding 1.5:1.0 had a corrected left atrial dimension of greater than 4.0 cm per M^2 body surface area.

When the defect is large, the mitral and tricuspid valves may appear without a septal echo separating them, as in single ventricle. Nonspecific findings dependent on the magnitude of the shunt include dilatation of the left and right ventricles. The direction of septal motion is normal.

Nanda et al. reported two cases of left ventricular–right atrial communication that appeared clinically to be uncomplicated ventricular septal defects.[34] The unique echocardiographic feature in these two cases was a marked systolic fluttering of the tricuspid valve, thought to be due to the passage of the blood shunting from the ventricle through a defect in the tricuspid valve into the right atrium.

Acute perforation of the interventricular septum most often occurs as a complication of myocardial infarction. While there have been no specific echocardiographic abnormalities identified, right ventricular dilatation is a characteristic finding.[35] (See Chapter 14 for further discussion.)

References

1. Gray H: Anatomy of the Human Body. Philadelphia, Lea & Febiger, 1962.
2. McDonald IG, Feigenbaum H, and Chang S: Analysis of the left ventricular wall motion by reflected ultrasound: Application to assessment of myocardial function. Circulation 46:14–25, 1972.
3. Abbasi AS, Eber LM, MacAlpin RN, and Kattus AA: Paradoxical motion of interventricular septum in left bundle branch block. Circulation 49:423–427, 1974.
4. Jacobs JJ, Feigenbaum H, Corya BC, and Phillips JF: Detection of left ventricular asynergy by echocardiography. Circulation 48:263–271, 1973.
5. Diamond MA, Dillon JC, Haine CL, Chang S, and Feigenbaum H: Echocardiographic features of atrial septal defect. Circulation 43:129–135, 1971.
6. Meyer RA, Schwartz DC, Benzing G, III, and Kaplan S: Ventricular septum in right ventricular volume overload: An echocardiographic study. Am J Cardiol 30:349–353, 1972.
7. Pearlman AS, Morganroth J, Henry WL, and Epstein SE: Determinants of ventricular septal motion (Abstr). Circulation (Suppl III) 49,50:239, 1974.
8. Tajik AJ, Gau GT, Ritter DG, and Schattenberg TT: Echocardiographic pattern of right ventricular diastolic volume overload in children. Circulation 46:36–43, 1972.
9. Kerber, RE, Dippel WF, and Abboud FM: Abnormal motion of the interventricular septum in right ventricular volume overload: Experimental and clinical echocardiographic studies. Circulation 48:86–96, 1973.

10. McCann WD, Harbold NB, Jr., and Giuliani ER: The echocardiogram in right ventricular overload. JAMA *221*:1243–1245, 1972.
11. Kamigaki M, and Goldschlager N: Echocardiographic analysis of mitral valve motion in atrial septal defect. Am J Cardiol *30*:343–348, 1972.
12. Tajik AJ, Gau GT, and Schattenberg TT: Echocardiogram in atrial septal defect. Chest *62*:213–214, 1972.
13. Hagan AD, Francis GS, Sahn DJ, Karliner JS, Friedman WF, and O'Rourke RA: Ultrasound evaluation of systolic anterior septal motion in paitents with and without right ventricular volume overload. Circulation *50*:248–254, 1974.
14. Smith McK, and Hood WP, Jr.: Echocardiographic patterns recorded from a patient with a peripheral arterio-venous shunt. J Clin Ultrasound *1*:288–293, 1973.
15. Sawaya J, Longo MR, and Schlant RC: Echocardiographic interventricular septal wall motion and thickness: A study in health and disease. Am Heart J *87*:681–688, 1974.
16. Chung KJ, Gramiak R, and Manning JA: The value of echocardiography in congestive cardiomyopathy in children (Abstr). *In* White D (Ed.): Ultrasound in Medicine. New York, Plenum Press, 1975, p. 93.
17. Abasi AS, Ellis N, and Child J: Echocardiographic features of infiltrative cardiomyopathy (Abstr). *In* White D (Ed.): Ultrasound in Medicine. New York, Plenum Press, 1975, p. 108.
18. Rossen RM, Goodman DJ, Ingham RE, and Popp RL: Ventricular systolic septal thickening and excursion in idiopathic hypertrophic subaortic stenosis. N Engl J Med *291*:1317–1319, 1974.
19. McDonald IG: Echocardiographic demonstration of abnormal motion of the interventricular septum in left bundle branch block. Circulation *48*:272–280, 1972.
20. Dillon JC, Chang S, and Feigenbaum H: Echocardiographic manifestations of left bundle branch block. Circulation *49*:876–880, 1974.
21. Weiss AN, Chaval S, and Ludbrook PA: Echocardiographic recognition of paradoxical interventricular septal motion associated with right ventricular premature beats (Abstr). Circulation (Suppl III) *49,50*:250, 1974.
22. DeMaria N, Vera Z, Neumann A, Awan N, and Mason DT: Alterations in ventricular contraction pattern in the Wolff-Parkinson-White syndrome: Detection by echocardiography (Abstr). Circulation (Suppl II) *51,52*:33, 1975.
23. Theroux P, Francis G, Hagan A, Johnson A, and O'Rourke R: Echocardiographic study of interventricular septal motion in the Wolff-Parkinson-White syndrome (Abstr). Circulation (Suppl II) *51,52*:70, 1975.
24. Kanakis C, Wyndham CRC, Younce C, Miller R, and Rosen K: Echocardiographic findings in the Wolff-Parkinson-White syndrome (Abstr). Circulation (Suppl II) *51,52*:200, 1975.
25. Feigenbaum H: Echocardiographic diagnosis of pericardial effusion. Am J Cardiol *26*:475–479, 1970.
26. Feigenbaum H: Echocardiography. Philadelphia, Lea & Febiger, 1972.
27. Yoshikawa J, Owaki T, Kato H, and Tanaka K: Abnormal motion of interventricular septum of patients with prosthetic valve. *In* White D (Ed.): Ultrasound in Medicine. New York, Plenum Press, 1975, p. 1.
28. Adams N, McFadden RB, Chambers J, Cornish D, and Vogel JK: Acquired paradoxic septal motion following successful coronary artery bypass surgery (Abstr). *In* White D (Ed.): Ultrasound in Medicine. New York, Plenum Press, 1975, p. 106.
29. Gibson TC, Grossman W, McLaurin LP, and Craige E: Echocardiography in patients with constrictive pericarditis (Abstr). Circulation (Suppl III) *49,50*:86, 1974.
30. Pool PE, and Seagren SC: Effects on abnormal septal motion of surgery for constrictive pericarditis (Abstr). *In* White D (Ed.): Ultrasound in Medicine. New York, Plenum Press, 1975, p. 104.
31. King DL, Steeg CN, and Ellis K: Visualization of ventricular septal defects by cardiac ultrasonography. Circulation *48*:1215–1220, 1973.
32. Carter WH, and Bowman CR: Estimation of shunt flow in isolated ventricular septal defect by echocardiogram (Abstr). Circulation (Suppl IV) *48*:64, 1973.
33. Laird WP, and Fixler DE: Use of ultrasound to define shunting in ventricular septal defects. *In* White D (Ed.): Ultrasound in Medicine. New York, Plenum Press, 1975, p. 43.
34. Nanda NC, Gramiak R, and Manning JA: Echocardiography of the tricuspid valve in congenital left ventricular–right atrial communication. Circulation *51*:268–272, 1975.
35. Chandraratna PAN, Balachandran PK, Shah PM, and Hodges M: Echocardiographic observations on ventricular septal rupture complicating acute myocardial infarction. Circulation *51*:506–510, 1975.
36. Chandra MS, Kerber RE, Brown DD, and Funk DC: Echocardiography in Wolff-Parkinson-White syndrome (Abstr). Circulation (Suppl II) *51,52*:49, 1975.
37. Lundström N: Echocardiography in the diagnosis of Ebstein's anomaly of the tricuspid valve. Circulation *47*:597–605, 1973.

8

The Left Ventricle

Left ventricular performance is the most important factor in both the therapeutic and the prognostic implications of the majority of adult cardiac diseases. Echocardiographic analysis of the left ventricle provides the clinician with a valuable tool for the assessment of left ventricular function. To date, however, the applications relative to the activity of the left ventricle in individual cases remain rather gross. The primary usefulness of routine left ventricular recordings lies at present in the detection of wall motion abnormalities, the measurement of chamber size, and the determination of circumferential muscle fiber shortening velocity. The ultimate value of the echocardiogram may derive from its ability to provide serial measurements of certain parameters of left ventricular function.[1] This provides a distinct advantage over invasive studies, which are limited in this regard because it is not practicable to perform them on a repetitive basis.

NORMAL ANATOMY AND PHYSIOLOGY

The left ventricular chamber is bordered by the interventricular septum on its anterior and medial aspects, and by the free wall of the left ventricle anteriorly, laterally, inferiorly, and posteriorly. The superior–posterior region is composed of the mitral valve orifice and the aortic outflow tract. The septum and posterobasal free wall are routinely seen on the echocardiogram, and in many cases, the anterior left ventricular wall is also visualized.[2] The lateral wall and the apex are seen infrequently with present recording techniques.

Two facts about the left ventricle highlight its performance: a high pressure is generated within the chamber during ventricular systole, and this pressure is produced in a very short period of time. The rapid generation of left ventricular pressure is accomplished by a large muscle mass that requires a high rate of oxygen consumption. In addition, a normally functioning mitral valve is necessary to prevent blood reflux into the low-pressure left atrial chamber.

NORMAL ECHOCARDIOGRAPHIC FEATURES

The left ventricular recordings should be performed as the last part of the echocardiographic examination, when the patient is most relaxed. This provides a more nearly basal state for measurements of left ventricular function.

The Posterior Wall

In recording the posterior wall of the left ventricle, it is best to localize the area just below the posterior mitral leaflet and above the posteromedial papillary muscle (Fig. 8–1). This is best accomplished by first locating the mitral valve and then directing the ultrasound beam into the left ventricle, generally in an inferior lateral direction (Fig. 8–2), ideally until the posterior wall loses the terminal diastolic dip reflected from the point of its attachment to the mitral annulus. When the beam is aimed farther inferiorly, it intersects the posteromedial papillary muscle. At this point, the systolic excursion of the posterior wall becomes more pronounced and the chordae tendineae disappear from view.

When the echo beam intersects the posterior left ventricular wall between the papillary muscle and mitral valve, it is traversing a minor axis of the left ventricle. This dimension is approximately one half the length of the long axis of the normal left ventricle. In this important view (Fig. 8–1), several structures will be visible, including the right ventricular anterior wall, the interventricular septum, some portions of the mitral leaflets (usually during diastolic opening), and the chordae tendineae, as well as the posterior left ventricular wall.

The posterior wall is composed of three tissue components, the endocardium, the myocardium, and the epicardial–pericardial interface, each of which has a distinct echocardiographic appearance (Fig. 8–3). The region of the posterior wall may present a confusing array of echoes of similar appearance, but recognition of certain characteristics is helpful in distinguishing their origin:

1. The chordae tendineae lie anterior to the posterior wall and reflect one or more echoes that exhibit an undulating, low-amplitude anterior motion during ventricular systole that becomes slowly posterior in direction during diastole.

2. The endocardial surface appears as a fainter echo, which can easily be missed without careful adjustment of the echo intensity. The endocardium moves anteriorly during ventricular systole and, of paramount importance, exhibits a more rapid rate of anterior motion than the other structures in this region. During diastole it has a fast posterior excursion followed by a slow one. When the segment of endocardium near the mitral annulus is recorded, the echocardiogram shows the distinctive late-diastolic notch, which probably occurs as a result of the myocardial fiber attachment to the cardiac skeleton.

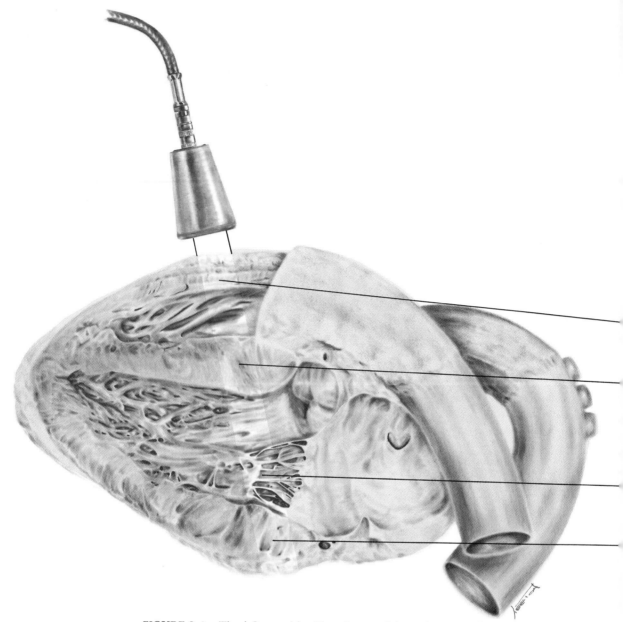

FIGURE 8-1. The left ventricle. The ultrasound beam intersects the muscular interventricular septum and the posterior left ventricular wall below the posterior mitral leaflet. Key: AWRV = Anterior wall of right ventricle. IVS = Interventricular septum. C = Chordae tendineae. PWLV = Posterior wall of left ventricle.

3. The myocardium between endocardium and epicardium often appears relatively echo-free, especially during ventricular systole.[3]

4. The epicardial–pericardial interface, which is the outer region of the myocardium and adjacent pericardium, reflects an echo denser than those from the myocardium (anterior) and the lung (posterior). The edge of the pericardial–epicardial interface is most obvious when a pericardial effusion is present. This echo also moves anteriorly during ventricular systole, but at a slower rate than the endocardial echo.

The posterior left ventricular wall has been subjected to close scrutiny by various investigators[1, 4–17] seeking to determine if the motion of this structure would provide information relative to the function of the ventricle as a whole.

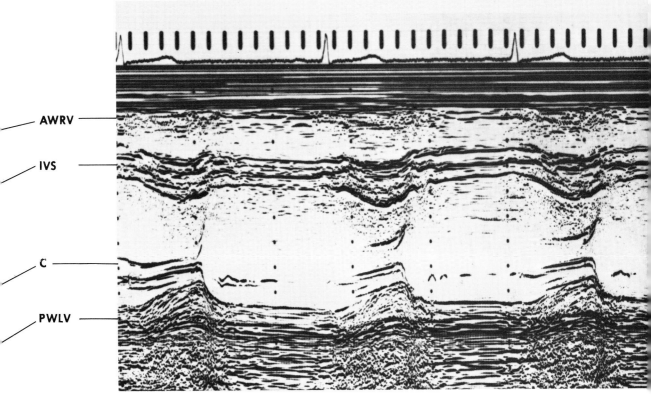

AWRV

IVS

C

PWLV

FIGURE 8–1. Continued.

From these studies, two important limitations have become apparent. First, certain of these measurements of posterior wall motion have proved difficult to reproduce. This is related in part to technical difficulties in obtaining posterior wall recordings. Furthermore, even the subtlest of many variables may effect small increments of change in posterior wall motion as measured with the echocardiogram. For example, changes in blood flow to the left heart due to respiration probably have a detectable effect. Therefore, to obtain valid data, it is necessary to record posterior wall motion for many consecutive beats.

Second, measurements of the motion of an isolated segment of myocardium cannot be assumed to be true for the other areas of the left ventricle. This is especially limiting in the study of segmental myocardial dyskinesia or akinesia, which commonly occur secondary to coronary artery disease.

The motion of the posterior left ventricular wall has been compared to an inverted ventricular volume curve[18] and may be divided into six phases (Fig. 8–4).

1. Isovolumetric contraction. This phase begins during the QRS complex of the electrocardiogram and ends with the onset of ventricular ejection. During this interval, the posterior wall moves slightly posteriorly. Sometimes no motion is evident; least often, a slight anterior excursion is observed. The posterior motion caused by atrial filling sometimes entirely obscures this phase.

2. Ventricular ejection. The posterior wall moves anteriorly as a result of myocardial fiber shortening and consequent chamber narrowing. An additional component of the anterior displacement results from the motion of the entire heart toward the anterior chest wall during ventricular systole. At approximately the peak of its forward excursion, the aortic valve closes, and left ventricular ejection is terminated.

3. Isovolumetric relaxation. During this phase, the left ventricle is a closed chamber as the pressure falls within it. At this time, the posterior wall exhibits a slow posterior excursion from the peak anterior position attained during systolic ejection.

4. Early diastolic filling. The beginning of this phase coincides with mitral valve opening. The posterior wall moves posteriorly at a more rapid rate than

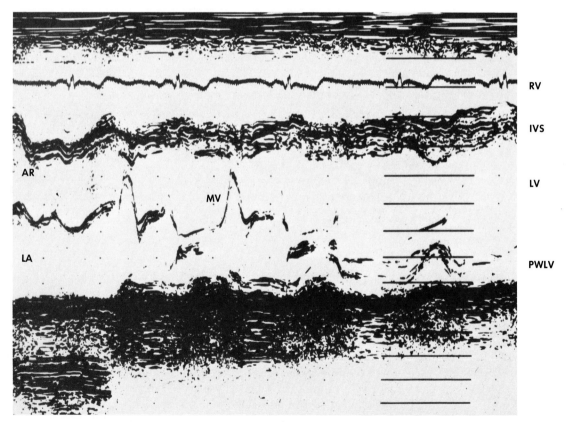

FIGURE 8–2. Scan from the mitral valve (MV) to the left ventricle (LV). From the mitral valve, the transducer has been angled inferiorly and laterally (AR = aortic root; LA = left atrium; RV = right ventricle; IVS = interventricular septum; PWLV = posterior wall of the left ventricle).

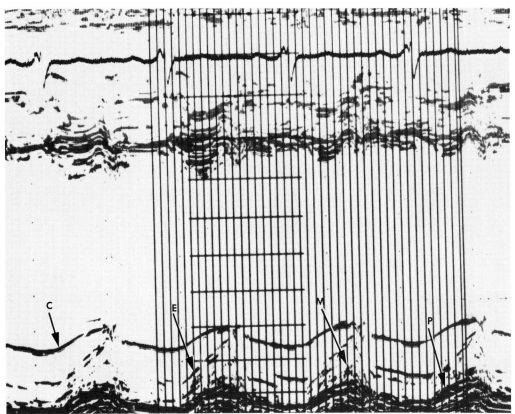

PWLV

FIGURE 8–3. The posterior wall of the left ventricle (PWLV). A chordal echo (c) is seen as a relatively heavy band with slight anterior systolic excursion. The endocardial echo (E) is less intense and exhibits the greatest systolic motion. The myocardium (M) immediately behind the endocardium is relatively echo-free, while the epicardial–pericardial area (P) reflects the most intense echo.

during isovolumetric relaxation as the ventricle expands to accommodate the blood entering from the left atrium.

5. Mid-diastole. Following the period of rapid filling, the wall moves slowly posteriorly as a slower rate of ventricular filling continues until the time of atrial contraction in late diastole.

6. Atrial filling. Atrial contraction following the P wave of the electrocardiogram causes an abrupt posterior displacement if the left ventricular posterior wall recording is made near its point of attachment to the mitral annulus. This motion appears to be a result of the influence of atrial motion on the cardiac skeleton and not of an actual increase in left ventricular volume at this time.

Parameters of Motion

In order to establish meaningful echocardiographic criteria of posterior left ventricular wall motion, several parameters have been carefully studied. At present, it appears that the most significant factors are amplitude of posterior wall excursion during ventricular systole, the posterior wall systolic velocity, and posterior wall early-diastolic velocity.

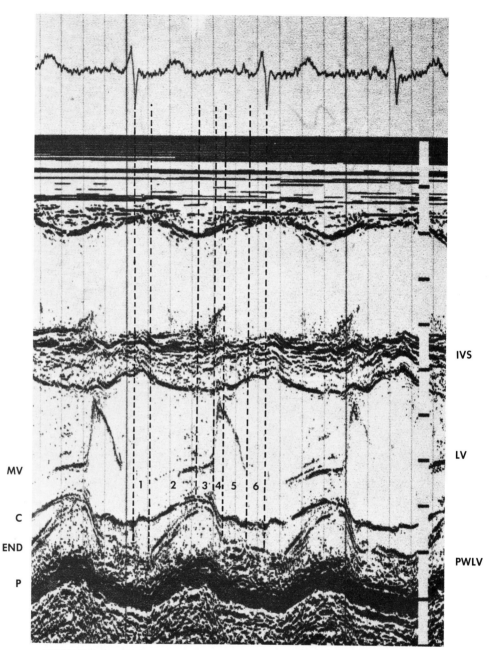

FIGURE 8-4. Motion of the posterior left ventricular wall (PWLV). (1) Isovolumetric contraction, (2) ventricular ejection, (3) isovolumetric relaxation, (4) early-diastolic filling, (5) mid-diastole, (6) atrial filling (IVS = interventricular septum; LV = left ventricle; MV = mitral valve; C = chordal echo; END = endocardium; P = pericardium).

Posterior Wall Excursion. The systolic anterior excursion of the posterior wall is actually a composite motion caused by myocardial contraction and, to a lesser extent, by the anterior displacement of the entire heart.[18]

There have been significant variations in the reported normal values for posterior wall systolic amplitude. In three separate studies, the normal mean amplitude of excursion at rest was found to be 0.4 cm,[8] 0.72 cm,[9] and 1.15

cm,[18] respectively. The greatest error in this measurement, especially in the early studies, lay in failure to record the endocardial surface properly on the echocardiogram. Eliciting this echo requires considerable technical skill and machine sensitivity. Without a clear recording of this fine echo, the true amplitude of posterior wall excursion is generally underestimated. Furthermore, the posterior wall amplitude of motion will be erroneous if the mitral annulus, the apical myocardium, or the posteromedial papillary muscle is mistaken for the posterobasal left ventricular wall.

Increased stroke volume is associated with an increase in the posterior wall excursion. This is seen in postexercise states[8, 9] and following administration of drugs that produce an inotropic effect.[16] On the other hand, drugs that increase cardiac output by increasing heart rate (chronotropic effect) do not in themselves increase posterior wall excursion. Increasing the heart rate by atrial pacing actually reduces posterior wall excursion.[8]

Posterior Wall Systolic Velocity. The posterior wall systolic velocity is the rate (cm/sec) at which the endocardial surface moves anteriorly during ventricular systole. This may be measured as the maximal velocity of excursion or as the mean velocity from the beginning of contraction to the peak systolic anterior position.

In one study, the mean maximal posterior wall velocity was found to be 4.1 ± 1.1 cm/sec.[9] After exercise this increased to 9.2 ± 2.8 cm/sec. (In 2 of 25 normals, the mean posterior wall velocity appeared to diminish following exercise.) This represents an average increase of approximately 130 percent in the maximal posterior wall velocity following exercise. In the same study, a similar increase was seen in the mean posterior wall velocity after exercise.

Direct and indirect effects on the posterior wall velocity have been observed with the administration of drugs that alter circulatory hemodynamics. Increased heart rate subsequent to atropine infusion also increases the mean posterior wall velocity.[19] The effect of isoproterenol infusion on posterior wall velocity is an increase in both the maximal and the mean velocities that is comparable to the response following exercise. However, methoxamine, which directly affects only the peripheral resistance, slightly diminishes the posterior wall velocity.[16] Increasing blood pressure by phenylephrine infusion decreases the posterior wall velocity.[19] Propranolol, with its negative inotropic effect, has also been found to reduce the posterior wall velocity.[20]

Others have found, however, that when the posterior wall velocity is compared with other parameters of left ventricular function, there is poor correlation of the posterior wall excursion rate during ventricular systole with the ejection fraction, the mean velocity of circumferential fiber shortening (V_{CF}) and the ratio of pre-ejection period to left ventricular ejection time (PEP/LVET).[4] Furthermore, measurements of the mean and maximal posterior wall velocities appear to be poorly reproducible, with variations of up to 52 percent in serial determinations in individual patients. Beat-to-beat changes in posterior wall velocity of almost 150 percent may occur. The epicardial velocity also exhibits a poor correlation with the endocardial measurements.

Variations in posterior wall velocity are most apparent in the presence of cardiac arrhythmias. In these cases, marked fluctuations in the left ventricular volume as well as alterations in electrical depolarization probably account for the posterior wall changes from beat to beat (Fig. 8–5). Becuase of these discrepancies, Quinones et al. have proposed that "normalized" posterior wall velocity may be more valid.[17]

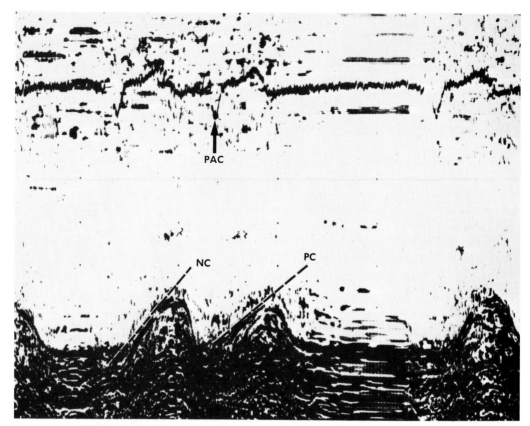

FIGURE 8–5. Effect of arrhythmia on posterior left ventricular wall motion. The second beat is a premature atrial contraction (PAC). The posterior wall velocity of the early beat (PC) is slowed in comparison with the previous normal contraction (NC).

Posterior Wall Diastolic Velocity.   Fogelman et al. have studied the rate of posterior excursion of the left ventricular posterior wall following systolic contraction and have proposed that this is a function of myocardial relaxation.[10] They found the maximal diastolic velocity to be 18.0 ± 3.0 cm/sec and the mean to be 9.4 ± 1.7 cm/sec. These values were found to increase with exercise but were abnormally reduced in the presence of ischemia. Kovick and associates reported that the diastolic endocardial velocity was significantly reduced in patients with muscular dystrophy.[21]

Posterior Wall Thickness

Precise measurement of the thickness of the posterior wall provides an excellent means for direct determination of an index of the left ventricular muscle mass. This measurement has assumed special importance in the echocardiographic diagnosis of asymmetric septal hypertrophy (see Chapter 13).

On the echocardiogram, the posterior wall width is measured during late diastole, either immediately prior to atrial systole[22] or at the time of the R wave of the electrocardiogram. Wall thickness is measured from the light endocardial echo to the epicardial–pericardial echo. If the posterior boundary of this echo is not readily separable from pulmonary tissue, an abrupt decrease in the gain (Fig. 8–6) may be helpful in its delineation, although the newer recorders seldom make this maneuver necessary (Fig. 8–7).

Feigenbaum and associates found that the echocardiographic left ventricular thickness was within 3 mm of the necropsy measurement.[23] Intraoperative measurement tended to be slightly larger than the echo determination, but correlation of the two measurements was within 5 mm in every case. Sjögren et al. found that the posterior wall thickness measurement was highly reproducible on repeat examinations.[14] The normal posterior wall diastolic width is 0.8 to 1.3 cm.

Bennett et al. have determined that the end-systolic width of the posterior wall may relate to the systolic pressure within the left ventricle.[24] They found that the normal left ventricular systolic width ranged from 1.3 to 1.9 cm in 15 subjects. Furthermore, they found a correlation between the end-systolic width relative to the end-systolic internal dimension of the left ventricle and the peak systolic intraventricular pressure.

Separate studies have determined that the posterior wall thickens by approximately 60 to 70 percent during ventricular systole.[14, 18, 25] This increase corresponds closely with systolic thickening of the interventricular septum.

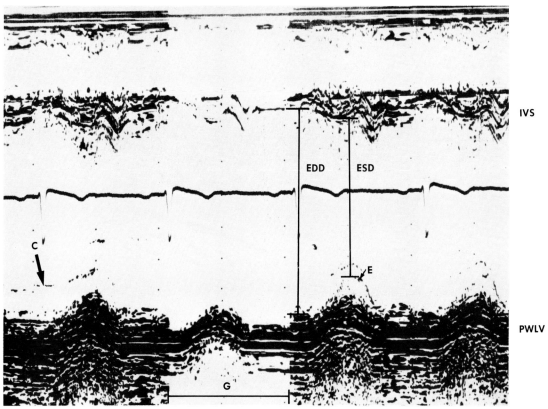

FIGURE 8–6. Dimensions of the left ventricle. The end-diastolic dimension (EDD) is measured at the time of the electrocardiographic QRS complex. The end-systolic dimension (ESD) is measured at peak posterior wall anterior motion from the endocardial (E) echo. In this example, the latter echo is seen adequately only in the third and fourth beats. The chordal echo (C) should not be mistaken for the endocardium. Gain reduction (G) is employed to assist in defining the posterior wall thickness (IVS = interventricular septum; PWLV = posterior wall of the left ventricle).

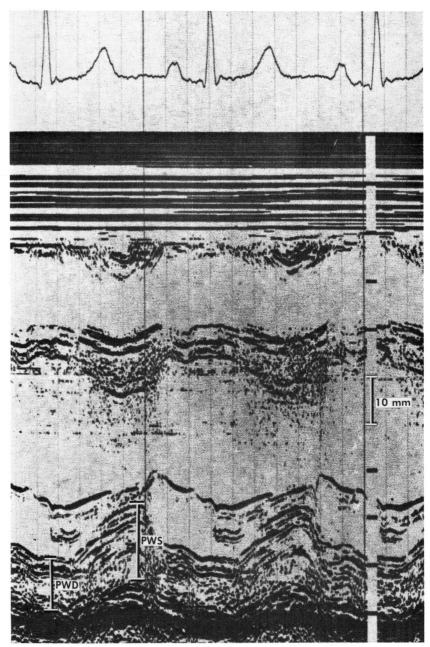

FIGURE 8–7. The posterior wall diastolic thickness (PWD) is measured at the time of the electrocardiographic QRS complex, in this case, 11 mm. The width increases to 18 mm at peak anterior systolic motion (PWS).

VENTRICULAR CHAMBER DIMENSIONS

The most reliable single echocardiographic measurement of the left ventricular size is the end-diastolic minor axis dimension (EDD) (Fig. 8–6). This may be measured at the time of the predominant R or S wave of the electrocardiogram, from the posterior edge of the septum to the endocardial echo of the posterior wall. Meyer et al. have pointed out, however, that because the posterior wall may move slightly posteriorly during the period of isovolumetric contraction, the measurement is best made at the beginning of the electrocardiographic QRS complex.[26] The left ventricular dimension is difficult to determine in that precise location if the posterior (left ventricular) edge of the septum is not distinct on the same recording that gives the optimal view of the posterior endocardium. (This is more often a problem in determining the end-systolic measurement.) In the event that the left ventricular septal echo is obscure, the dimension may be estimated by first measuring the septal thickness in its best view. The septal thickness is then subtracted from the distance between the right ventricular septal edge and the posterior wall endocardium to obtain the left ventricular dimension.

At the time of the maximal excursion of the posterior wall, its end-systolic dimension (ESD) is measured from its endocardial echo to the left ventricular edge of the septum. (The septal edge is usually maximally posterior slightly before this time.) As an index of overall ventricular size, the end-systolic dimension is less reliable than the diastolic measurement in that a dyskinetic area within the ventricle will cause geometric distortion during contraction. Consequently, when the beam is intersecting a localized area of diseased septum or posterior wall, the left ventricle will appear spuriously large during systole. On the other hand, if a diseased area is present but is not within the beam target area, the systolic dimension measured will be smaller than is truly representative of the left ventricular systolic size.

The end-systolic and end-diastolic dimensions vary according to such factors as flow rate and diastolic filling time. In one study of the effects of acute changes on the left ventricle,[27] elevation of the patient's head caused detectable reductions of the end-systolic dimension (3.2 cm to 2.8 cm) and the end-diastolic dimension (4.8 cm to 4.2 cm). Similar changes in end-systolic and end-diastolic dimensions following nitroglycerin administration have been observed in this study and in reports by DeMaria et al.[28] and by Burggraf and Parker.[29] These effects have been attributed to reduced venous return to the heart. Phenylephrine, which increases the afterload, increases the end-diastolic dimension but has no significant effect on the end-systolic dimension.[27]

VENTRICULAR VOLUMES

Extrapolation of one-dimensional echocardiographic measurements to left ventricular volume determinations requires the assumption that the left ventricular chamber is a certain shape. While exact conformation does not exist, the left ventricle normally has a shape that, for practical purposes, resembles a prolate ellipse,[30] i.e., a cylinder with a diameter equal to twice its longitudinal axis. Thus, the left ventricular volume can be estimated by measuring the dimension of the minor axis (D) traversed by the echo beam. The formula for the volume of a prolate ellipse is

$$V = \frac{\pi}{6} D_1 D_2 L$$

where D_1 and D_2 are the two minor axes, and L is the dimension of the long axis.[36] If D_1 and D_2 are assumed to be equal, and L is equal to twice the minor axis ($2D$), the formula becomes

$$V = \frac{\pi}{6}D^2 = \frac{\pi}{3}D^3$$

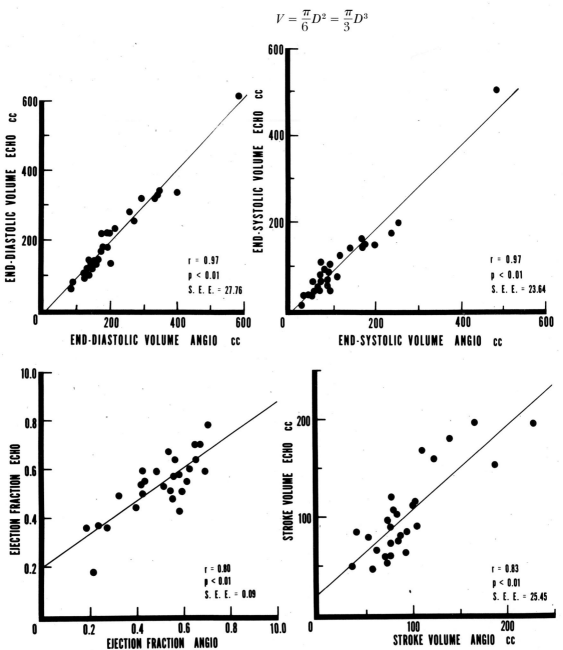

FIGURE 8–8. *Top,* Comparison of end-diastolic volume and of end-systolic volume by echocardiographic and angiocardiographic methods. For end-diastolic volume, the regression equation is $y = -12 - 1.04x$. For end-systolic volume the regression equation is $y = -6 + 0.96x$. In both, y = echocardiographic volume and x = angiocardiographic volume. The correlation coefficient is $r = 0.97$ for both, and the standard error of the estimate (SEE) is small in each comparison. *Bottom,* Comparison of ejection fraction and of total left ventricular stroke volume by echocardiography and angiocardiography. For ejection fraction the regression equation is $y = 0.20 + 0.68x$. For stroke volume the regression is $y = 21 + 0.86x$. SEE is relatively larger for these two derived parameters. (From Pombo et al.: Circulation, *43*, April, 1971, p. 484, by permission of the American Heart Association, Inc.)

By assuming the algebraic cancellation of $\frac{\pi}{3}$, the formula becomes

$$V = D^3$$

Therefore, the volume of the left ventricle is approximately equal to the cube of the minor axis dimension. The end-diastolic volume (EDV) is determined by cubing the minor end-diastolic dimension, and the end-systolic volume (ESV) is calculated by cubing the minor end-systolic dimension. The volumes determined in this way have shown significant correlation with angiographic volume estimations (Fig. 8–8).[31, 32]

This method of left ventricular volume determination is inaccurate in cases of chamber enlargement.[32] In these instances, the volume size will be progressively overestimated as the left ventricular dimensions increase. The error occurs because the long axis becomes less than twice the minor axis determination as the ventricle assumes a more nearly spherical shape.[33, 34]

For enlarged ventricles, additional formulae have been derived.[34]

$$ESV = 47ESD - 120$$
$$EDV = 59EDD - 153$$

Meyer et al. have observed a good correlation between the angiographic volume determination and the echocardiographic calculation at end-diastole in children.[26] They found this correlation to be true for end-diastolic dimensions between 2 and 5 cm, and derived the following linear regression equation:

$$EDV = 27.7\ EDD - 42.2$$

Localized areas of akinesia or dyskinesia of any portion of the ventricle, including the septum, also invalidate these methods for volume estimation, as symmetrical contraction is lost.[33] This error is especially true for systolic volume estimations, because geometrical distortions are maximal during ventricular systole.[35, 36] This method also becomes invalid in the event that septal motion is abnormal for any other reason, including right ventricular volume overload and left bundle branch block.

Arrhythmias must also be taken into account in the calculation of left ventricular volumes (Fig. 8–9). Redwood and associates, for example, found that changes in the R-R interval in patients with atrial fibrillation correlated positively with the end-diastolic left ventricular dimension.[27]

Morganroth and associates studied the echocardiographic left ventricular dimensions in trained athletes.[37] Those who were engaged in isotonic forms of exercise (i.e, running) had significantly larger end-diastolic dimensions with normal posterior wall thicknesses, whereas those involved in isometric types of exercise had normal end-diastolic dimensions but increased wall thickness measurements. In another study, left ventricular volumes were not found to change immediately after isometric exercise.[38]

The amount of blood ejected from the left ventricle in one cardiac cycle is termed the stroke volume (SV). The echocardiogram may be utilized to calculate the stroke volume by first determining end-systolic and end-diastolic volumes and then calculating their difference as the stroke volume (Fig. 8–8).

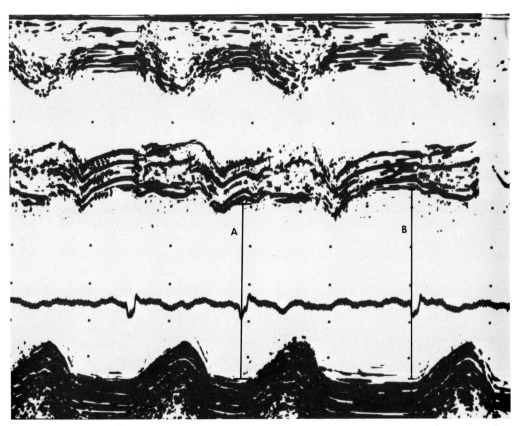

FIGURE 8–9. The effect of varying diastolic filling times on the ventricular dimension. The rhythm is atrial fibrillation. Following a short R-R interval, the end-diastolic dimension (A) is 4.4 cm, but after the completion of the next cardiac cycle, this dimension has increased to 5.0 cm (B) as a result of the longer period of ventricular filling.

This is expressed as

$$SV = EDV - ESV$$

Popp and Harrison found an excellent correlation between the echo stroke volume and that derived by the Fick method.[39] As the ventricle enlarges, however, the stroke volume determination by this means becomes progressively less accurate as ESV and EDV become overestimated (resulting in inordinately large stroke volume calculations).

VENTRICULAR FUNCTION

The echocardiogram has provided the cardiologist with new hopes for a simple but accurate means for the objective assessment of the efficiency with which the left ventricle delivers blood to the systemic circulation. Some of the indices of the left ventricular function include the ejection fraction, cardiac output, circumferential muscle fiber shortening velocity, normalized posterior wall and septal velocity, mitral valve motion, and aortic valve motion.

Ejection Fraction

The ejection fraction (EF) is that amount of blood ejected from the ventricle during one systolic contraction and is expressed as

$$EF = \frac{SV}{EDV}$$

(Multiplied by 100, the EF may also be expressed as the percent of blood ejected.) The ejection fraction determined echocardiographically has been found to correlate well with angiographic studies (Fig. 8–8),[1, 17, 31, 32, 34, 40] although the echocardiogram does tend to overestimate this value in some cases.[17]

The ejection fraction determined in this way is normally approximately 60 percent and is significantly reduced in patients with mitral stenosis, compensated volume overload, and congestive failure.[40] It is increased in patients with the obstructive form of asymmetric septal hypertrophy. The ejection fraction calculated from the echocardiogram is also increased in the case of compensated aortic regurgitation or mitral regurgitation, as the volume of blood ejected from the left ventricle is equal to the regurgitant volume plus the amount delivered to the peripheral tissues. Qualitatively, this is manifested by the prominent septal and posterior wall systolic motion observed on the echocardiogram in these two types of valvular regurgitation.

Cardiac Output

The cardiac output (CO) is the effective volume of blood ejected in one minute, expressed in cubic centimeters (or milliliters) per minute. Thus it is a product of the stroke volume and heart rate (HR).

$$CO = SV \times HR$$

Because the calculation of the cardiac output is dependent on the accuracy of the stroke volume determination, echocardiographic estimation of cardiac output is erroneously high in cases of moderate or severe left ventricular dilatation.

Circumferential Muscle Fiber Shortening Velocity

Determination by cineangiogram of the mean velocity of shortening of a minor internal equator of the left ventricle (V_{CF}, expressed in circumferences per second) is an expression of myocardial contractility.[41] It normally is greater than 1.10 circumferences per second. The V_{CF} may be calculated from the echocardiogram[42] when it is assumed that the echocardiographic minor axis dimension of the left ventricle is equal to the diameter across the minor internal equator. Several studies have shown a significant correlation between the V_{CF} calculated from the echocardiogram and that determined from the cineangiogram.[1, 7, 17]

The mean V_{CF} is derived from the echocardiogram by the formula

$$\text{Mean } V_{CF} = \text{EDD} - \text{ESD/EDD} \times \text{ET}$$

where ET equals the ejection time of the left ventricle.[7] The ET is the time from the QRS peak to the maximum anterior displacement of the posterior wall in systole, minus 50 msec, to correct for the pre-ejection period. Calculation of the ET may also be accomplished by measuring the time from the beginning of posterior wall movement anteriorly to its maximal anterior position.[40]

The accuracy of V_{CF} determination by these methods is obviously dependent on technically excellent left ventricular posterior wall recordings. For example, in calculating the ejection time, precise location of the most anterior position of the posterior wall may be difficult because it often does not appear to be a single point in time. The method is also limited by the same factors that affect the validity of the end-systolic and end-diastolic dimensions.

Studies of myocardial contractility are easily carried out utilizing echocardiographic V_{CF} calculations. For example, reduction of the preload by the administration of nitroglycerin and by head-up tilting causes a slight decrease in the V_{CF} determined in this way.[28] In other studies, however, acute changes in preload did not significantly affect the V_{CF}.[43, 44] It has been observed that the V_{CF} decreases with the augmentation of afterload by increasing the blood pressure with the infusion of either phenylephrine[19] or angiotensin.[44] Quinones et al. have pointed out that the sensitivity of the V_{CF} to acute changes in afterload must be taken into consideration in its application in the clinical setting.[44] Increasing heart rate by atropine infusion has the effect of increasing V_{CF}.[19] Alcohol decreases the mean V_{CF} by about 5 percent from 30 to 60 minutes after ingestion.[45]

Sahn et al. studied the V_{CF} in newborns and found a range from 0.92 to 2.2 circumferences per second (average 1.51 ± 0.4).[46] Although the V_{CF} was slightly depressed during the first 30 minutes of life, it rose and remained unchanged thereafter for the first 6 days.

A number of diseases that affect myocardial contractility have been found to alter the V_{CF}. From the formulae, it is apparent that a shortened left ventricular ejection time and reduced ejection fraction both result in a decrease in the V_{CF}. Therefore, the V_{CF} is abnormally low in left ventricular failure.[40, 47] Conversely, obstructive asymmetric septal hypertrophy in the absence of failure may result in an increased V_{CF} as the ejection time is relatively shortened and the ejection fraction is increased. Changes in V_{CF} as well as the percent change in the minor axis diameter have been found to correlate with abnormal changes in systolic time intervals in patients with coronary artery disease.[48]

Normalized Posterior Wall and Septal Velocity

The velocities of contraction of the septum and posterior wall corrected for the left ventricular ejection time and end-diastolic dimension have been proposed as additional indices of left ventricular function.[17] Termed the "normalized velocities," their formulae are

$$V_{PW} \text{ (sec}^{-1}) = \text{PWE/LVET} \times \text{EDD}$$

and

$$V_{IVS} \ (sec^{-1}) = IVSE/LVET \times EDD$$

where V_{PW} = normalized mean posterior wall velocity
     V_{IVS} = normalized mean interventricular septal velocity
     PWE = posterior wall systolic excursion
     IVSE = interventricular septum systolic excursion.

In this study, both V_{PW} and V_{IVS} were found to correlate well with echocardiographic and angiographic mean V_{CF} in patients without coronary artery disease.

Mitral Valve Motion

When the mitral valve apparatus itself is functioning normally, the motion of the valve leaflets may be regarded as a reflection of the pressure–volume relationships between the left atrium and the left ventricle. (The flow rate of blood across the mitral valve relative to mitral valve motion is discussed in Chapter 4.) Because the left ventricle is by far the dominant of the two left

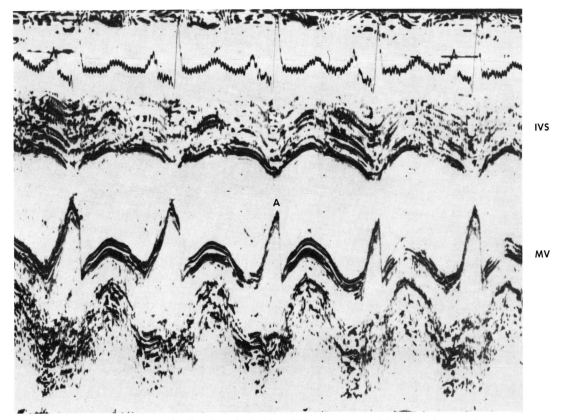

FIGURE 8-10. Absent early-diastolic mitral valve (MV) opening resulting from increased left ventricular end-systolic pressure. There is no E wave, as mitral valve opening occurs only after atrial contraction (A) (IVS = interventricular septum).

heart chambers in terms of the internal pressures generated, the motion of a normal mitral valve may be assumed to be primarily a manifestation of left ventricular pressure and volume.

Mitral opening occurs at the time the left ventricular pressure falls below the pressure within the left atrium. Echocardiographic detection of the onset of rapid anterior excursion of the anterior mitral leaflet (D′ point) follows the hemodynamic pressure crossover between atrium and ventricle by approximately 30 msec.[49, 50] Mitral valve closure (C_0 point), defined as the termination of the last rapid posterior motion in end-diastole on the echocardiogram, also follows closely (by approximately 25 msec) the point at which the left ventricular pressure exceeds the left atrial pressure.[49, 50] The isovolumetric relaxation period of the left ventricle is the interval from aortic valve closure to mitral opening; the period of isovolumetric contraction is the interval from the onset of the QRS complex to aortic valve opening.

The rate of mitral opening (DE slope) varies inversely with the end-systolic left ventricular pressure, which normally approaches zero after aortic valve closure. Koencke et al. found that a DE slope of less than 25 cm/sec correlated with an initial left ventricular diastolic pressure exceeding 12 mm Hg.[51] Rarely, a markedly elevated left ventricular end-systolic pressure may result in mitral opening only in late diastole following atrial contraction (Fig. 8–10). The total mitral leaflet diastolic opening amplitude of excursion (DE amplitude) is in part

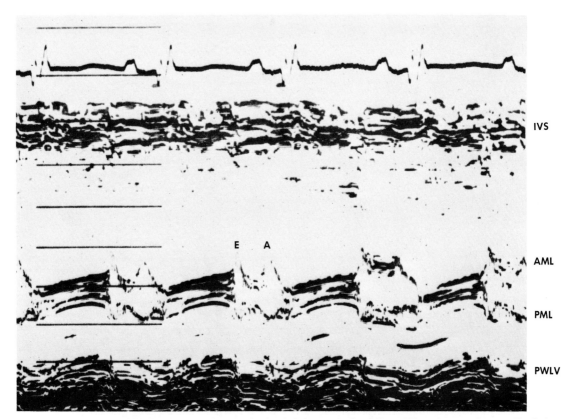

FIGURE 8–11.   The mitral valve in left ventricular failure. The valve opening amplitude has become reduced and the anterior (AML) and posterior (PML) leaflets appear as mirror images. The E and A waves are equal in amplitude, with a fine diastolic fluttering. The entire mitral apparatus is removed from the posterior left ventricular wall (PWLV) (IVS = interventricular septum).

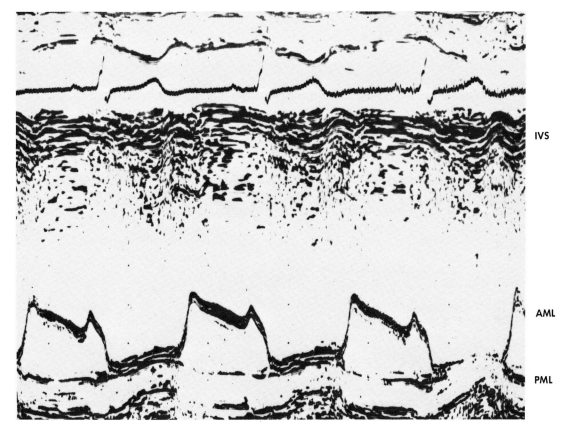

IVS

AML

PML

FIGURE 8–12. Reduced left ventricular compliance. The mitral EF slope is diminished to 20 mm per sec because of the decrease in flow to the left ventricle. The valve itself, however, is thin and pliable as manifested by the sharp A wave (IVS = interventricular septum; AML = anterior mitral leaflet; PML = posterior mitral leaflet).

a function of the flow into the ventricle. Early diastolic flow is influenced both by the end-systolic left ventricular volume and by left ventricular compliance. For this reason, the E wave and A wave become of similar magnitude when the flow during early diastole approaches the flow during atrial systole, as occurs in left ventricular failure. In severe left ventricular failure, the flow across the mitral valve is so reduced that the small mitral opening of the E and A waves of the two mitral leaflets takes on a "fishmouth" appearance on the echocardiogram (Fig. 8–11).

The EF slope is primarily a function of left ventricular compliance, provided the mitral leaflets possess normal pliability. Compliance refers to the distensibility of the ventricle and is defined in terms of the relationship between the pressure within the ventricle and its volume. In other words, a decreased compliance indicates a lesser volume for a given pressure. As the left ventricular compliance decreases, as occurs in the myocardial infiltrative diseases,[52] left ventricular hypertrophy and coronary disease,[53] the flow rate across the mitral valve decreases. Consequently, the mitral valve maintains a longer period of opening during diastole to accommodate the slower flow rate into the "stiff" ventricle. In these disease states, reduced left ventricular compliance may therefore be manifested on the echocardiogram as a diminished EF slope (Fig. 8–12). In a series of 32 patients without mitral disease, a slope of less than 60 mm/sec showed significant correlation with diminished left ventricular compliance, regardless of cause.[53]

The time from maximal mitral valve opening during atrial systole (A point) to complete mitral closure (C point) is a function both of the time elapsed between the completion of atrial contraction and the beginning of ventricular contraction (a function of the PR interval) and of the relative pressure differential between the two chambers at end-diastole.[51] In the event that the pressure in a diseased left ventricle rises abnormally following atrial systole (decreased compliance), then mitral valve closure begins earlier (i.e., the A point occurs sooner). The result is that the AC interval becomes prolonged. It may be even further prolonged when complete mitral closure (C point) is delayed because of the time expended by an abnormally functioning left ventricle in raising its pressure above that in the left atrium. Among 14 patients with left ventricular end-diastolic pressures over 19 mm Hg and an 8 mm Hg or greater rise during atrial systole, the PR–AC intervals were less than 0.06 second.[51] That is, the AC interval was prolonged and, therefore, the PR–AC interval was shortened.

When the left ventricle fails, there are certain qualitative changes in the appearance of the mitral valve on the echocardiogram (Figs. 8–11 and 8–13). As the left ventricle dilates, the mitral leaflets become removed from the expanding posterior wall. Thus, the mitral valve appears more centrally located between the septum and the posterior wall of the ventricle. Failure of the ventricle also may be associated with a fine fluttering of both the anterior and the

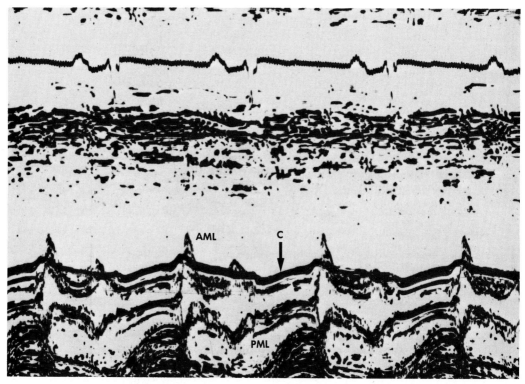

FIGURE 8–13. The mitral valve in left ventricular failure. Heavy echoes from the chordae tendineae (C) are frequently visible. The anterior (AML) and posterior (PML) mitral leaflets exhibit similar reduced opening amplitudes, with fluttering throughout diastole.

posterior leaflets during the diastolic opening, perhaps a result of stretching of the chordae tendineae as the papillary muscles are pulled away from the valve leaflets. The chordae themselves often appear much more prominent in patients with left ventricular failure. The anterior and posterior leaflets appear as mirror images of each other as the anterior leaflet excursion is reduced, and the E and A waves are also of equal amplitude. Rothbaum et al. have reported a patient with a rapidly rising left ventricular diastolic pressure causing complete mid-diastolic mitral valve closure.[54]

Aortic Valve Motion

Weissler et al., using external carotid pulse tracings and simultaneous phonocardiograms, have shown that noninvasive techniques can measure such parameters of left ventricular function as the duration of left ventricular ejection.[55, 56] Left ventricular ejection time indices may be correlated with intracardiac hemodynamic measurements and therefore are of value in assessing left ventricular performance. Systolic time intervals can also be measured echocardiographically for the study of both the left[57-59] and right[58] ventricles. In determining left ventricular systolic time intervals from the echocardiogram, the opening and closing movements of at least one normal aortic valve leaflet must be recorded, along with a simultaneous electrocardiogram. With this method, the left ventricular ejection time (LVET) and total electromechanical systole (EMS) can be measured (see Fig. 5–8), and the pre-ejection period (PEP) can be derived according to the formula

$$PEP = EMS - LVET$$

Stefadouros and Witham[57] and Vredevoe et al.[59] found an excellent degree of correlation between those values determined from the echocardiogram and those calculated from phonocardiogram–carotid pulse tracings. Hirschfeld and associates made similar measurements of both the right and the left ventricular systolic time intervals by recording the pulmonic and aortic valves.[58] They, too, found that both methods exhibited a high degree of correlation and that the echocardiographic technique was actually considerably more practical when performed on infants who were critically ill. Furthermore, they observed that the left ventricular ejection time is normally shorter than that of the right ventricle (LVET/RVET = 0.80 in normals) and that reversal of this ratio is characteristic of transposition of the great vessels (see Chapter 12).

ACQUIRED ABNORMALITIES

Congestive cardiomyopathy is characterized by ventricular dilatation (Fig. 8–14). It may be differentiated from coronary artery disease by an associated reduction in myocardial contractility that is more generalized than the segmental abnormal contractility characteristic of coronary artery disease. Echocardiographically, the differentiation usually can be made by analysis of motion of the septum and the left ventricular posterior wall. The amplitude of motion of both these structures is reduced in congestive cardiomyopathy, whereas in cor-

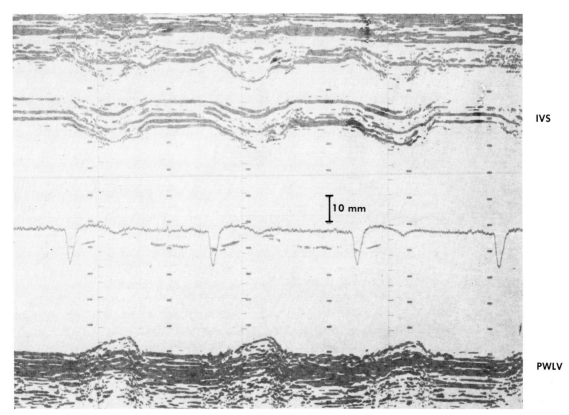

IVS

10 mm

PWLV

FIGURE 8-14. The left ventricle in congestive cardiomyopathy. The internal dimensions are markedly increased (ESD = 7.5 cm, EDD = 8.9 cm). The posterior wall of the left ventricle (PWLV) exhibits diminished amplitude of excursion (5 mm) as does the septum (IVS) (6 mm).

onary disease, the motion of one wall is usually preserved or even exaggerated, while the opposite wall motion is abnormally reduced or absent.[60] An exception is found in the patient who has sustained infarctions of both the anterior and the posterior myocardial walls, resulting in diminished or absent contractile motion of both the septum and the posterior left ventricular wall. Corya et al. found that the sum of the amplitude of motion of the left ventricular surface of the septum and the posterior wall endocardial surface provides an excellent means for differentiating the two groups.[60] They found that among patients with coronary disease, the sum generally exceeded 1.5 cm, whereas in the cardiomyopathy group, it was usually 1.2 cm or less. The presence of a compensatory, exaggerated motion of the noninvolved myocardium in coronary disease accounts for the difference.

Among patients with congestive cardiomyopathies, the flattened (type B) systolic motion also may occur,[61] most likely as a result of the net effect of diminished contraction offset by the anterior systolic cardiac motion. Reversed (type A) motion, however, is rare in these patients, unless left bundle branch block is present.

Six patients with primary myocardial disease studied by McDonald et al. had increased internal left ventricular dimensions, decreased mean V_{CF} and reduced posterior wall systolic thickening.[18]

Kovick and associates studied 22 patients with documented muscular dystrophy.[21] In this group, they found that both the maximal systolic endocardial velocity and the maximal diastolic endocardial velocity were significantly reduced, suggesting abnormalities of the myocardium that affect both contraction and relaxation. Lies et al. revealed that the mean V_{CF} is decreased in most patients with muscular dystrophy and subclinical cardiomyopathy.[62]

Finally, it should be noted that the echocardiogram is particularly useful in differentiating pericardial effusion from chamber dilatation in patients with an enlarged cardiac silhouette on the chest x-ray. It is also helpful in the identification of those cases in which there is concomitant chamber dilatation and pericardial effusion (see Chapter 12).

SECONDARY LEFT VENTRICULAR DILATATION

Because the left ventricle may be dilated in numerous disease states in which the myocardium is normal, the routine measurement of the minor axis dimension is of considerable value in all patients studied echocardiographically. For example, in patients with aortic regurgitation due to infective endocarditis, echocardiography provides a good objective means of observing progressive left ventricular enlargement (see Chapter 6).

INFILTRATIVE DISEASE OF THE MYOCARDIUM

Infiltrative disease of the myocardium constitutes a secondary form of cardiomyopathy occurring in association with amyloidosis, hemochromatosis, mucopolysaccharidosis, and idiopathic hypereosinophilia. In such cases, the echocardiogram may show abnormalities, despite the absence of other clinical evidence of cardiac involvement. Commonly, the echocardiogram shows symmetrical thickening of the septum and left ventricular free wall, reduction in the mitral EF slope (a result of decreased ventricular compliance), normal ejection fraction, and reduced septal and posterior left ventricular wall motion.[52, 63]

CONGENITAL MALFORMATION OF THE LEFT VENTRICLE

Single Ventricle

In the congenital anomaly known as single ventricle, the heart has two atria and one ventricle, most commonly the left ventricle.[64] The tricuspid and mitral valves may both be intact, but occasionally there is only a single atrioventricular valve. Transposition of the great vessels is frequently observed in association with single ventricle. A right ventricular infundibulum, which invariably communicates with the aorta, is present, and pulmonary stenosis may or may not be present.

The most characteristic echocardiographic feature of single ventricle is the absence of an interventricular septum.[65, 66] In most cases a single valve leaflet is apparent, with marked diastolic anterior excursion. This leaflet exhibits diastolic apposition to the anterior cardiac wall in most cases. When there are two atrioventricular valves, a second, parallel-moving leaflet may be seen at a deeper level in the chamber, either on the same view or with slight changes in the transducer angle. In individual cases it has not been possible to determine whether a single leaflet recording represents a common atrioventricular valve or only one of two separate valves. In most cases, posterior leaflets have not been recorded.

Present knowledge does not permit echocardiographic differentiation of single ventricle from corrected transposition of the great vessels with a large ventricular septal defect. The utmost care, with multiple transducer positions and angles, must be taken in searching for a septal echo in all cases.

Single ventricle may also be confused with similar echocardiographic findings in tricuspid atresia with severe hypoplasia of the right ventricle (see Chapter 9).[65]

Primary Endocardial Fibroelastosis

In a small series, Chung et al. found changes in endocardial fibroelastosis to be the same as those described for other causes of congestive car-

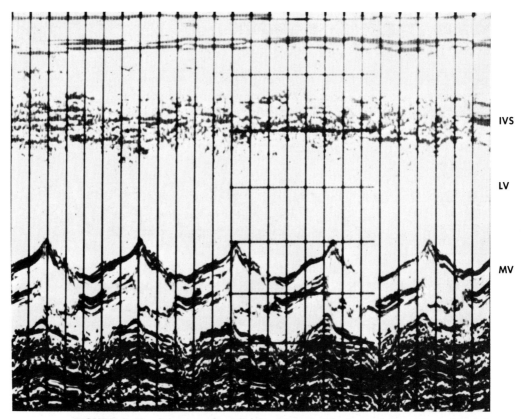

FIGURE 8–15.   Primary endocardial fibroelastosis. The internal dimensions of the left ventricle are increased (end-diastolic dimension = 3.8 cm) in this 10-month-old child. The mitral valve motion is characteristic of decreased flow due to left ventricular failure (IVS = interventricular septum; LV = left ventricle; MV = mitral valve).

diomyopathy.[66] These include marked dilatation of the left ventricle, diminished mitral valve motion, and normal thickness but decreased motion of the septum and posterior left ventricular wall (Fig. 8–15).

Hypoplasia of the Left Heart

Underdevelopment of the left atrium, mitral valve, left ventricle, aortic valve, and ascending aorta may occur singly or in various combinations. Hypoplasia of the left ventricle is characterized by a small left ventricle and an enlarged right ventricle.[67] Because the mitral valve is usually stenotic or atretic, its echo is grossly deformed, with low amplitude when a recognizable motion is present.

The aortic root is not identifiable when aortic atresia is present (see Chapter 5). As contrasted to the case of single ventricle, however, a septum should be recorded in the hypoplastic left heart.

_____ *References*

1. Belenkie I, Nutter DO, Clark DW, McCraw DB, and Raizner AE: Assessment of left ventricular dimensions and function by echocardiography. Am J Cardiol *31*:755–762, 1973.
2. Corya BC, Feigenbaum H, Rasmussen S, and Black MJ: Anterior left ventricular wall echoes in coronary artery disease: Linear scanning with a single element transducer. Am J Cardiol *34*:642–657, 1974.
3. Feigenbaum H, Stone JM, Lee DA, Nasser WK, and Chang S: Identification of ultrasound echoes from the left ventricle by use of intracardiac injections of indocyanine green. Circulation *41*:615–621, 1970.
4. Ludbrook P, Karliner JS, London A, Peterson KL, Leopold GR, and O'Rourke RA: Posterior wall velocity: An unreliable index of total left ventricular performance in patients with coronary artery disease. Am J Cardiol *33*:475–482, 1974.
5. Jacobs JJ, Feigenbaum H, Corya BC, and Phillips JF: Detection of left ventricular asynergy by echocardiography. Circulation *48*:263–271, 1973.
6. Rees G, Bristow JD, Kremkau EL, Green GS, Herr RH, Griswold HE, and Starr A: Influence of aortocoronary bypass surgery on left ventricular performance. N Engl J Med *284*:1116–1120, 1971.
7. Cooper RH, O'Rourke RA, Karliner JS, Peterson KL, and Leopold GR: Comparison of ultrasound and cineangiographic measurements of the mean rate of circumferential fiber shortening in man. Circulation *46*:914–923, 1972.
8. Smithen CS, Wharton CFP, and Sowton E: Independent effects of heart rate and exercise on left ventricular wall movement measured by reflected ultrasound. Am J Cardiol *30*:43–47, 1972.
9. Kraunz RF, and Kennedy JW: Ultrasonic determination of left ventricular wall motion in normal man: Studies at rest and after exercise. Am Heart J *79*:36–43, 1970.
10. Fogelman AM, Abbasi AS, Pearce ML, and Kattus AA: Echocardiographic study of the abnormal motion of the posterior left ventricular wall during angina pectoris. Circulation *46*:905–913, 1972.
11. Inoue K, Smulyan H, Mookherjee S, and Eich RH: Ultrasonic measurement of left ventricular wall motion in acute myocardial infarction. Circulation *43*:778–785, 1971.
12. Stefan G, and Bing RJ: Echocardiographic findings in experimental myocardial infarction of the posterior left ventricular wall. Am J Cardiol *30*:629–639, 1972.
13. Kerber RE, and Abboud FM: Echocardiographic detection of regional myocardial infarction: An experimental study. Circulation *48*:997–1005, 1973.
14. Sjögren A-L, Hytönen I, and Frick MH: Ultrasonic measurements of left ventricular wall thickness. Chest *57*:37–40, 1970.
15. Pauley P-E, and Pedersen JF: Myocardial contraction velocity and acceleration in man measured by ultrasound echocardiography differentiation. Cardiovasc Res *7*:266–276, 1973.
16. Kraunz RF, and Ryan TJ: Ultrasound measurements of ventricular wall motion following administration of vasoactive drugs. Am J Cardiol *27*:464–473, 1971.
17. Quinones MA, Gaasch WH, and Alexander JK: Echocardiographic assessment of left ventricular function: With special reference to normalized velocities. Circulation *50*:42–51, 1974.

18. McDonald IG, Feigenbaum H, and Chang S: Analysis of left ventricular wall motion by reflected ultrasound: Application to assessment of myocardial function. Circulation *46*:14–25, 1972.

19. Hirshleifer J, Crawford M, O'Rourke RA, and Karliner JS: Influence of acute alterations in heart rate and systemic arterial pressure on echocardiographic measures of left ventricular performance in normal human subjects. Circulation *52*:835–841, 1975.

20. Frishman W, Smithen C, Befler B, Kligfield P, and Killip T: Noninvasive assessment of clinical response to oral propranolol therapy. Am J Cardiol *35*:635–644, 1975.

21. Kovick RB, Fogelman AM, Abbasi AS, Peter JB, and Pearce ML: Echocardiographic evaluation of posterior left ventricular wall motion in muscular dystrophy. Circulation *52*:447–454, 1975.

22. Morganroth J, Henry WL, Maron BJ, Clark CE, and Epstein SE: Idiopathic left ventricular hypertrophy: Echocardiographic evidence against its existence. N Engl J Med *290*:1047–1050, 1974.

23. Feigenbaum H, Popp RL, and Chip JN: Left ventricular wall thickness measured by ultrasound. Arch Intern Med *121*:391–395, 1968.

24. Bennett DH, Evans DW, and Ray VJ: Echocardiographic left ventricular dimensions in pressure and volume overload: Their use in assessing aortic stenosis. Br Heart J *37*:971–977, 1975.

25. Cohen MV, Cooperman LB, and Rosenblum R: Regional myocardial function in idiopathic hypertrophic subaortic stenosis: An echocardiographic study. Circulation *52*:842–847, 1975.

26. Meyer RA, Stockert J, and Kaplan S: Echographic determination of left ventricular volumes in pediatric patients. Circulation *51*:297–303, 1975.

27. Redwood DR, Henry WL, and Epstein SE: Evaluation of the ability of echocardiography to measure acute alterations in left ventricular volume. Circulation *50*:901–904, 1974.

28. DeMaria AN, Vismara LA, Auditore K, Amsterdam EA, Zelis R, and Mason DT: Effects of nitroglycerin on left ventricular cavitary size and cardiac performance determined by ultrasound in man. Am J Med *57*:754–760, 1974.

29. Burggraf GW, and Parker JO: Left ventricular volume following amyl nitrite and nitroglycerin in man as measured by ultrasound (Abstr). Circulation (Suppl IV) *7,8*:49, 1973.

30. Dodge HT, Sandler H, Ballew DW, and Lord JD, Jr.: The use of biplane angiocardiography for the measurement of left ventricular volume in man. Am Heart J *60*:762–776, 1960.

31. Pombo JF, Troy BL, and Russell RO: Left ventricular volumes and ejection fraction by echocardiography. Circulation *43*:480–490, 1971.

32. Murray JA, Johnston W, and Reid JM: Echocardiographic determination of left ventricular dimensions, volumes and performance. Am J Cardiol *30*:252–257, 1972.

33. Gibson DG: Estimation of left ventricular size by echocardiography. Br Heart J *35*:128–134, 1973.

34. Fortuin NJ, Hood WP, Jr., Sherman ME, and Craige E: Determination of left ventricular volumes by ultrasound. Circulation *44*:575–584, 1971.

35. Ratshin RA, Boyd CN, Jr., Rackley CE, Moraski RE, and Russell RO, Jr.: Quantitative echocardiography: Correlations with ventricular volumes by angiocardiography in patients with coronary artery disease with and without wall motion abnormalities (Abstr). Circulation (Suppl IV) *7,8*:49, 1973.

36. Russell RO, Moraski RE, and Rackley CE: Comparison of left ventricular volumes obtained by biplane angiography and echocardiography in patients with abnormally contracting segments (Abstr). Circulation (Suppl IV) *7,8*:116, 1973.

37. Morganroth J, Maron BJ, Henry WL, and Epstein SE: Comparative left ventricular dimensions in trained athletes. Ann Intern Med *82*:521–524, 1975.

38. Stefadouros M, El Shahawy M, Witham AC, and Grossman W: Noninvasive study of the effect of isometric exercise on the size and performance of the normal left ventricle (Abstr). Circulation (Suppl IV) *7,8*:48, 1973.

39. Popp RL, and Harrison DC: An atraumatic method for stroke volume determination using ultrasound (Abstr). Clin Res *17*:258, 1969.

40. Fortuin NJ, Hood WP, Jr., and Craige E: Evaluation of left ventricular function by echocardiography. Circulation *46*:26–35, 1972.

41. Karliner JS, Gault JH, Eckberg D, Mullins CB, and Ross J, Jr.: Mean velocity of fiber shortening: A simplified measure of left ventricular myocardial contractility. Circulation *44*:323–333, 1971.

42. Paraskos J, Grossman W, Saltz S, Dalen S, and Dexter L: A noninvasive technique for the determination of velocity of circumferential fiber shortening in man. Circ Res *29*:610, 1971.

43. Rankin LS, Moos S, and Grossman W: Effects of altered preload on V_{CF} and other left ventricular ejection phase indices (Abstr). Am J Cardiol *35*:164, 1975.

44. Quinones MA, Gaasch WH, Cole JS, and Alexander JK: Echocardiographic determination of left ventricular stress-velocity relations in man: With reference to the effects of loading and contractility. Circulation *51*:689–700, 1975.

45. Delgado C, Fortuin NJ, and Ross RS: Acute effects of low doses of alcohol on left ventricular function by echocardiography. Circulation *51*:535–540, 1975.

46. Sahn DJ, Deely WJ, Hagan AD, and Friedman WF: Echocardiographic assessment of left vening (V$_{CF}$) by echocardiography (Abstr). Circulation (Suppl II) *43*:34, 1971.

47. Fortuin NJ, and Hood WP, Jr.: Determination of mean velocity of circumferential fiber shortening (V$_{CF}$) by echocardiography (Abstr). Circulation (Suppl II) *43,44*:34, 1971.

48. Reddy BP, Lee CC, Stack R, Taylor M, and Weissler AM: Left ventricular performance in coronary artery disease by systolic time intervals and echocardiography (Abstr). Circulation (Suppl III) *49,50*:60, 1974.

49. Pohost GM, Dinsmore RE, Rubenstein JJ, O'Keefe DD, Granthan RN, Scully HE, Beierholm EA, Frederiksen JW, Weisfeldt ML, and Daggett WM: The echocardiogram of the anterior leaflet of the mitral valve. Circulation *51*:88–97, 1975.

50. Rubenstein JJ, Pohost GM, Dinsmore RE, and Harthorne JW: The echocardiographic determination of mitral valve opening and closure. Circulation *51*:98–103, 1975.

51. Konecke LL, Feigenbaum H, Chang S, Corya BC, and Fischer JC: Abnormal mitral valve motion in patients with elevated left ventricular diastolic pressures. Circulation *47*:989–996, 1973.

52. Borer JS, Henry WL, and Epstein SE: Echocardiographic characteristics of infiltrative cardiomyopathy (Abstr). Circulation (Suppl III) *49,50*:217, 1974.

53. Quinones MA, Gaasch WH, Waisser E, and Alexander JK: Reduction in the rate of diastolic descent of the mitral valve echogram in patients with altered left ventricular diastolic pressure-volume relations. Circulation *49*:246–254, 1974.

54. Rothbaum DA, DeJoseph RL, and Tavel M: Diastolic heart sound produced by mid-diastolic closure of the mitral valve. Am J Cardiol *34*:367–370, 1974.

55. Weissler AM: Noninvasive methods for assessing left ventricular performance in man. Am J Cardiol *34*:111–114, 1974.

56. Weissler AM, Harris WS, and Schoenfeld CD: Systolic time intervals in heart failure in man. Circulation *37*:149–159, 1968.

57. Stefadouros MA, and Witham AC: Systolic time intervals by echocardiography. Circulation *51*:114–117, 1975.

58. Hirschfeld S, Meyer R, Schwartz DC, Korfhagen J, and Kaplan S: Measurement of right and left ventricular systolic time intervals by echocardiography. Circulation *51*:304–309, 1975.

59. Vredevoe LA, Creekmore SP, and Schiller NB: The measurement of systolic time intervals by echocardiography. J Clin Ultrasound *2*:99, 1974.

60. Corya BC, Feigenbaum H, Rasmussen S, and Black MJ: Echocardiographic features of congestive cardiomyopathy compared with normal subjects and patients with coronary artery disease. Circulation *49*:1153–1159, 1974.

61. Sawaya J, Longo MR, and Schlant RC: Echocardiographic interventricular septal wall motion and thickness: A study in health and disease. Am Heart J *87*:681–688, 1974.

62. Lies JE, Bonanno JA, DeMaria A, and Mason DT: Echographic detection of subclinical cardiomyopathy (Abstr). Circulation (Suppl IV) *48*:192, 1973.

63. Abbasi AS, Ellis N, and Child J: Echocardiographic features of infiltrative cardiomyopathy (Abstr). In White D (Ed.): Ultrasound in Medicine. New York, Plenum Press, 1975, p. 108.

64. Perloff JK: The Clinical Recognition of Congenital Heart Disease. Philadelphia, W. B. Saunders Company, 1970.

65. Chesler E, Joffe HS, Vecht R, Beck W, and Schrire V: Ultrasound cardiography in single ventricle and the hypoplastic left and right heart syndromes. Circulation *42*:123–129, 1970.

66. Chung KJ, Gramiak R, and Manning JA: The value of echocardiography in congestive cardiomyopathy in children (Abstr). In White D (Ed.): Ultrasound in Medicine. New York, Plenum Press, 1975, p. 93.

67. Meyer RA, and Kaplan S: Echocardiography in the diagnosis of hypoplasia of the left or right ventricles in the neonate. Circulation *46*:55–64, 1972.

9

The Right Ventricle

Among adults, abnormalities of the right ventricle are almost exclusively secondary either to disorders of the pulmonary circulation or to left-heart abnormalities. Even in the presence of primary right ventricular disease, as in the cardiomyopathies, the right ventricular hemodynamic alterations are usually overshadowed by concomitant involvement of the left ventricle. Nonetheless, routine recording of the right ventricle is easily accomplished and is of potential benefit in every echocardiographic examination.

ANATOMY AND PHYSIOLOGY

The right ventricle is the most anterior of the four cardiac chambers. Its anterior wall comprises the anterior surface of the myocardium and lies a few centimeters beneath the chest wall, from which it is separated by areolar and connective tissue of variable thickness. The right ventricle is anterior, superior, and slightly medial of the left ventricle.

The right ventricular chamber may be considered to have two portions, the body of the main pumping chamber and the outflow tract, or *conus arteriosus.* Viewed in cross section, the main chamber has a crescent shape, with its anteroposterior and longitudinal dimensions greater than the transverse dimension. The conus arteriosus lies superior to the main chamber and joins it to the pulmonary artery.

The right ventricle is a low-pressure chamber whose function is to deliver blood to the low-resistance pulmonary circulation. The systolic pressure ranges from 15 to 28 mm Hg, with a mean of 24 mm Hg.[1]

ECHOCARDIOGRAPHIC FINDINGS

The right ventricular anterior myocardium is the first cardiac structure encountered by the ultrasound beam. Its echo lies near the heavy echo of the chest wall and may be continuous with the chest wall or may be continuously or intermittently separated by an echo-free space. Some posterior excursion during ventricular systole is usually observed, although occasionally no motion is apparent, depending on transducer angulation (Fig. 9–1).

The posterolateral boundary of the right ventricle is the interventricular septum, which also normally moves posteriorly during ventricular systole. A small-amplitude anterior motion of the septum can often be seen beginning immediately before the QRS complex of the electrocardiogram.

The internal dimension of the right ventricular chamber (RVID) is measured at the onset of the QRS complex, from either the anterior (epicardial) or the posterior edge of the anterior myocardium to the anterior edge of the interventricular septum (Fig. 9–2). This dimension varies considerably among normal persons and is easily affected by cardiac rotation, transducer angulation, and perhaps by respiration as well.[2] The recording technique used for obtaining this measurement is the same beam angle as that employed for left ven-

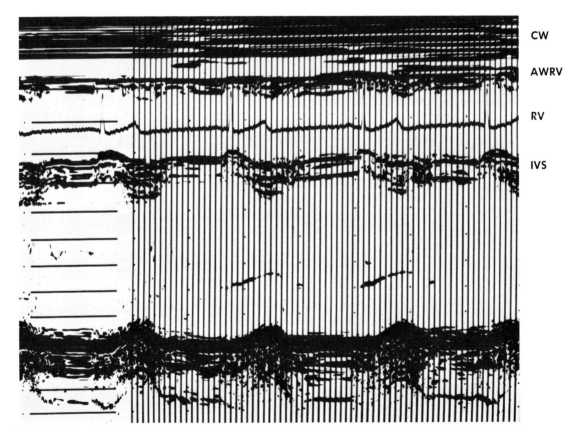

FIGURE 9–1. The normal right ventricle (RV). The heavy echo of the chest wall (CW) is adjacent to that from the anterior right ventricular myocardium (AWRV), the thickness of which is indistinct in this example. There is slight posterior systolic motion of the anterior myocardium, in parallel with the interventricular septum (IVS) during ventricular systole. Note the low-amplitude anterior motion of the septum immediately prior to and during the QRS complex of the electrocardiogram.

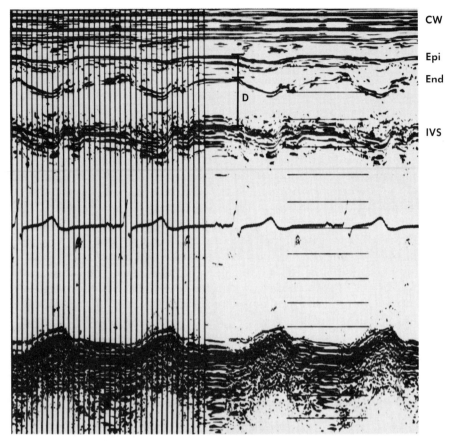

FIGURE 9-2. The normal right ventricle. The anterior myocardial thickness can be measured, as both its epicardial (Epi) and endocardial (End) surfaces are distinct. The internal dimension of the right ventricle (D) may be measured from either of these edges to the right ventricular edge of the interventricular septum (IVS) at the time of the electrocardiographic QRS complex. The echo-free space between the chest wall (CW) and the anterior myocardium is representative of subcutaneous tissue and is not evidence of a pericardial effusion.

tricular measurements. Although the left and right ventricles normally have approximately the same capacity (approximately 75 cc in adults), their internal dimensions on the anteroposterior beam axis are different because the two chambers have vastly different shapes.

In a study by Popp et al. of 26 normal adults, the right ventricular dimension measured from the epicardial surface of the right ventricular anterior wall to the interventricular septum ranged from 0.5 to 2.1 cm (mean 1.5 ± 0.39 cm).[3] The ratio of the left ventricular end-diastolic dimension to the right ventricular dimension was approximately 3:1. Diamond et al.[4] corrected the right ventricular dimension for body surface area (right ventricular dimension index or RVDI), and found this to range from 0.3 to 1.1 cm per M² (mean 0.7 cm per M²). In 28 normal children, Tajik et al.[5] found the RVDI varied from 0.8 cm per M² for those with a body surface area of 1.0 cm per M² or greater, and 1.3 cm per M² for those with a body surface area less than 1.0 cm per M².

Additional studies involving larger numbers of persons in the adult population are needed to provide a better definition of the normal range of right ventricular dimension. Furthermore, a better understanding is needed of the optimal view through this chamber, analogous to the criteria used for similar measurements of the left ventricle. We have found that changes in transducer angulation that maintain satisfactory left ventricular recordings may result in significant variations in right ventricular recordings with dimensions of up to 3.0 cm in normal adults.

The right ventricular outflow tract is apparent on the echocardiogram as an echo-free space anterior to the aortic root (Fig. 9–3). The size of the right ventricular outflow (RVO) tract has been compared with the size of the left atrium (LA). The RVO–LA ratio is 1.5 in normals.[6]

The right ventricular myocardial thickness is generally regarded as the thickness of the anterior wall (see Fig. 9–2), although the interventricular septum is, in fact, also one of its walls, and any study of the right ventricle must include assessment of the septum. The anterior wall thickness is sometimes impossible to measure, either because its anterior border is inseparable from the chest wall echoes or because the endocardial surface is indistinct. In 200 normal newborns, Hagan and associates found a rather wide range for both the end-diastolic thickness (range 2.0 to 4.7 mm, mean 3.0 mm) and the end-systolic thickness (range 3.3 to 7.3 mm, mean 5.0 mm).[7] These were very close to the posterior left ventricular wall widths. In another study of newborns, Solinger et al. found the anterior wall end-diastolic dimension to range from 1.1 to 2.9 mm.[8] Epstein et al. found that the width of the anterior wall increases by only about 0.5 from age 6 months to 18 years.[9] Similar studies have not been reported in adults.

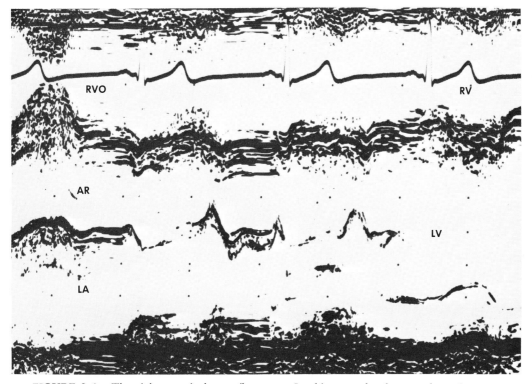

FIGURE 9-3. The right ventricular outflow tract. In this example, the transducer has scanned from the aortic root (AR) and the right ventricular outflow tract (RVO), lying anteriorly, to the body of the right ventricle (RV) and left ventricle (LV) (LA = left atrium).

RIGHT VENTRICULAR DILATATION

Increased volume of the right ventricle is easily detected echocardiographically as an increase in the RVID. Diamond et al. found that all their patients with atrial septal defects had an increased RVID index (Fig. 9–4).[4] Furthermore, the RVID index showed an excellent linear correlation when it was plotted against the pulmonary–systemic blood flow ratio. Paquet and Gutgesell studied seven patients with total anomalous pulmonary drainage and found that the right ventricular dimension was increased in all these as well.[10] When the right ventricle dilates without concomitant left ventricular enlargement or pulmonary hypertension, the septal motion is usually abnormal, as in left-to-right shunting from an atrial septal defect (see Chapter 7). However, a dilated right ventricle with normal septal motion does not exclude a left-to-right shunt (Fig. 9–5).

The right ventricle also is often dilated secondary to left ventricular failure and mitral valve disease (Fig. 9–6). Congestive cardiomyopathies also cause dilatation of both ventricles. Primary pulmonary hypertension and pulmonary stenosis cause right ventricular dilatation and hypertrophy.

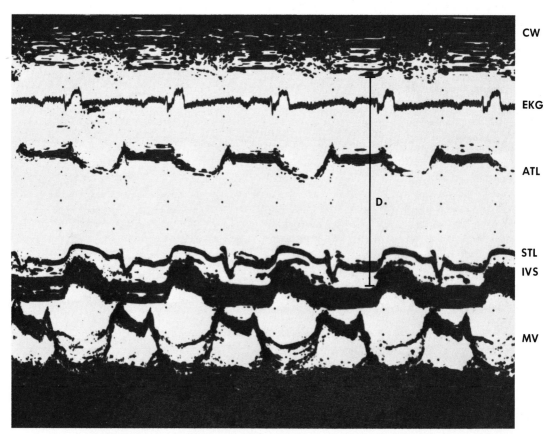

FIGURE 9–4. Right ventricular dilatation in atrial septal secundum defect. The internal dimension (D) is about 8.0 cm. Echoes from the anterior (ATL) and septal (STL) tricuspid leaflets are also present, and the interventricular septum (IVS) shows paradoxical motion. The mitral valve (MV) echo indicates systolic prolapse (CW = chest wall).

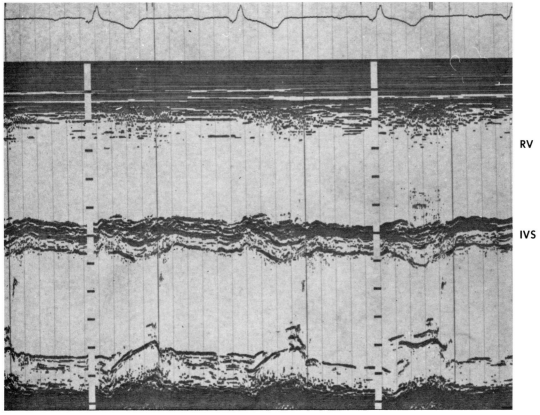

RV

IVS

FIGURE 9-5. Right ventricular dilatation in atrial septal secundum defect. In this example, the right ventricle (RV) is over 3.5 cm in its internal dimension. The motion of the interventricular septum (IVS) however, is posterior during ventricular systole.

RIGHT VENTRICULAR HYPERTROPHY

Right ventricular hypertrophy occurs secondary to pulmonary hypertension and right ventricular outflow stenosis. This may be recognized on the echocardiogram as thickening of the interventricular septum, and therefore is a cause of a form of secondary asymmetric septal hypertrophy.[11-13] We have observed that in some instances of primary asymmetric septal hypertrophy, the anterior myocardium appears to have a markedly increased systolic thickness and amplitude of motion (Fig. 9-7). The internal dimension also may be reduced in some cases of asymmetric septal hypertrophy, as it is impinged upon by the thickened septum (Fig. 9-8). Change in the thickness of the anterior myocardium has been correlated with the severity of cystic fibrosis.[2]

HYPOPLASTIC RIGHT VENTRICLE

Congenital hypoplasia of the right ventricle is almost always associated with tricuspid atresia, which is discussed in Chapter 10. A very small anterior chamber is present, as opposed to the entity of single ventricle, in which no an-

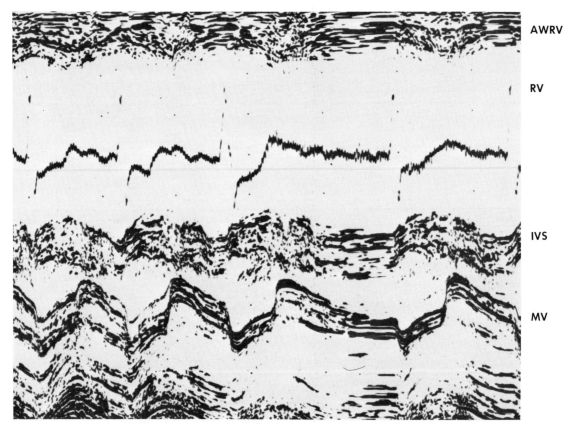

FIGURE 9-6. The right ventricle (RV) in mitral stenosis. The right ventricular internal dimension measures approximately 5.0 cm. The mitral valve (MV) is thickened, with a reduced EF slope (AWRV = anterior wall of right ventricle; IVS = interventricular septum).

terior chamber can be detected. The right ventricular outflow tract also appears small (Fig. 9–9).

UHL'S ANOMALY

French and associates have reported the echocardiographic features of a single case of Uhl's anomaly or congenital hypoplasia of the right ventricular myocardium.[14] They found the tricuspid valve closure to be delayed to 0.07 second after mitral closure in this patient. Other features included abnormal early pulmonic valve opening, right ventricular dilatation, and mitral valve prolapse.

RIGHT VENTRICULAR TUMORS

DeMaria and associates described a single case of myxoma arising in the right ventricle causing a continuous band of echoes in the right ventricular

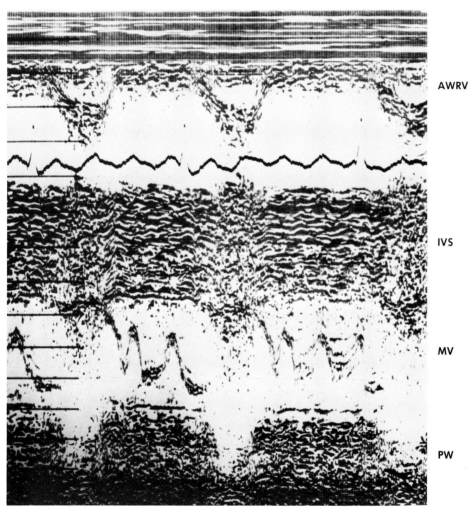

FIGURE 9-7. The anterior right ventricular myocardium (AWRV) in a patient with asymmetrical septal hypertrophy with obstruction shows increased (1.2 cm) posterior excursion and thickening during ventricular systole (IVS = interventricular septum, MV = mitral valve, PW = posterior wall).

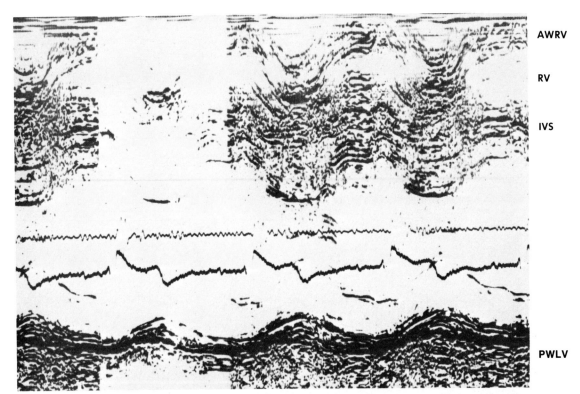

AWRV

RV

IVS

PWLV

FIGURE 9-8. The right ventricle (RV) in asymmetric septal hypertrophy. The greatly thickened interventricular septum (IVS) has caused a significant reduction in the right ventricular internal dimension (AWRV = anterior wall of right ventricle, PWLV = posterior wall of left ventricle).

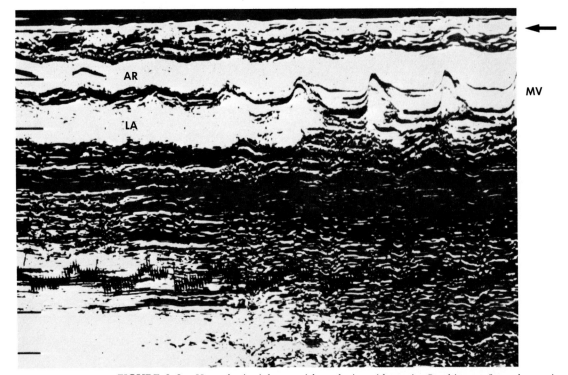

MV

AR

LA

FIGURE 9-9. Hypoplastic right ventricle and tricuspid atresia. On this scan from the aortic root (AR) to the mitral valve (MV), only a rudimentary right ventricular chamber is present (arrow). There is no apparent right ventricular outflow tract anterior to the aortic root (LA = left atrium).

outflow tract.[15] Tumor echoes were also observed within the body of the right ventricle during diastole.

A single case of a rhabdomyosarcoma within the right ventricle has been reported. In this case, tumor echoes were visualized within the dilated right ventricle, and the motion of the interventricular septum was paradoxical.[16]

_____ *References*

1. Hurst JW, and Logue RB (Eds.): The Heart. New York, McGraw-Hill Book Company, 1970.
2. Goldberg SJ, Allen HD, and Sahn DJ: Pediatric and Adolescent Echocardiography. Chicago, Year Book Medical Publishers, 1975.
3. Popp RL, Wolfe SB, Hirata T, and Feigenbaum H: Estimation of right and left ventricular size by ultrasound: A study of the echoes from the interventricular septum. Am J Cardiol 24:523–530, 1969.
4. Diamond MA, Dillon JC, Haine CL, Chang S, and Feigenbaum H: Echocardiographic features of atrial septal defect. Circulation 43:129–135, 1971.
5. Tajik AJ, Gau GT, Ritter DG, and Schattenberg TT: Echocardiographic pattern of right ventricular diastolic volume overload in children. Circulation 46:36–43, 1972.
6. Chung KJ, Nanda NC, Manning JA, and Gramiak R: Echocardiographic findings in tetralogy of Fallot (Abstr). Am J Cardiol 31:126, 1973.
7. Hagan AD, Deely WJ, Sahn D, and Friedman WF: Echocardiographic criteria for normal newborn infants. Circulation 48:1221–1226, 1973.
8. Solinger R, Elbl F, and Minhas K: Echocardiography in the normal neonate. Circulation 47:108, 1973.
9. Epstein ML, Goldberg SJ, Allen HD, Konecke L, and Wood J: Great vessel, cardiac chamber, and wall growth patterns in normal children. Circulation 51:1124–1129, 1975.
10. Paquet M, and Gutgesell H: Echocardiographic features of total anomalous pulmonary venous connection. Circulation 51:599–605, 1975.
11. Henry WL, Clark CE, and Epstein SE: Asymmetric septal hypertrophy (ASH): The unifying link in the IHSS disease spectrum. Circulation 47:827–832, 1973.
12. Brown OR, Harrison DC, and Popp RL: Echocardiography study of right ventricular hypertension producing asymmetrical septal hypertrophy (Abstr). Circulation (Suppl IV) 48:47, 1973.
13. Goodman DJ, Harrison DC, and Popp RL: Echocardiographic features of primary pulmonary hypertension. Am J Cardiol 33:438–443, 1974.
14. French JW, Baum D, and Popp RL: Echocardiographic findings in Uhl's anomaly: Demonstration of diastolic pulmonary valve opening. Am J Cardiol 36:349–353, 1975.
15. DeMaria AN, Vismara LA, Miller RR, Neumann A, and Mason DT: Unusual echographic manifestations of right and left heart myxomas. Am J Med 59:713–720, 1975.
16. Sassé L, Lorentzen D, and Alvarez H: Paradoxical septal motion secondary to right ventricular tumor. JAMA 234:955–956, 1975.

10

The Tricuspid Valve

In the overall spectrum of cardiac diseases, those that primarily affect the tricuspid valve are relatively unimportant. This is true because such abnormalities are uncommon, but more importantly, because they have far less severe hemodynamic consequences than valvular involvement in the higher pressure left heart. Where the echocardiographer is concerned, the relative unimportance of tricuspid disease is fortunate because a recording of the complete motion of that structure in adults is unusual. In spite of these considerations, the routine attempt to visualize the tricuspid valve is worthwhile because the structure usually can be recorded when the right ventricle is dilated and when the valve itself is abnormal. Also, failure to record the valve in newborns and in infants is in itself an indication of possible tricuspid maldevelopment.

ANATOMY AND PHYSIOLOGY

The tricuspid orifice lies medial and slightly inferior and anterior of the mitral orifice. It is inferior, anterior, and medial of the aortic root as well.

The valve is composed of leaflets, orifice ring, chordae tendineae, and papillary muscles. The three leaflets are designated the anterior, the posterior, and the septal (or medial). They are unequal in size, and the anterior leaflet is the longest from its attachment at the annulus to its free surface.[1] The posterior leaflet also attaches to the annulus, whereas the septal leaflet attaches to the septum and the posterior wall of the right ventricle.[2]

The tricuspid valve leaflets are attached to chordae tendineae of varying lengths and thicknesses. The chordae extend from two principal papillary muscles in the right ventricle, the anterior and posterior papillary muscles, and from a small medial papillary muscle as well.

The tricuspid annulus forms part of the fibrous skeleton of the heart and merges with the membranous interventricular septum on its medial aspect. It also inserts into connective tissue that is continuous with the aortic valve ring.

Because the normal peak right ventricular systolic pressure does not exceed 25 mm Hg (vs. a pressure up to 150 mm Hg in the left ventricle), the tricuspid valve is subject to much less strain than its bicuspid (mitral) left-heart counterpart.

ECHOCARDIOGRAPHIC FEATURES

Of the three tricuspid leaflets, the anterior leaflet is the most commonly recorded. It possesses a pattern of motion virtually identical to that of the anterior mitral leaflet.[2] Because it resembles the mitral leaflet, a sector scan from the leaflet superiorly to the aortic root, with which the tricuspid annulus is continuous at the anterior wall, is a useful means of proving that the tricuspid valve and not the mitral valve is being recorded (Fig. 10–1). Portions of the tricuspid valve are sometimes seen simultaneously with the aortic root, probably in part

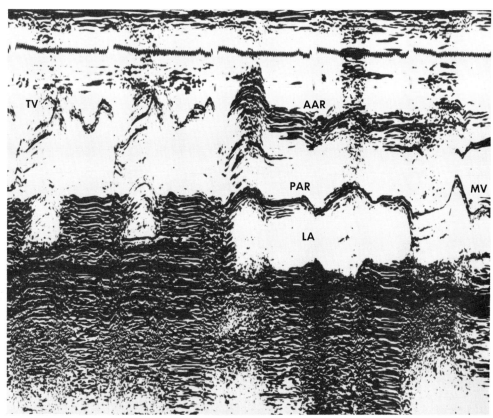

FIGURE 10-1. The normal tricuspid valve (TV). Positive identification is made by angling the transducer superiorly to the aortic root with which the tricuspid valve is continuous to the anterior wall (AAR). The mitral valve anterior leaflet (MV) is continuous with the aortic root posterior wall (PAR) (LA = left atrium).

as a result of beam width (Fig. 10–2). Positive identification of the tricuspid valve may also be made by locating the mitral valve, from which it is separated by the interventricular septum. The mitral valve may appear on the same view as the tricuspid valve (Fig. 10–3). If this is not the case, angulation of the transducer slightly laterally and superiorly from the tricuspid valve will bring the mitral apparatus into view.

The tricuspid valve is exceptionally well seen in patients with right ventricular dilatation from any cause. This is a result of the leftward anatomical rotation of the right ventricle that occurs with dilatation. This rotation displaces the tricuspid valve from its normal position behind the sternum into a more lateral position. In infants, the cartilaginous sternum does not obstruct the echo beam, so the tricuspid valve is routinely recorded, regardless of whether there is right ventricular enlargement.[3]

In adult patients without right ventricular hypertension or volume distention, the anterior tricuspid leaflet is seldom seen during all phases of the cardiac cycle. Most often the leaflet is discernible only during its diastolic phases of opening. Occasionally, a second leaflet, probably the septal leaflet, also may be seen moving posteriorly during the diastolic filling phases of the right ventricle. It is doubtful whether the tricuspid posterior leaflet can be recorded by echocardiography except in the presence of bizarre anatomical derangements.

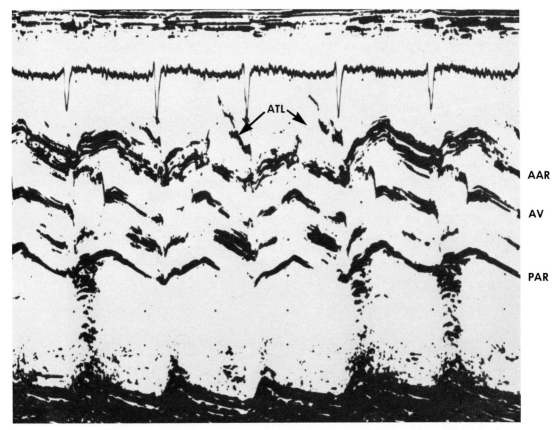

FIGURE 10–2. Tricuspid valve relationship to the aortic root. Sometimes the anterior tricuspid leaflet (ATL) is recorded along with the anterior wall of the root of the aorta (AAR) (AV = aortic valve; PAR = posterior aortic root wall).

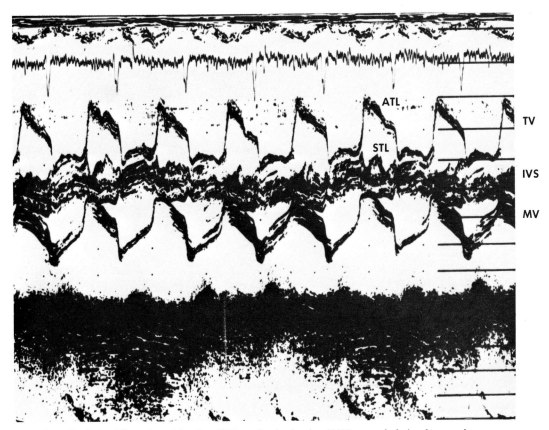

FIGURE 10–3. The tricuspid valve (TV) and mitral valve (MV) recorded simultaneously. Both the tricuspid anterior (ATL) and the septal (STL) leaflets are recorded; their motions are mirror images of each other. The mitral valve is slightly thickened and is mildly stenotic. The right ventricle is dilated (IVS = interventricular septum).

Transducer angulation is usually medial and inferior from the aortic root recording. The tricuspid valve may also be seen from the subxiphoid approach,[4] and this transducer placement should be attempted when the valve cannot be visualized from the precordial position.

Either the interventricular septum or the posterior right atrial wall may be seen behind the tricuspid valve, depending on transducer angle.[5] The right atrial chamber is most often seen from a transducer position below the tricuspid valve, with the transducer angled superiorly, as from the subxiphoid approach. In this position the right atrium appears behind the tricuspid valve. A study by Kawai et al. indicates that the right atrial dimension determined by echocardiography is sensitive for volume changes in this chamber.[39] However, further studies, especially regarding standardization of measurement, are needed.

Tricuspid valve opening slightly precedes that of the mitral valve, and its closing occurs just after (less than 0.03 sec) mitral closure. In right bundle branch block, the difference may be slightly increased.[3] The point of tricuspid closure (C point) coincides with the second group of high-frequency vibrations of the first heart sound.[6–8] The tricuspid anterior leaflet diastolic motion pattern is similar to the mitral motion, with an early diastolic E wave during rapid filling and a smaller-amplitude, late-diastolic A wave at the time of right ventricular filling during right atrial systole (Fig. 10–4).

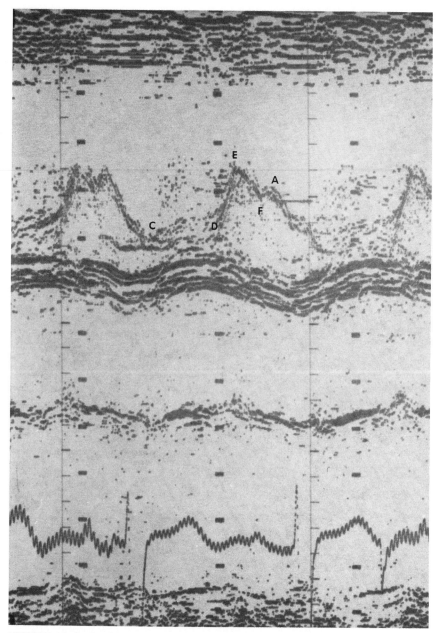

FIGURE 10-4. In this example of the normal adult tricuspid valve, only the anterior leaflet is visualized, with initial diastolic opening to the E point. Late diastolic opening at the A point occurs during atrial contraction (C = valve closure; D = valve opening; F = mid-diastolic closure).

Tricuspid Abnormalities

Tricuspid Stenosis

Whereas tricuspid stenosis is rarely detected clinically, it is found somewhat more frequently at autopsy.[9] It is usually secondary to rheumatic valvular disease, but in very rare instances it may occur as a congenital anomaly.[10] Tricuspid stenosis sometimes is associated with malformation of the right ventricle.

In a series of 6 patients[11] with documented tricuspid stenosis who were examined by echocardiography, the tricuspid EF slope was markedly reduced (Fig. 10–5), ranging from 8 to 30 mm per sec (normal 60 to 125 mm per sec). The stenotic tricuspid valve may also appear thickened.

Until there are more extensive studies of the tricuspid valve in normal adults as well as in those with tricuspid stenosis, however, the reliability of the EF slope in the diagnosis of tricuspid stenosis remains uncertain. The criteria for optimal tricuspid recordings have not yet been developed sufficiently to know when such technical errors as transducer angulation are having a significant effect. Nevertheless, the finding of a normal or increased EF slope probably excludes the diagnosis of tricuspid stenosis. Finally, reduction in right ventricular compliance, as in pulmonary hypertension, also affects the tricuspid closure rate (analogous to the reduced mitral EF slope in decreased left ventricular compliance).[3]

In the presence of mitral stenosis, the tricuspid valve usually can be well visualized because of right ventricular enlargement (Fig. 10–3). Often the two valves may be recorded simultaneously in such patients, and this affords an excellent opportunity to exclude the diagnosis of tricuspid stenosis when the tricuspid EF slope is normal. The tricuspid valve may exhibit diastolic flutter-

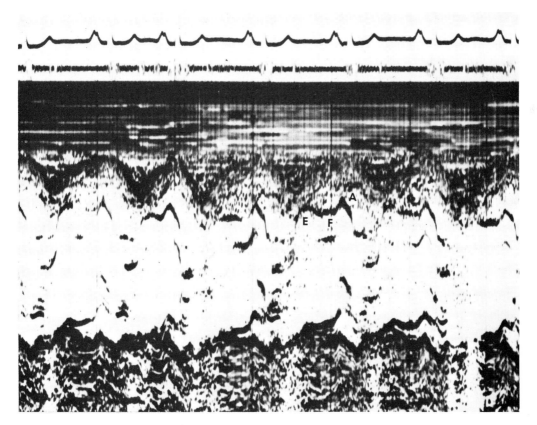

FIGURE 10–5. Tricuspid stenosis. The anterior leaflet has a markedly reduced EF slope. The A point remains well preserved.

ing due to pulmonic regurgitation secondary to pulmonary hypertension (clinically associated with the Graham Steell murmur) in patients with mitral stenosis.

Tricuspid Regurgitation

The echocardiographic criteria for the diagnosis of tricuspid regurgitation are also inadequately developed. Although an increased amplitude of excursion has been noted in some cases (Fig. 10–6),[11] the amplitude of anterior tricuspid leaflet excursion is highly variable, at least in part as a result of variations in transducer angulation. Furthermore, increased flow from any cause, including left-to-right heart shunting and high cardiac output states, probably causes increased amplitude of opening and diastolic closure rate as well. Enlargement of the right atrium may be helpful in the echocardiographic diagnosis of tricuspid regurgitation, but to date this can only be grossly estimated. As in all other right ventricular volume overload states, the systolic motion of the interventricular septum is often paradoxical.

Significant chronic tricuspid regurgitation probably can be reliably excluded if the right ventricular internal dimension is normal. The echocardiographic features of one case of surgically created tricuspid insufficiency (valv-

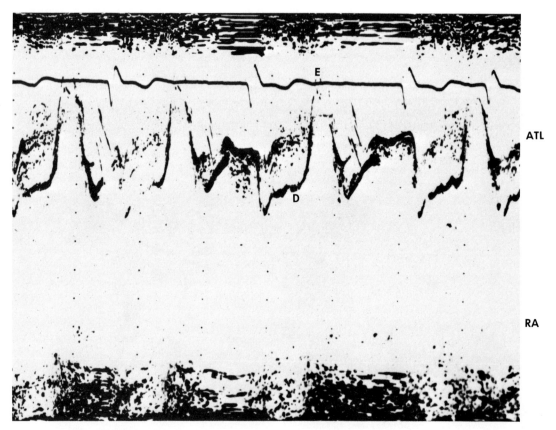

FIGURE 10–6.   The anterior leaflet (ATL) in tricuspid regurgitation exhibits marked excursion, measuring approximately 40 mm from the D to E points. The right atrium (RA) also appears greatly dilated.

otomy for intractable tricuspid endocarditis) has been reported.[12] In this instance, after valvotomy, the right ventricular dimension progressively increased from 1.8 cm to 3.5 cm, and the motion of the interventricular septum became paradoxical. Following insertion of a prosthetic tricuspid valve, the right ventricular dimension decreased to within the normal range, and normal septal motion was restored.

Secondary tricuspid regurgitation may occur in patients with right ventricular hypertension. Diamond et al.[13] described the echocardiographic findings in six such cases. All six had increased right ventricular internal dimensions (mean 2.6 cm per M^2 of body surface area, range 1.9 to 3.9 cm per M^2), and five of the six exhibited abnormal (type A) septal motion. For this reason, secondary tricuspid regurgitation should be considered in any patient with pulmonary hypertension in whom paradoxical motion of the septum is demonstrated.

Tricuspid prolapse has also been associated with regurgitation[14, 15] and may be associated with concomitant mitral valve prolapse[16, 17] In a series of 12 cases with echocardiographic features of prolapse of the tricuspid valve described by Chandraratna and associates,[16] eight also had mitral valve prolapse. One patient had Ebstein's anomaly. In only one instance, however, was there clinical evidence of tricuspid regurgitation. Because two of these patients were found at operation to have myxomatous degeneration of the mitral valve, it was assumed that this was also the cause of the tricuspid prolapse in those cases. The characteristic echocardiographic appearance of tricuspid prolapse perhaps resembles the same abnormality of the mitral valve. Normally the tricuspid leaflets move slowly anteriorly during ventricular systole, whereas prolapse is suggested by an abrupt posterior motion that begins either in early-systole or in mid-systole. It must be added, however, that to date, tissue documentation of myxomatous degeneration in such patients is too limited to be certain of prolapse when the tricuspid valve has this appearance.

Ebstein's Anomaly

Ebstein's anomaly is a congenital abnormality in which either or both the septal and the posterior tricuspid leaflets attach to the right ventricular myocardium, rather than to the valve annulus. The anterior leaflet, although large, maintains its normal attachment. The entire tricuspid valve apparatus is thus displaced inferiorly and toward the left.[18] The malposition of the valve results in an "atrialization" of a portion of the right ventricle and a reduction in the size of the functioning right ventricle.[19] The right atrium is massively dilated. The syndrome is also of interest in that in many cases, it is associated with the pre-excitation (Wolff-Parkinson-White) syndrome. The abnormality is detected in both pediatric and adult age groups.

One of the echocardiographic hallmarks of Ebstein's anomaly is the ease with which the anterior tricuspid leaflet can be recorded as a result of its lateral displacement.[3, 20, 21] Farooki et al. found that in most patients it could be recorded from the left of the midclavicular line, and that often it was actually difficult to avoid the anterior tricuspid leaflet echo from any transducer angle.[20] The leaflet echo also appears in a more anterior position than normal, and it may merge with the anterior myocardial and chest wall echoes.[3, 5, 22, 23]

Another very characteristic feature of the tricuspid motion in Ebstein's

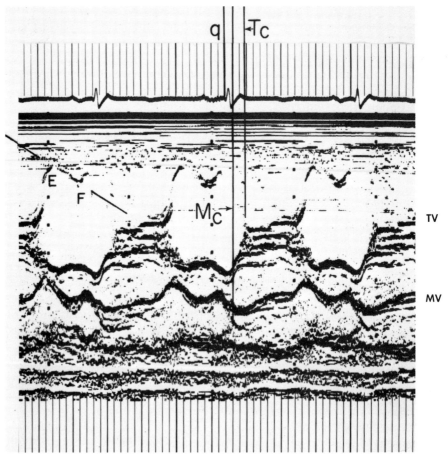

FIGURE 10–7.   Ebstein's anomaly of the tricuspid valve. Tricuspid valve closure (T_c) occurs about 70 msec after mitral valve closure (M_c) (time lines = 40 msec; TV = tricuspid valve; MV = mitral valve). (Recording courtesy of Dr. Richard Meyer.)

anomaly is its marked delay in closure relative to closure of the mitral valve (Fig. 10–7). This correlates with the auscultatory features of a widely split first heart sound in these patients. In a series of 19 patients studied by Tajik and associates,[22] in no case was the interval from mitral to tricuspid closure less than 0.06 sec (normal, less than 0.03 sec), and this ranged to as long as 0.17 sec. Milner and associates established that in their series of ten cases with Ebstein's anomaly, an interval of greater than 0.08 sec from tricuspid to mitral closure was diagnostic of that condition.[26] Series by Crews et al.[24] and Farooki et al.[20] showed similar results. The delay in tricuspid closure cannot be attributed primarily to increased flow, as patients with atrial septal defects and total anomalous venous drainage do not exhibit such mitral–tricuspid asynchrony.[3] Furthermore, abnormal delay in right ventricular depolarization is unlikely to be the cause.[22] One plausible explanation is that the abnormal tricuspid location profoundly alters right ventricular hemodynamics (delayed onset in the rise of right ventricular pressure in ventricular systole), causing retarded tricuspid valve closure.[22]

Lundström found that the anterior leaflet opens rapidly, but rather than showing the normal mid-diastolic closure, remains in an almost fully open position throughout diastole so that a distinctive A wave may be absent.[3] Others, however, have found the EF slope to be preserved or only slightly reduced in this entity.[20, 25, 26]

Because the abnormal tricuspid valve results in tricuspid regurgitation, a functional state of right ventricular overload exists. As a consequence, the motion of the interventricular septum is almost always paradoxical, exhibiting either the type A or type B pattern.[3, 5] The right atrium is enlarged,[5, 23] but the left ventricle and the mitral valve are normal.

Tricuspid Atresia

In tricuspid atresia, no tricuspid orifice or tricuspid valvular tissue is present. Blood enters the left heart through an interatrial septal defect and is then delivered to both the pulmonary and the systemic circulations through various communications among the great vessels. The right ventricle is hypoplastic.

In this instance, the echocardiogram will reveal a normal mitral valve which may exhibit increased amplitude of motion.[28] The tricuspid echo, however, is missing, and the right ventricle is either very small or may not be identified at all (Fig. 10–8).[29–31] The left ventricular chamber is dilated.

Secondary Alterations in Tricuspid Motion

Any adult patient in whom a good recording of one or more of the tricuspid leaflets is obtained must be suspect for right ventricular volume or

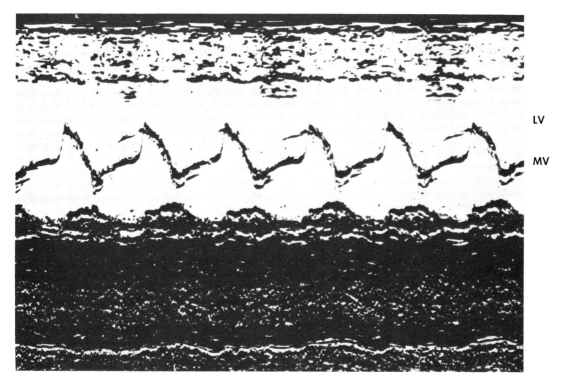

FIGURE 10–8.   Tricuspid atresia in a newborn. There is no discernible right ventricular chamber or tricuspid valve tissue. The left ventricle (LV) is large, with prominent mitral valve (MV) motion.

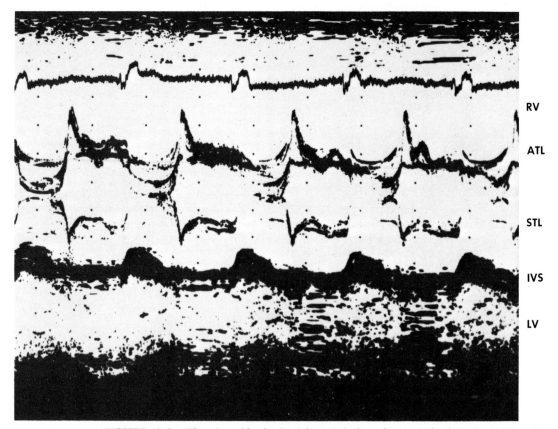

FIGURE 10-9.   The tricuspid valve in right ventricular volume overload. In this patient with an atrial septal defect, the right ventricle (RV) is greatly dilated, and both the anterior (ATL) and the septal (STL) tricuspid leaflets are recorded. The motion of the interventricular septum (IVS) is paradoxical (LV = left ventricle).

pressure overload (Fig. 10–9). This is a result of right ventricular chamber expansion, which displaces the tricuspid valve to a relatively more lateral position from its usual location behind the sternum. The right ventricular overload states are discussed in detail in Chapter 7.

Patients with ventricular septal defects may exhibit systolic fluttering of the tricuspid valve. Nanda and associates reported two cases of communication from the left ventricle to the right atrium through defects in the septum and tricuspid valve.[15] Tricuspid leaflet fluttering in systole was observed in both patients.

Diastolic tricuspid fluttering has been observed to occur in pulmonary regurgitation,[32] atrial septal defect,[33] transposition of the great vessels,[34] and congenital communication from the left ventricle to the right atrium.[15] Delayed tricuspid closure has been associated with Uhl's anomaly (see Chapter 9).

A right atrial tumor may appear during diastole as an echo density in the area of the tricuspid valve.[35–37] A similar appearance of a mass protruding through the tricuspid orifice has been identified in a case of a sinus of Valsalva aneurysm extending into the right atrium.[38]

1. Gray H: Anatomy of the Human Body. Philadelphia, Lea & Febiger, 1962.
2. Silver MD, Lam JHC, Ranganathan N, and Wigle ED: Morphology of the human tricuspid valve. Circulation *43*:333–348, 1971.
3. Lundström N-R: Echocardiography in the diagnosis of Ebstein's anomaly of the tricuspid valve. Circulation *47*:597–605, 1973.
4. Chang S, and Feigenbaum H: Subxiphoid echocardiography. J Clin Ultrasound *1*:14–20, 1973.
5. Yuste P, Minguez I, Aza V. Señor J, Asin E, and Martinez-Bordiu C: Echocardiography in the diagnosis of Ebstein's anomaly. Chest *66*:273–277, 1974.
6. Burggraf GW, and Craige E: The first heart sound in complete heart block. Circulation *50*:17–24, 1974.
7. Waider W, Madry R, McLaurin L, and Craige E: Genesis of right sided heart sounds (Abstr). Circulation (Suppl IV) *7,8*:63, 1973.
8. Waider W, and Craige E: First heart sound and ejection sounds: Echocardiographic and phonocardiographic correlation with valvular events. Am J Cardiol *35*:346–356, 1975.
9. El-Sherif N: Rheumatic tricuspid stenosis. Br Heart J *33*:16–31, 1971.
10. Steelman RB, Perloff JK, Cochran PT, and Ronan JA: Congenital stenosis of the pulmonic and tricuspid valves. Am J Med *54*:788–792, 1973.
11. Joyner CR, Hey EB, Johnson J, and Reid JM: Reflected ultrasound in the diagnosis of tricuspid stenosis. Am J Cardiol *19*:66–73, 1967.
12. Seides SF, DeJoseph RL, Brown AE, and Damato AN: Echocardiographic findings in isolated, surgically created tricuspid insufficiency. Am J Cardiol *35*:679–682, 1975.
13. Diamond MA, Dillon JC, Haine CL, Chang S, and Feigenbaum H: Echocardiographic features of atrial septal defect. Circulation *43*:129–135, 1971.
14. Ainsworth RP, Hartmann AF, Aker U, and Schad N: Tricuspid valve prolapse with late systolic tricuspid insufficiency. Radiology *107*:309–311, 1973.
15. Nanda NC, Gramiak R, and Manning JA: Echocardiography of the tricuspid valve in congenital left ventricular–right atrial communication. Circulation *51*:268–272, 1975.
16. Chandraratna PAN, Lopez JM, Fernandez JJ, and Cohen LS: Echocardiographic detection of tricuspid valve prolapse. Circulation *51*:823–826, 1975.
17. Gooch AS, Maranhão V, Scampardones G, Cha SD, and Yang SS: Prolapse of both mitral and tricuspid leaflets in systolic murmur–click syndrome. N Engl J Med *287*:1218–1222, 1972.
18. Hagan A, Sahn DJ, and Friedman WF: Cross-sectional echocardiographic features of Ebstein's malformation (Abstr). Circulation (Suppl III) *50*:17, 1974.
19. Perloff, JK: The Clinical Recognition of Congenital Heart Disease. Philadelphia, WB Saunders Company, 1970.
20. Farooki ZQ, Henry JG, and Green EW: Echocardiographic spectrum of Ebstein's anomaly of the tricuspid valve. Circulation *53*:63–68, 1976.
21. Lundström N-R, and Edler I: Ultrasoundcardiography in infants and children. Acta Paediatr Scand *60*:117–128, 1971.
22. Tajik AJ, Gau GT, Giuliani ER, Ritter EG, and Schattenberg TT: Echocardiogram in Ebstein's anomaly with Wolff-Parkinson-White preexcitation syndrome, Type B. Circulation *47*:813–815, 1973.
23. Kotler MN, and Tabatznik B: Recognition of Ebstein's anomaly by ultrasound technique. Circulation (Suppl II) *43,44*:34, 1971.
24. Crews TL, Pridie RB, Benham R, and Leatham A: Auscultatory and phonocardiographic findings in Ebstein's anomaly: Correlation of first heart sound with ultrasonic records of tricuspid valve movement. Br Heart J *34*:681–687, 1972.
25. Kotler MN: Tricuspid valve in Ebstein's anomaly (Letter to the Editor). Circulation *49*:194, 1974.
26. Milner S, Meyer RA, Venables AW, and Kaplan S: The tricuspid valve in children—an echocardiographic and phonocardiographic study (Abstr). Am J Cardiol *35*:157, 1975.
27. Waxler EB, Kawai N, and Kasparian H: Right atrial myxoma: Echocardiographic, phonocardiographic, and hemodynamic signs. Am Heart J *83*:251–257, 1972.
28. Chesler E, Joffe HS, Vecht R, Beck W, and Schrire V: Ultrasound cardiography in single ventricle and the hypoplastic left and right heart syndromes. Circulation *42*:123–129, 1970.
29. Murphy KF, Kotler MN, Reichek N, and Perloff JK: Ultrasound in the diagnosis of congenital heart disease. Am Heart J *89*:638–656, 1975.
30. Chesler E, Joffe H, Beck W, and Schrire V: Echocardiography in the diagnosis of congenital heart disease. Pediatr Clin North Am *18*:1163–1190, 1971.
31. Meyer RA, and Kaplan S: Echocardiography in the diagnosis of hypoplasia of the left or right ventricles in the neonate. Circulation *46*:55–64, 1972.
32. Gramiak R, and Shah PM: Cardiac ultrasonography: A review of current applications. Radiol Clin North Am *9*:469, 1971.
33. Nanda NC, Gramiak R, and Manning JA: Echocardiographic studies of the tricuspid valve in atrial septal defect. *In* White D (Ed.): Ultrasound in Medicine. New York, Plenum Press, 1975, pp. 11–17.

34. Chung KJ, Nanda NC, Manning JA, and Gramiak R: Echocardiographic findings in tetralogy of Fallot (Abstr). Am J Cardiol *31*:126, 1973.
35. Wolfe SB, Popp RL, and Feigenbaum H: Diagnosis of atrial tumors by ultrasound. Circulation *39*:615–622, 1969.
36. Kleid JJ, Klugman J, Hass J, and Battock D: Familial atrial myxoma. Am J Cardiol *32*:361–364, 1973.
37. Farooki ZQ, Henry JG, and Green EW: Echocardiographic diagnosis of right atrial extension of Wilm's tumor. Am J Cardiol *36*:363–367, 1975.
38. Weyman AE, Dillon JC, Feigenbaum H, and Chang S: Premature pulmonic valve opening following sinus of Valsalva aneurysm rupture into the right atrium. Circulation *51*:556–560, 1975.
39. Kawai N, Gewitz M, Eshaghpour E, and Linhart JW: Echocardiographic determination of right atrial dimensions and volume (Abstr). Circulation (Suppl III) *49,50*:28, 1974.

11

The Pulmonary Artery and Pulmonic Valve

Because the motion of the pulmonic valve is a direct reflection of the hemodynamics within the pulmonary circulation and the right ventricle, its potential value in echocardiography is far greater than is generally appreciated. Furthermore, the frequency of congenital anomalies involving the pulmonic valve and the pulmonary artery makes the study of these structures especially important in pediatrics.

ANATOMY AND PHYSIOLOGY

The pulmonic valve is composed of the anterior, right, and left semilunar cusps. The valve orifice lies anterior, superior, and slightly to the left of the aortic valve. It separates the outflow tract of the right ventricle, termed the *conus arteriosus*, from the main pulmonary artery.

In contrast to the aortic valve, the pulmonic valve is subjected to the low pressures of the right heart, with the mean pulmonary artery systolic pressure at about 24 mm Hg.[1]

ECHOCARDIOGRAPHIC FEATURES

Pulmonic valve recording has met with variable success, becoming progressively easier with decreasing age and increasing pulmonary artery size.[2] In one series, the structure was recorded satisfactorily in greater than 90 percent of pediatric cases.[3] On the other hand, in an early study it was recorded in only 25 percent of adults,[2] but this improved to 55 percent in a later report.[4]

The pulmonic valve may be detected echocardiographically by placing the transducer high near the left sternal border and rotating it laterally and superiorly from the angle at which the aortic valve is observed. The space posterior to the pulmonary artery is the lateral aspect of the left atrium.[2] Another method for its detection is first to locate the mitral valve and then to angle the transducer superiorly and very slightly medially so that the aorta is not seen. The pulmonary artery lies anterior of the dense echoes emanating from the infundibulum and the space between the pulmonary artery and the left atrium.[5, 6] A third method is simply to place the transducer directly over the pulmonary artery impulse when it can be palpated.[5]

The pre-ejection and opening systolic movements of the left cusp are often the only discernible portions of the valve motion (Fig. 11-1). Accurate recording therefore requires extreme care on the part of a technologist who is intimately familiar with this motion. Sometimes the anterior cusp, moving in an opposite direction during ventricular systole, is also seen (Fig. 11-2). After the QRS complex, the left cusp opens in a posterior and superior direction at a rate

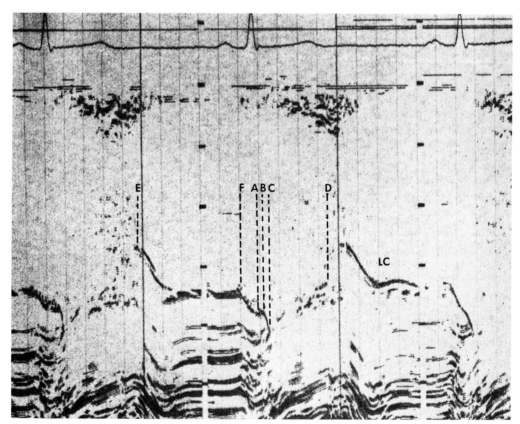

FIGURE 11-1. The normal pulmonic valve. In this example only the left cusp (LC) is recorded and the pulmonary artery walls are not visualized. Full pulmonic valve opening occurs at the C point. The amplitude of excursion during the open position cannot be determined in this example. Valve closure is at the D point. The maximal anterior position (E point) is followed by a slow posterior motion which occurs only during early diastole when the heart rate is slow, as in this case. Displacement of the valve during right atrial systole begins at the F point and reaches its maximum posterior position at the A point. The cusp then moves anteriorly for a short distance to the B point until right ventricular ejection begins.

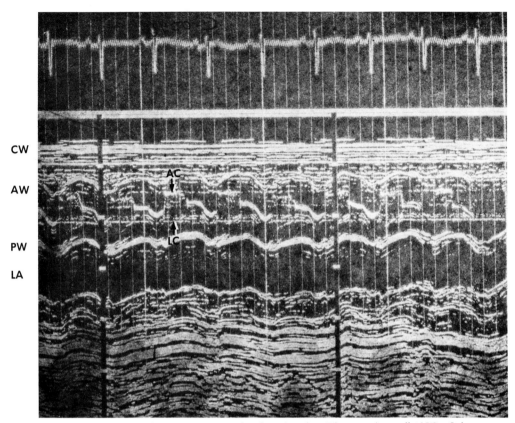

FIGURE 11–2. The pulmonary artery and pulmonic valve. The anterior wall (AW) of the vessel lies just beneath the chest wall (CW). In this example, both the anterior (AC) and left (LC) valve cusps are seen during right ventricular ejection (PW = posterior pulmonary artery wall; LA = left atrium).

of less than 300 mm per sec (B-C segment)[4] and remains proximate to the posterior pulmonary artery–left atrial wall separation (C-D segment) until the end of right ventricular systole, when it closes to its diastolic position (D-E segment) with a forward and inferior motion. It then moves slowly posteriorly until late diastole (E-F segment). Weyman et al. have determined the average normal pulmonic valve EF slope to be 36.9 ± 25.4 mm per sec with a wide range, from 6 to 115 mm per sec.[5] Immediately after the P wave of the electrocardiogram, the left cusp exhibits a short posterior motion, termed the *a* wave. This short pre-systolic motion has been attributed to the rise in right ventricular pressure that occurs during right atrial contraction, displacing the pulmonic valve away from the right ventricle into the low-pressure pulmonary artery. Consequently, the pre-systolic motion is absent in atrial fibrillation. Because the depth of the *a* wave is amplified by the increased blood flow to the right heart during inspiration, it has been proposed that this measurement should be the maximum observed during quiet breathing at the time of inspiration.[6] The normal *a* wave deflection averaged 4.4 mm (range 3 to 12 mm) in the series reported by Nanda et al.[4] and 3.7 mm (range 2 to 7 mm) in the report by Weyman et al.[5]

Right ventricular systolic time intervals can be calculated directly from recordings of the pulmonic valve (Fig. 11–3).[7] The right ventricular ejection time (RVET) is measured from the time of pulmonic leaflet opening to closure (CD interval), and the pre-ejection period (RPEP) extends from the electrocar-

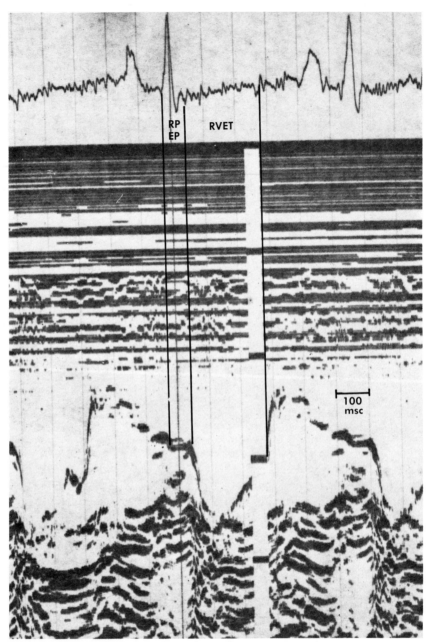

FIGURE 11-3. Calculation of right ventricular ejection time indices. The pre-ejection period (RPEP) is measured from the beginning of the QRS complex of the electrocardiogram to the cusp opening. The ejection time (RVET) is measured from the point of valve opening to that of valve closure.

diographic Q wave of the QRS complex to the time of valve opening. The RPEP/RVET is an index of right ventricular performance, as it is affected by afterload (pulmonary artery pressure), the diastolic volume, the contractile state of the myocardium, and electrical depolarization.[8] Hirschfeld and associates found the mean RPEP/RVET to be 0.24, with a range from 0.16 to 0.28 in normals.[8] This index, however, is invalid in the presence of complete right bundle branch block. With simultaneous echocardiograms and phonocardiograms, the time of pulmonic valve closure has been related to the occurrence of the pulmonic component of the second heart sound (P_2). Pulmonic valve closure precedes P_2 by 30 to 75 msec (mean 56 msec),[9] which lends evidence to the contention that valve closure itself does not directly produce the pulmonic component of the second heart sound.

PULMONARY HYPERTENSION

Abnormal elevation in the pulmonary artery pressure, whether secondary to left heart disease or primary in the pulmonary circulation itself, results in characteristic alterations in the echocardiographic appearance of the pulmonic valve as well as nonspecific secondary changes in the interventricular septum, the right ventricle, the mitral valve, the tricuspid valve, and the left ventricle.

Pulmonic Valve

The specific echocardiographic features of pulmonary hypertension pertain to pulmonic valve motion (Figs. 11–4 and 11–5).[4, 5, 8] These include:

1. Reduced diastolic (EF) slope. Nanda described the diastolic motion in

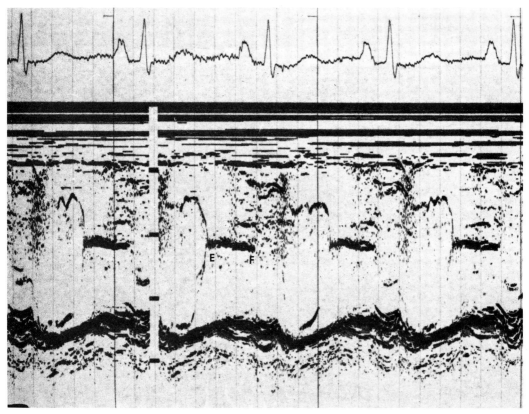

FIGURE 11–4. Severe pulmonary hypertension. The EF slope is virtually flat and there is coarse fluttering of the anterior cusp during ejection. (The pre-ejection period is obscure and cannot be assessed for an *a* wave.)

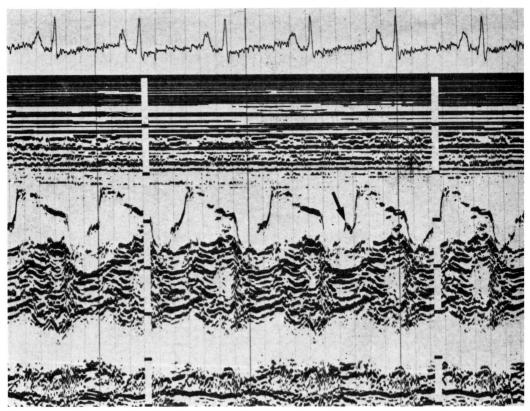

FIGURE 11-5. Severe pulmonary hypertension. The *a* wave is absent during most beats. There is a notch (arrow) and fine leaflet fluttering during right ventricular ejection.

pulmonary hypertension as "flat" as opposed to the normal "oblique" motion during diastole.[4] Weyman and associates quantified this change and found the EF slope to average only 5.2 mm per sec in patients with pulmonary hypertension.[5] Furthermore, they found that a negative (i.e., anterior and inferior diastolic excursion) EF slope was seen only in patients with pulmonary hypertension.

2. Decreased *a* wave. The increased pulmonary artery pressure appears to reduce or eliminate the effect of right atrial contraction on the pre-systolic motion of the pulmonic valve. In one series, 19 of 24 patients with pulmonary hypertension had no *a* wave; the remainder had *a* waves less than 2 mm in depth.[5] Mean pulmonary artery pressures in excess of 40 mm Hg have been correlated with total loss of the *a* wave, whereas it was present but diminished in those persons with less severe pulmonary artery hypertension (mean less than 40 mm).[4]

3. Prolonged pre-ejection period (RPEP). Corrected for heart rate (RPEP/R-R, where R-R is the time interval between the two preceding QRS complexes), this was found to be significantly prolonged (mean 110 msec) compared to normals (mean 85 msec).[4] In an extensive study of right ventricular ejection time indices in patients with pulmonary hypertension, Hirschfeld et al. correlated the RPEP/RVET with the pulmonary artery diastolic pressure (PADP) and with the mean pulmonary artery pressure (MPAP).[8] They found

that when the RPEP/RVET is less than 0.30, the PADP is likely to be 15 mm Hg or less. In addition, their studies correlated the RPEP/RVET of less than 0.30 with a MPAP less than 35 mm Hg and the RPEP/RVET of greater than 0.40 with a MPAP over 45 mm Hg.

4. Opening (BC) slope. This has been described in the cases of pulmonary hypertension as being approximately double (mean 420 mm per sec) the slope in normals (mean 211 mm per sec).[4] The validity of this measurement has been questioned because it has been observed that the opening slope is not constant, with the rate of opening accelerating in its late phase.[5]

5. Opening amplitude. In their study, Nanda et al.[4] found this to be slightly decreased in the pulmonary hypertensive group, but there was no significant difference from the normals in the series reported by Weyman et al.[5] Furthermore, the exact position of maximal opening is frequently impossible to delineate.

6. Abnormal systolic motion. A mid-systolic notch was observed in 18 of 20 patients with pulmonary hypertension and was never recorded in normal persons. A fluttering motion of the valve leaflet was also seen in 22 of 24 patients with pulmonary hypertension.[5]

Interventricular Septum

Because the septum is a functional part of the right ventricle (as well as of the left ventricle), it hypertrophies in conditions of increased right ventricular pressure.[10] Thus, in these instances, the septal thickness becomes significantly greater than that of the posterior left ventricular free wall and must be differentiated from primary asymmetric septal hypertrophy. Goodman et al. found that of nine cases of primary pulmonary hypertension, the septum was thickened in six (up to 19 mm) and was at the upper limit of normal thickness in the other three.[11] The posterior left ventricular wall thickness was normal in all cases. Four of these patients had flattened (type B) septal motion, and in all these cases, tricuspid or pulmonic regurgitation appeared to have supervened. In the absence of right ventricular volume overload, however, the septal direction of motion usually remains normal in right ventricular hypertension.[12]

Right Ventricle

In the series reported by Goodman and associates,[11] the right ventricular internal dimension was increased in all cases, ranging from 22 to 45 mm (mean 30 mm; normal less than 22 mm).

Mitral Valve

The mitral valve exhibits a reduction in the EF slope in conditions of right ventricular hypertension (Fig. 11–6).[11, 13] This may be due to reduced left ventricular filling resulting from the altered cardiac geometry or reduced left ventricular compliance in right ventricular pressure overload. Diminution in the size of the left ventricle may also be a contributing factor.[11] Goodman et al. found that the mitral EF slope was uniformly reduced, ranging from 0 to 57

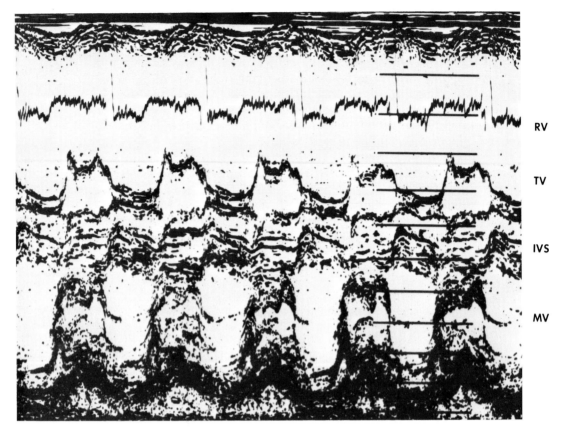

RV

TV

IVS

MV

FIGURE 11-6.   The mitral valve (MV) and tricuspid (TV) valve in pulmonary hypertension. The mitral valve is thickened with increased echoes behind it during diastolic opening, bearing some resemblance to a left atrial myxoma. The mitral EF slope is reduced and there is a suggestion of holosystolic prolapse. The tricuspid valve is easily recorded within a dilated right ventricle (RV) (IVS = interventricular septum).

mm per sec (mean 27 mm per sec). The DE slope (rate of mitral opening) may also be reduced, probably also a result of decreased left ventricular filling rate. This was found to be true in eight of their nine cases.[11]

These changes may be confused with mitral stenosis, which in itself is a cause of secondary pulmonary hypertension. Useful points of differentiation on the echocardiogram are the appearance of mitral leaflet thickening, parallel motion of the posterior mitral leaflet, and frequently, concomitant aortic valve disease in patients with mitral stenosis.

Another change occurring in some cases of pulmonary hypertension is a posterior systolic motion of the mitral valve characteristic of mitral valve prolapse.[11, 14, 15] Occasionally there is a resemblance to a left atrial myxoma when the mitral leaflet tissue becomes sufficiently redundant. It has been suggested that the common denominator in cases of primary pulmonary hypertension and mitral valve prolapse may be a connective tissue disorder.[11]

Tricuspid Valve

The tricuspid valve can be recorded in most patients with primary pulmonary hypertension and appears normal except for possible reduction in the EF slope. Tricuspid leaflet fluttering may occur if pulmonic regurgitation is present.

Left Ventricle

In the presence of primary pulmonary hypertension, the left ventricle is normal in size or may actually be smaller than normal. This may cause the mitral anterior leaflet to appear closer to the septum during diastole.[11]

VALVULAR PULMONIC STENOSIS

With rare exceptions, valvular pulmonic stenosis has a congenital origin. Its severity is dependent on the degree of commissural fusion of the valve leaflets.[16] Valvular stenosis sometimes is associated with other congenital cardiac anomalies, including atrial and ventricular septal defects.

Weyman and associates[6] found that a pressure gradient of over 50 mm Hg across a stenotic pulmonic valve was associated with an increased depth of the *a* wave, which in their series had an average depth of 10 mm (range 8 to 13 mm). Furthermore, in most of their patients with severe pulmonic stenosis, the valve leaflet echo never returned to the baseline between the *a* wave and the onset of systolic opening. In normal persons, because the *a* wave depth is increased during inspiration, failure to return to the baseline may be seen during that phase of the respiratory cycle only. Mild pulmonic stenosis (pressure gradient less than 50 mm Hg) is associated with a normal *a* wave. These investigators attributed the increased *a* wave depth to an increased right ventricular end-diastolic pressure, which accentuates the pre-systolic pulmonic valve displacement normally seen at the time of atrial contraction.

Dillon et al. have suggested that valvular pulmonic stenosis might be differentiated from the infundibular form of right ventricular outflow obstruction by the presence of gross, chaotic systolic leaflet fluttering in cases with infundibular pulmonic stenosis.[17] They also found that one case of severe infundibular stenosis showed no *a* wave on the echocardiogram.

TRUNCUS ARTERIOSUS

In the congenital anomaly known as truncus arteriosus, a single great vessel arising from the base of the heart supplies the pulmonary, systemic, and coronary circulations. There is a single semilunar valve. A ventricular septal defect is also present.

In a series of five proven cases of truncus arteriosus, the aortic root was found to be large, and the aortic valve was easily detected by echocardiography.[3] The aorta was seen to override the interventricular septum where continuity of the anterior aortic wall and the septum could not be demonstrated. Because there is only a single semilunar valve, a pulmonic valve could not be detected in these patients.

In a single case report[18] of a young adult with a proven truncus arteriosus, the anterior mitral leaflet exhibited fluttering typical of regurgitation through the semilunar valve, although in the series of Chung et al.,[3] both the mitral and the tricuspid valves were normal in all cases. In such instances septal motion may be paradoxical, with a dilated right ventricle, presumably the result of right ventricular volume overload.

TETRALOGY OF FALLOT

The overriding aorta of tetralogy results in septum–anterior aortic wall discontinuity.[3, 19–24] In this anomaly, however, rather than a single great vessel exiting from both right and left ventricles as is the case in truncus arteriosus, a hypoplastic pulmonary artery is present. Echocardiographic differentiation between truncus and tetralogy is difficult and rests primarily on whether a pulmonic valve can be detected.[3] If a second semilunar valve is observed in the presence of anterior aortic wall–septum discontinuity, the diagnosis of tetralogy may be presumed. Conversely, however, failure to detect the pulmonic valve in this setting is an inadequate basis for excluding the diagnosis of tetralogy, because the valve may be present but insufficiently developed for detection by echocardiography.

In a series of 25 patients studied by Morris and associates, five echocardiographic features were described: (1) Increased right ventricular internal dimension, which was especially marked in adults. The right ventricular to left ventricular dimension ratio (normal = 0.33) was increased in every case and was as great as 1.45 in one patient. (2) Hypertrophy of the interventricular septum in 20 of the 25 cases. (3) Narrowed right ventricular outflow tract. (4) Enlarged aortic root dimension. (5) Septum–anterior aortic root discontinuity, which was detected in all 25 patients.[23]

COMPLETE TRANSPOSITION OF THE GREAT VESSELS

In patients with transposition of the great vessels, the pulmonary artery originates from the left ventricle, and the aorta arises from the right ventricle. Communication between the right and left hearts, such as ventricular septal defect, or between the great vessels, is necessary for survival.

The alteration in anatomic relationship between the aorta and the pulmonary artery provides the basis for one of the echocardiographic characteristics of this entity.[25] Normally the pulmonic valve is recorded superior and to the left of the aortic valve. In transposition, however, the two valves lie more nearly in the same horizontal plane, and they may be recorded simultaneously. This occurs because the pulmonic valve lies in a position slightly inferior of its usual location. When the pulmonary artery and the aorta lie in more or less adjacent positions, it may not be possible to record the valves at the same time. In this case, however, transposition may be suspected because only by angling the transducer in a medial–lateral rotation can both valves be identified without having to angle superiorly as well. Considerable technical expertise is necessary to accomplish this maneuver.

A second echocardiographic feature of transposition is the alteration in the relative position of the great vessels themselves, even when valvular tissue is not visualized.[25–27] In an ultrasound scan of a normal heart from the aorta to the pulmonary artery, the right ventricular outflow tract suddenly expands posteriorly and the aorta disappears from view. At the depth at which the aortic valve is visualized, a heavy echo thought to represent the crista supraventricularis will appear, and the pulmonic valve will be seen at the approximate depth of the anterior wall of the aorta.[25] At this position, the pulmonary artery appears to be coursing posteriorly just before the point at which it passes behind the aorta. In transposition, however, the anterior great vessel (aorta) is seen in its usual position in front of the pulmonary artery as the transducer is rotated superiorly. The two great vessels therefore are superimposed, without an intervening crista supraventricularis.

Hirschfeld and associates have found that the systolic time intervals of the left and right ventricles are changed in transposition.[7] Because the left ventricle ejects blood into the low-resistance pulmonary circulation, its ejection time (LVET) is lengthened as the valve opens earlier due to the reduced afterload. This is associated with corresponding shortening of the pre-ejection period (LPEP). The right ventricle, ejecting against the high-resistance peripheral circulation, however, has a prolonged pre-ejection period (RPEP) and a shorter ejection time (RVET). The LVET–RVET ratio in patients with transposition was found to be 1.22 (normal 0.80), and the LPEP–RPEP ratio was 0.52 (normal 1.25).

Nanda et al. have studied 11 patients with *d*-transposition and subpulmonic obstruction.[27] In addition to the echocardiographic features of *d*-transposition described, 10 of these patients showed prolonged diastolic apposition of the mitral valve with the septum, and four had systolic anterior mitral motion (SAM) resembling the mitral pattern characteristic of obstructive asymmetric septal hypertrophy. In these four, there was premature pulmonary valve closure coincident with the SAM. In addition, the pulmonary artery was smaller than the aorta in ten cases, and the subpulmonic area was smaller in five.

Because a number of other congenital anomalies may occur in association with transposition of the great vessels, the remainder of the echocardiographic examination shows highly variable features which are mentioned throughout Part II of this text.

DOUBLE-OUTLET RIGHT VENTRICLE

In rare instances, both the pulmonary artery and the aorta arise from the right ventricle, and frequently there is concomitant pulmonic stenosis.

Patients with this syndrome characteristically fail to exhibit the normal continuity of the anterior mitral valve leaflet to the posterior aortic wall.[28, 29] On the other hand, this continuity is present in cases of tetralogy of Fallot, from which it must be differentiated. French and Popp have pointed out that technical factors may complicate the sign of discontinuity and that therefore caution must be taken in arriving at a diagnosis based on whether such continuity is present.[30]

References

1. Hurst JW, and Logue RB (Eds.): The Heart. New York, McGraw-Hill Book Company, 1970.
2. Gramiak R, Nanda NC, and Shah PM: Echocardiographic detection of the pulmonary valve. Radiology *102*:153–157, 1972.
3. Chung KJ, Alexson CG, Manning JA, and Gramiak R: Echocardiography in truncus arteriosus: The value of pulmonic valve detection. Circulation *48*:281–286, 1973.
4. Nanda NC, Gramiak R, Robinson TI, and Shah PM: Echocardiographic evaluation of pulmonary hypertension. Circulation *50*:575–581, 1974.
5. Weyman AE, Dillon JC, Feigenbaum H, and Chang S: Echocardiographic patterns of pulmonic valve motion with pulmonary hypertension. Circulation *50*:905–910, 1974.
6. Weyman AE, Dillon JC, Feigenbaum H, and Chang S: Echocardiographic patterns of pulmonary valve motion in valvular pulmonary stenosis. Am J Cardiol *34*:644–651, 1974.
7. Hirschfeld S, Meyer R, Schwartz DC, Korfhagen J, and Kaplan S: Measurement of right and left ventricular systolic time intervals by echocardiography. Circulation *51*:304–309, 1975.
8. Hirschfeld S, Meyer R, Schwartz DC, Korfhagen J, and Kaplan S: The echocardiographic assessment of pulmonary artery pressure and pulmonary vascular resistance. Circulation *52*:642–650, 1975.
9. Chandraratna PAN, Lopez JM, and Cohen LS: Echocardiographic observations on the mechanism of the second heart sound. Circulation *51*:292–296, 1975.
10. Henry WL, Clark CE, and Epstein SE: Asymmetric septal hypertrophy (ASH): The unifying link in the IHSS disease spectrum. Circulation *47*:827–832, 1973.
11. Goodman DJ, Harrison DC, and Popp RL: Echocardiographic features of primary pulmonary hypertension. Am J Cardiol *33*:438–443, 1974.
12. Diamond MA, Dillon JC, Haine CL, Chang S, and Feigenbaum H: Echocardiographic features of atrial septal defect. Circulation *43*:129–135, 1971.
13. McLaurin LP, Gibson TC, Waider W, Grossman W, and Craige E: An appraisal of mitral valve echocardiograms mimicking mitral stenosis in conditions with right ventricular pressure overload. Circulation *43*:801–809, 1973.
14. Phillips B, Diethrich EB, Friedewald VE, and Ellis J: Calcified intra-atrial mass detected by M-mode echocardiography and multi-head transducer scanning: A case report *In* White, D (Ed.): Ultrasound in Medicine. New York, Plenum Press, 1975, p. 49.
15. Watts LE, Nomeir AM, and DeMelo RA: Echocardiographic findings in patients with mitral valve prolapse mimicking left atrial tumor (Abstr). *In* White D, (Ed.): Ultrasound in Medicine. New York, Plenum Press, 1975, p. 100.
16. Selzer A: Principles of Clinical Cardiology: An Analytical Approach. Philadelphia, W. B. Saunders Company, 1975.
17. Dillon JC, Weyman AE, Feigenbaum H, and Chang S: Echocardiographic differentiation of infundibular from valvular pulmonic stenosis (Abstr). Circulation (Suppl III) *49,50*:223, 1974.
18. Chandraratna PAN, Bhaduri U, Littman BB, and Hildner FJ: Echocardiographic findings in persistent truncus arteriosus in a young adult. Br Heart J *36*:732–736, 1974.
19. Tajik AJ, Gau GT, Ritter DG, and Schattenberg TT: Echocardiogram in tetralogy of Fallot. Chest *64*:107–108, 1973.
20. Allen HD, and Goldberg SJ: Echocardiography in congenital heart disease. Ariz Med *31*:571–575, 1974.
21. Murphy KF, Kotler MN, Reichek N, and Perloff JK: Ultrasound in the diagnosis of congenital heart disease. Am Heart J *89*:638–656, 1975.
22. Chung KJ, Nanda NC, Manning JA, and Gramiak R: Echocardiographic findings in tetralogy of Fallot (Abstr). Am J Cardiol *31*:126, 1973.
23. Morris DC, Felner JM, Schlant RC, and Franch RH: Echocardiographic diagnosis of tetralogy of Fallot. Am J Cardiol *36*:908–913, 1975.
24. Goodman MJ, Tham P, and Kidd BSL: Echocardiography in the evaluation of the cyanotic newborn infant. Br Heart J *36*:154–166, 1974.
25. Dillon JC, Feigenbaum H, Konecke LL, Keutel J, Hurwitz RA, Davis RH, and Chang S: Echocardiographic manifestations of *d*-transposition of the great vessels. Am J Cardiol *32*:74–78, 1973.
26. Gramiak R, Chung KJ, Nanda N, and Manning J: Echocardiographic diagnosis of transposition of the great vessels. Radiology *106*:187–189, 1973.
27. Nanda NC, Gramiak R, Manning JA, and Lipchik EO: Echocardiographic features of subpulmonic obstruction in dextro-transposition of the great vessels. Circulation *51*:515–521, 1975.
28. Chesler E, Joffe HS, Beck W, and Schrire V: Echocardiographic recognition of mitral–semilunar valve discontinuity: An aid in the diagnosis of origin of both great vessels from the right ventricle. Circulation *43*:725–732, 1971.
29. Hallermann FJ, Kincaid OW, Ritter DG, and Titus JL: Mitral–semilunar valve relationships in the angiography of cardiac malformations. Radiology *94*:63–68, 1970.
30. French JW, and Popp R: Variability of echocardiographic discontinuity in double outlet right ventricle and truncus arteriosus. Circulation *51*:848–854, 1975.

12

The Pericardium

The detection of pericardial effusion was among the first clinical applications of cardiac ultrasound and was reported extensively in the mid to late 1960's.[1-12] More than any other of the uses of echocardiography, the assessment for pericardial fluid is responsible for the rapid growth of this diagnostic method.[13] The current technique is the most sensitive, the most convenient, and the safest means available to the clinician for the diagnosis of pericardial effusion. Unfortunately, the echocardiographic criteria for the diagnosis of pericardial thickening and constrictive pericarditis have not been as well developed.

ANATOMY

The pericardium forms a closed cavity that surrounds the heart and normally contains only a few cubic centimeters of fluid. It is composed of two layers, the visceral pericardium, which is adherent to the epicardial surface of the myocardium, and the parietal pericardium. These two serous layers are continuous with each other at the pericardial reflections, of which the most important in echocardiography is at the atrioventricular groove. The anterior pericardium is adjacent to the connective tissue layer beneath the anterior chest wall, the posterior pericardium is next to the mediastinum, and the posterolateral pericardium borders the pleura and lung tissue.

ECHOCARDIOGRAPHIC FEATURES

The standard view for the assessment of the pericardium is through the right and left ventricles, slightly lateral of the optimal view of the mitral valve. The interface between the pericardium and the lung provides one of the most intense echoes reflected from the heart (Fig. 12–1).[5] As the gain is reduced, this echo persists after all others from the heart and lung have disappeared (Fig.

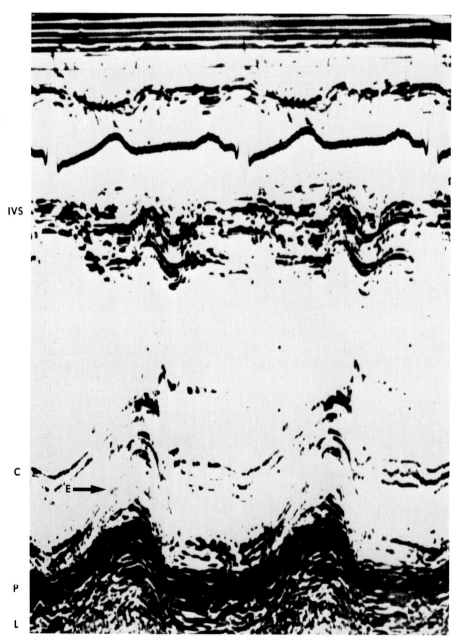

FIGURE 12–1. The intense echo from the pericardium-lung interface (P) moves anteriorly during ventricular ejection, paralleling the motion of the chordae tendineae (C). The faint endocardial echo (E) has the greatest motion of any structure in this region (IVS = interventricular septum; L = lung).

12–2). The dimension across the pericardium–lung interface echo is greater than the actual width of the pericardium itself, and therefore this does not provide a measure of pericardial thickness. Nevertheless, this echo will be referred to as the pericardial echo.

The anterior pericardium is often indistinct on the echocardiogram because it is adjacent to the intense chest wall echoes and to the underlying connective tissue, which does not provide a strong interface with the pericardium. The distance between the chest wall and the anterior ventricular myocardium is highly variable, depending both on the thickness of the interposing connective tissue and on the shape of the chest wall itself.

Both the anterior and posterior pericardium move in parallel with the adjacent myocardium, but with a lower systolic amplitude and rate of excursion than the endocardium (Fig. 12–1). Slight separation of the epicardium from the parietal pericardium during ventricular systole, and often into early diastole, is a normal variation when the pericardial motion continues to parallel that of the epicardium (Fig. 12–3).[14] Horowitz and associates have also pointed out that the parietal pericardium probably cannot move quite as freely as the visceral pericardium because it has a posterior connection to the mediastinum.[14]

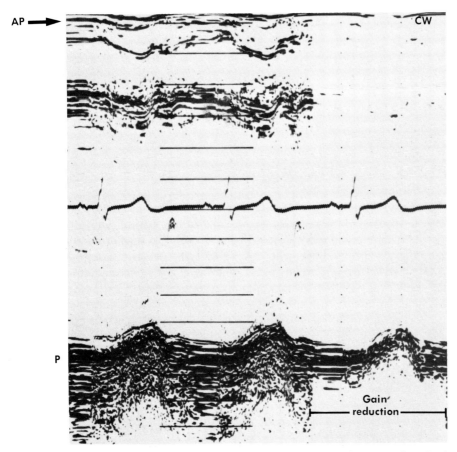

FIGURE 12-2. The pericardium-lung interface (P) echo persists with severe gain reduction. The anterior pericardial (AP) echo is less intense because of its weaker acoustical interface with the adjacent chest wall and connective tissue (CW).

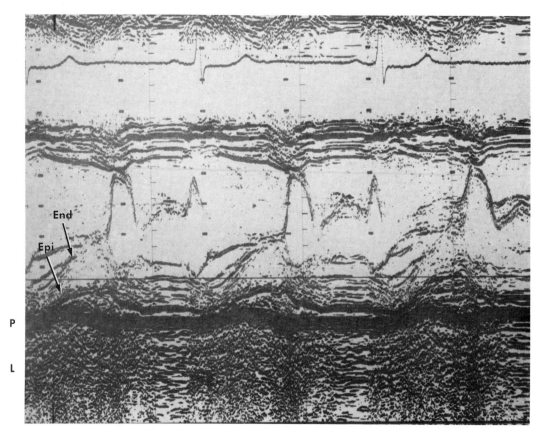

FIGURE 12-3. A slight separation between the epicardium (Epi) and parietal pericardium (P) is sometimes seen in patients without pericardial effusion. Note that the pericardium continues to show anterior excursion during ventricular systole (End = endocardium; L = lung).

PERICARDIAL EFFUSION

Fluid may accumulate within the pericardial sac under a variety of circumstances, most often as a result of pericardial inflammation with effusion. The increasing frequency of cardiac surgery has resulted in the common occurrence of hemopericardium. Echocardiographic identification of pericardial fluid is not only more accurate than any other method, it is also associated with greater facility than radiographic and isotopic techniques because it is accomplished at the bedside. Its obvious advantage over diagnostic pericardiocentesis is its safety.

Echocardiographic detection of pericardial fluid is contingent on the premise that the fluid can move freely within the pericardial sac. Therefore, with the patient in the supine position, even a small abnormal accumulation of fluid can be detected posterior of the left ventricle. The fluid may be even more apparent with the patient in the semirecumbent position.[15]

Two features mark the presence of pericardial effusion: (1) separation between the visceral and parietal pericardium and (2) failure of the parietal pericardium to move with the myocardium (Fig. 12-4). It must be emphasized, however, that pulsations of the parietal pericardium may continue in the presence of an effusion, especially in children.[15] These pulsations are usually dampened, however.

Another indication of a pericardial effusion is the absence of an echo-free space posterior of the left atrium that is continuous with the fluid-filled space posterior of the left ventricle. The pericardial reflection at the atrioventricular groove prevents extension of the effusion behind the left atrium. This is demonstrable on a sector scan from the aortic root to the mitral valve (Fig. 12–5).

An isolated echo-free space anterior of the right ventricular myocardium cannot be reliably interpreted as a result of pericardial fluid accumulation because a large anterior space is often seen in normal persons (Fig. 12–6). Most commonly this occurrence in the normal situation indicates increased connective tissue in front of the heart or, as in one case report, a diaphragmatic hernia.[14] Furthermore, with free communication within the pericardial sac, a large posterior echo-free space should be evident if effusion is detected anteriorly. If the fluid has become loculated anteriorly, however, a posterior echo-free space may not be visualized. We have observed one patient who developed a large loculated anterior hemopericardium following cardiac surgery. Diagnosis was possible in this instance only by comparison with a preoperative echocardiogram that did not show an anterior echo-free space.

Quantification of pericardial fluid from echocardiographic data is difficult. The dimension across the posterior space appears to correlate with the size of the effusion in only a gross way.[3, 8] Horowitz and associates have explained that the inability to predict the extent of an effusion from the size of the posterior

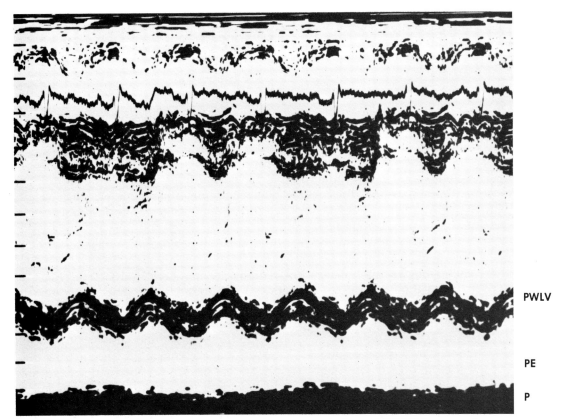

PWLV

PE

P

FIGURE 12-4.   Pericardial effusion. The posterior left ventricular wall (PWLV) is separated from the motionless parietal pericardium (P) by an echo-free space representing the effusion (PE).

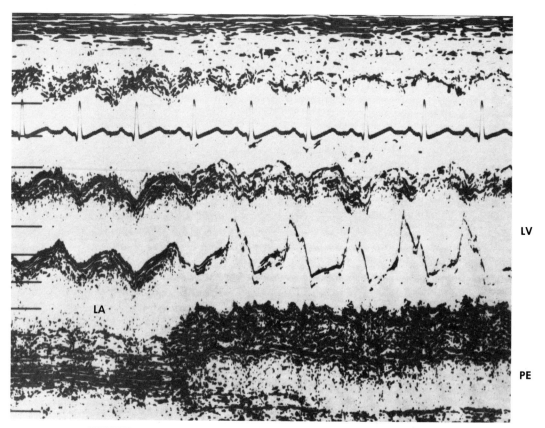

FIGURE 12–5. Pericardial effusion on aortic root–mitral valve sector scan. The pericardial effusion (PE) does not extend beyond the junction between the left ventricle (LV) and left atrium (LA).

echo-free space is most likely because the total cardiac size is not taken into account with this method.[14] Therefore, they have proposed that calculation of the difference between the volumes of two spheres, the heart (diameter from anterior epicardium to posterior epicardium) and the pericardial sac (diameter from anterior pericardium to posterior pericardium), will provide an estimate of the volume of the pericardial fluid within 100 ml of accuracy. These measurements have been correlated with those obtained following aspiration of pericardial fluid at operation.

Early reports estimated that the volume of pericardial fluid would have to exceed 40 cc for ultrasonic detection.[7, 9, 10] However, a recent study of patients undergoing cardiac surgery showed that in some cases as little as 15 cc of pericardial fluid could be detected with ultrasound.[14]

Different investigators have found that when the technique is carefully employed, the diagnosis of pericardial effusion by echocardiography is both sensitive and specific. Feigenbaum et al. found only one false-negative result among 200 patients examined for pericardial effusion, and in this case the fluid was loculated.[5] In the same series there were three false-positive diagnoses, one of which proved to be fibrinous thickening of the pericardium. Casarella and Schneider found an overall accuracy of 90 percent, with two false-positives among 21 patients diagnosed by echocardiography as having an effusion and 2 false-negatives in 15 cases in which effusion was documented by other means.[16]

In the study by Horowitz et al., of 39 patients with satisfactory echocardiograms who underwent pericardial aspiration at the time of cardiac surgery, 25 had negative echocardiograms, and only 0 to 16 ml of pericardial fluid were aspirated at operation. In 13 patients who had echocardiographic evidence of an effusion, from 15 to 775 ml of fluid were aspirated at operation.[14]

The most significant factor associated with failure to detect pericardial fluid by echocardiography is loculation. This is most likely to occur in the presence of adhesions secondary to previous infections or cardiac surgery.

False-positive diagnosis is almost invariably a result of misidentification of the posterior left ventricular wall. The mitral annulus is among the structures that can simulate the posterior wall (Figs. 12–7 and 12–8), but a hypertrophied papillary muscle, thickened chordae, or a thickened posterior mitral valve leaflet (Fig. 12–9) can also be mistaken for the posteior wall in some instances. Occasionally, the endocardium may appear as a heavier echo than usual, with the echo-free space between it and the pericardium simulating an effusion (Fig. 12–10). Popp and Harrison have pointed out that this error may be avoided by increasing the gain, thereby filling in this space.[17] Abnormal thickening of the pericardium can lead to the same error.[5, 14]

Pleural fluid may be mistaken for a pericardial effusion, although differentiation should not be a problem if the echocardiographic recording is of ade-

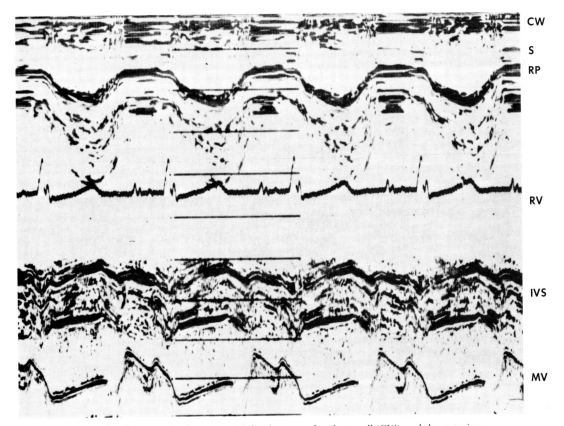

FIGURE 12-6. A large echo-free space (S) lies between the chest wall (CW) and the anterior right ventricular pericardium (RP) in a person without pericardial effusion. (As an incidental finding, note the abnormal posterior deflection of the interventricular septum (IVS) at the time of the QRS complex, as a result of left bundle branch block.) (MV = mitral valve; RV = right ventricle.)

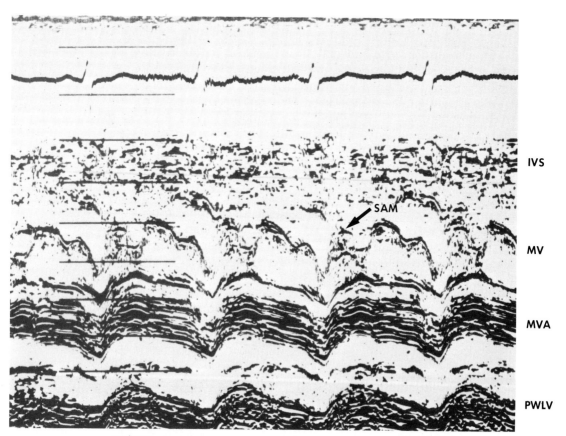

FIGURE 12–7. The space between the mitral annulus (MVA) and the true left ventricular posterior wall (PWLV) may be mistaken for a pericardial effusion. The preservation of the motion of the posterior wall is good evidence that this is not separated pericardium. The identification of the structures was further verified on sector scan to the left atrium (see Fig. 12–8). (Note: The patient has ASH with systolic anterior mitral valve motion (SAM).) (IVS = interventricular septum; MV = mitral valve.)

quate quality. The best means for distinguishing a pleural effusion from a pericardial effusion is a scan to the left atrium. The echo-free space representative of a pericardial effusion ends at the left ventricular–left atrial junction (see Fig. 12–6), whereas the space caused by a pleural effusion extends behind the left atrium. Simultaneous pleural and pericardial effusions cause the parietal pericardial–pleural echo to appear isolated in an echo-free space between the myocardium and lung (Fig. 12–11).[12]

Associated Findings

Motion of the anterior and posterior cardiac walls is often exaggerated in the presence of a large effusion.[6, 9, 13] Sometimes, as the heart apparently becomes freely suspended within the pericardial sac, the wall motion and that of the interventricular septum become parallel (Figs. 12–12 and 12–13).[9, 13, 18, 19] This is sometimes associated with the electrocardiographic phenomenon known as electrical alternans in which the frequency of this anterior–posterior motion becomes one half the heart rate.[4, 19] Diastolic notching of the posterior

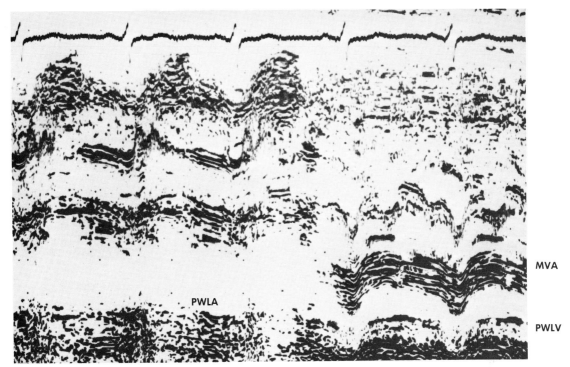

MVA

PWLA

PWLV

FIGURE 12–8. Same patient as Figure 12–7. Sector scan between the left atrium and left ventricle establishes that the true posterior left ventricular wall (PWLV) is continuous with the posterior left atrial wall (PWLA) (MVA = mitral valve annulus).

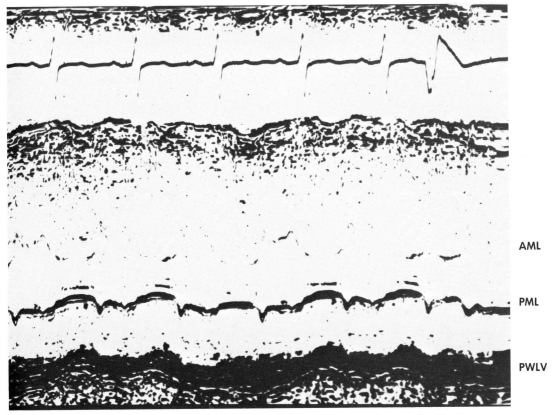

AML

PML

PWLV

FIGURE 12–9. Thickened posterior mitral valve leaflet (PML) with only faint visualization of the anterior leaflet (AML) creates the false impression of an effusion (PWLV = posterior wall of left ventricle).

225

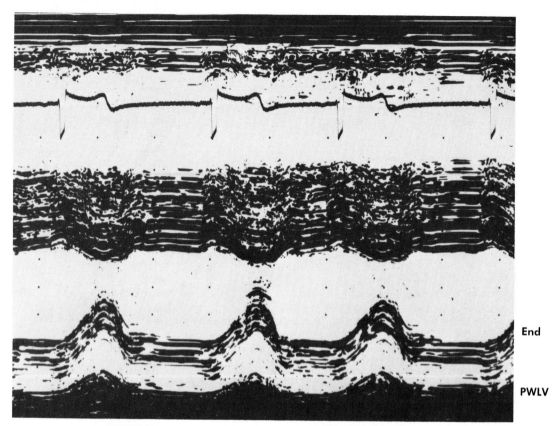

FIGURE 12–10. Thickened endocardium (End) in a patient with asymmetric septal hypertrophy may create the impression of a pericardial effusion (PWLV = posterior wall of left ventricle).

left ventricular wall is also sometimes observed in association with a large effusion (Fig. 12–12).

The mitral valve motion also may be exaggerated in the presence of a large effusion. Levisman and Abbasi have observed that a false impression of mitral valve prolapse may be created in the case of "swinging heart" and should be suspected whenever simultaneous systolic posterior motion of the anterior wall, septum, and posterior wall occurs (Fig. 12–13).[20]

CARDIAC TAMPONADE

When pericardial fluid accumulates rapidly, the pericardium may not expand sufficiently to accommodate the increase without a commensurate increase in the intrapericardial pressure (normally equal to pleural pressure). An excessive rise in the pressure within the pericardial sac interferes with diastolic filling of the heart and results in the clinical entity known as *cardiac tamponade*. This is suspected clinically by a falling, paradoxical blood pressure, rising venous pressure, and quiet heart sounds. The cardiac silhouette may or may not appear enlarged on the chest x-ray. Tamponade may occur in any setting in which pericardial fluid is present.

The principal value of the echocardiogram in suspected tamponade is to confirm the presence of pericardial fluid. Although the diagnosis of cardiac tamponade is based entirely on clinical evidence, certain features of the echocardiogram may be helpful. Feigenbaum and associates have described two patients with tamponade in whom the motion of both the anterior and posterior walls was markedly diminished.[4] In both cases the wall motion increased following removal of the pericardial fluid. D'Cruz et al. studied three such patients and found that during inspiration the opening amplitude and EF slope of the mitral valve decreased.[18] Also, during inspiration, the internal dimension of the right ventricle increased while that of the left ventricle decreased. They explained these changes as a result of expansion of the right ventricle on inspiration, which directly impedes left ventricular filling, accounting for both the reduced left ventricular dimension and the alterations of the mitral valve motion.

More extensive studies are necessary for better definition of the echocardiographic changes that occur prior to and during tamponade. For example, serial studies of patients with accumulating pericardial fluid might be particularly useful to the clinician in deciding when to intervene to avoid the development of tamponade.

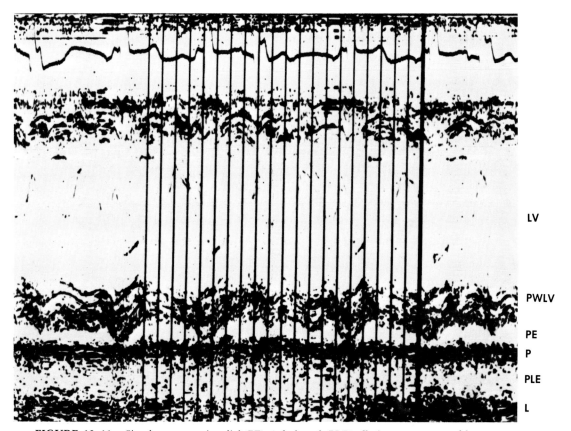

FIGURE 12-11. Simultaneous pericardial (PE) and pleural (PLE) effusions are separated by an echo (P) from the parietal pericardium and parietal pleura (PWLV = posterior wall of left ventricle; LV = left ventricle; L = lung).

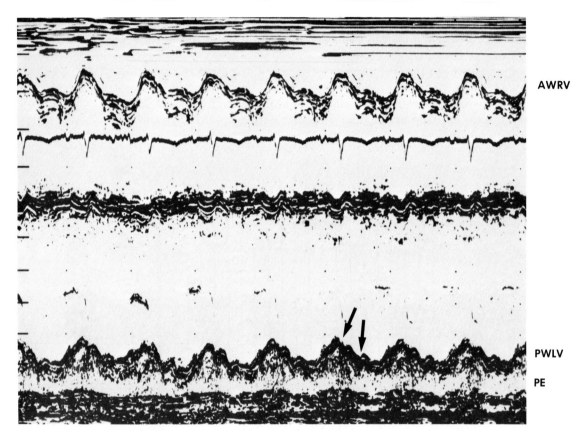

AWRV

PWLV

PE

FIGURE 12–12.   Parallel motion of the anterior right ventricular wall (AWRV) and the posterior wall of the left ventricle (PWLV) in the presence of a pericardial effusion (PE). A notching (arrows) of the posterior wall motion is also sometimes observed.

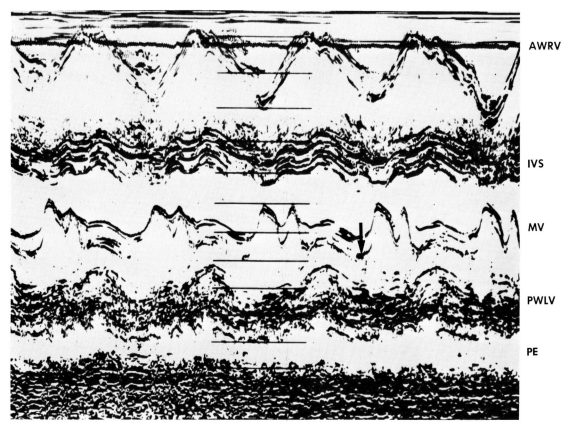

AWRV

IVS

MV

PWLV

PE

FIGURE 12–13. A large pericardial effusion (PE) has caused parallel motion of the anterior wall (AWRV), interventricular septum (IVS), and posterior left ventricular wall (PWLV). This swinging motion of the entire heart has also caused an impression of a late systolic prolapse (arrow) of the mitral valve (MV). Note also the exaggerated motion of the anterior wall.

PERICARDIAL FIBROSIS

There have been isolated reports of thickening of the pericardium detected by echocardiography. Pate et al. described four cases of pericardial fibrosis in which the myocardium and pericardium were distinctly separated.[7] Feigenbaum et al. reported one case of pericardial thickening.[5] Horowitz and colleagues found that the visceral and parietal pericardium in two patients with pericardial fibrosis could be identified as two separate echoes with constant separation, moving in parallel, presumably as a result of adhesions between the two pericardial layers. They felt that this could be a specific sign of pericardial adhesions.

Constrictive pericarditis occurs when the rigid pericardium impairs cardiac function. Gibson et al. reported that in eight patients with constrictive pericarditis, the only consistent finding was abnormal motion of the interventricular septum in diastole.[21] They did not find measurement of the pericardial thickness to be of value. Horowitz et al.[22] studied four such patients and found that the end-diastolic dimension was significantly reduced when compared to that of patients with restrictive cardiomyopathy. Systolic septal thickening was normal in the patients with constrictive pericarditis as compared to those with

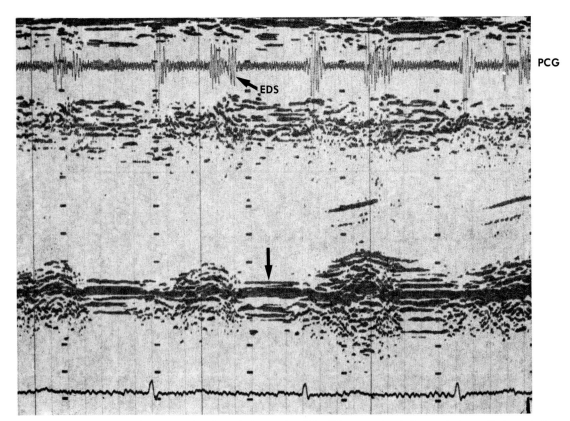

FIGURE 12-14. Constrictive pericarditis. The posterior left ventricular wall (arrow) does not exhibit the normal slow posterior excursion during diastolic filling of the left ventricle. The phonocardiogram (PCG) records an early diastolic sound (EDS) characteristic of constrictive pericarditis and occurring at the termination of the rapid posterior motion of the posterior wall following left ventricular ejection.

cardiomyopathy. They also noted a flattened motion of the left ventricular posterior wall in diastole, which corresponds to the restriction on ventricular filling that occurs in constrictive pericarditis (Fig. 12–14).

References

1. Feigenbaum H, Waldhausen JA, and Hyde LP: Ultrasound diagnosis of pericardial effusion. JAMA *191*:107–110, 1965.
2. Soulen RL, Lapayowker MS, and Gimenez JL: Echocardiography in the diagnosis of pericardial effusion. Radiology *86*:1047–1051, 1966.
3. Feigenbaum H, Zaky A, and Waldhausen JA: Use of ultrasound in the diagnosis of pericardial effusion. Ann Intern Med *65*:443–452, 1966.
4. Feigenbaum H, Zaky A, and Grabhorn LL: Cardiac motion in patients with pericardial effusion: A study using reflected ultrasound. Circulation *34*:611–619, 1966.
5. Feigenbaum H, Zaky A, and Waldhausen JA: Use of reflected ultrasound in detecting pericardial effusion. Am J Cardiol *19*:84–90, 1967.
6. Rothman J, Chase NE, Kricheff II, Mayoral R, and Beranbaum ER: Ultrasonic diagnosis of pericardial effusion. Circulation *35*:358–364, 1967.
7. Pate JW, Gardner HC, and Norman RS: Diagnosis of pericardial effusion by echocardiography. Ann Surg *165*:826–829, 1967.
8. Goldberg BB, Ostrum BJ, and Isard HJ: Ultrasonic determination of pericardial effusion. JAMA *202*:927–930, 1967.

9. Klein JJ, and Segal BL: Pericardial effusion diagnosed by reflected ultrasound. Am J Cardiol 22:57–64, 1968.

10. Klein JJ, Raber G, Shimada H, Kingsley B, and Segal BL: Evaluation of induced pericardial effusion by reflected ultrasound. Am J Cardiol 22:49–56, 1968.

11. Pridie RB, and Turnbull TA: Diagnosis of pericardial effusion by ultrasound. Br Med J 3:356–357, 1968.

12. Feigenbaum H: Ultrasonic cardiology: Diagnostic ultrasound as an aid to the management of patients with pericardial effusion. Dis Chest 55:59–62, 1969.

13. Feigenbaum H: Echocardiographic diagnosis of pericardial effusion. Am J Cardiol 26:475–479, 1970.

14. Horowitz MS, Schultz CS, Stinson EB, Harrison DC, and Popp RL: Sensitivity and specificity of echocardiographic diagnosis of pericardial effusion. Circulation 50:239–247, 1974.

15. Abbasi AS, Ellis N, and Flynn JJ: Echocardiographic M-scan technique in the diagnosis of pericardial effusion. J Clin Ultrasound 1:300–305, 1973.

16. Casarella WJ, and Schneider BO: Pitfalls in the ultrasonic diagnosis of pericardial effusion. Radiology 119:760–767, 1970.

17. Popp RL, and Harrison DC: Echocardiography. *In* Weissler AM (Ed.): Noninvasive Cardiology. New York, Grune & Stratton, 1974.

18. D'Cruz IA, Cohen HC, Prabhu R, and Glick G: Diagnosis of cardiac tamponade by echocardiography: Changes in mitral valve motion and ventricular dimensions, with special reference to paradoxical pulse. Circulation 52:460–465, 1975.

19. Gabor GE, Winsberg F, and Bloom HS: Electrical and mechanical alternation in pericardial effusion. Chest 59:341–344, 1971.

20. Levisman JA, and Abbasi AS: Abnormal motion of the mitral valve with pericardial effusion: Pseudo-prolapse of the mitral valve. Am Heart J 91:18–20, 1976.

21. Gibson TC, Grossman W, McLaurin LP, and Craige E: Echocardiography in patients with constrictive pericarditis (Abstr). Circulation (Suppl III) 50:86, 1974.

22. Horowitz MS, Rossen RM, Harrison DC, and Popp RL: Ultrasonic evaluation of constrictive pericardial disease. Circulation (Suppl III) 49, 50:87, 1974.

Part III

Pathological States of Special Importance to Echocardiography

13

Asymmetric Septal Hypertrophy

Since the original descriptions of left ventricular outflow tract obstruction caused by hypertrophy of the interventricular septum,[1, 2] the echocardiogram has become the best means for the diagnosis of this entity.[3] Recent observations utilizing the echocardiogram have provided further insight into the mechanism of obstruction[4-6] as well as the familial link in asymptomatic persons who have thickened septums without obstruction.[3]

Terminology in this syndrome is confusing and still debated.[7] At present the term "asymmetric septal hypertrophy" (ASH) encompasses all patients with primary septal thickening, regardless of whether there is left ventricular outflow obstruction. When obstruction exists, the terms "idiopathic hypertrophic subaortic stenosis" (IHSS) and "hypertrophic obstructive cardiomyopathy" (HOCM) are widely used. "Asymmetric septal hypertrophy with obstruction," although more cumbersome, is a more precise definition.

CLINICAL FEATURES

Asymmetric septal hypertrophy may become clinically manifest at any age. While it is most frequently diagnosed after the first decade of life, it can develop in infancy and is a recognized cause of infant death.[8] The first clinical evidence of disease, however, is usually a murmur, ordinarily developing in an asymptomatic individual in the second or third decade of life. Over 90 percent of these patients eventually develop symptoms, generally 10 years after the murmur is first heard.[9] In order of frequency, exertional dyspnea, angina pec-

235

toris, fatigue, palpitations, presyncope, and syncope are the most common symptoms of ASH. Sudden death may occur before any symptoms develop. Many persons, however, have nonobstructive asymmetric septal hypertrophy for an entire lifetime without ever developing a murmur or symptoms.[10]

Physical findings characteristic, but not diagnostic, of ASH include a double apical impulse with a nonradiating thrill; a systolic ejection murmur at the apex and left sternal border, which may not radiate; paradoxical splitting of the second heart sound; and a brisk peripheral pulse, which may be bifid. The chest x-ray may show cardiac enlargement, especially of the left ventricle, with pulmonary congestion.

Numerous electrocardiographic abnormalities in association with ASH have been described. The most common of these is left ventricular hypertrophy; arrhythmias and conduction abnormalities may also occur.

It must be emphasized that the clinical, x-ray, and electrocardiographic findings vary considerably among patients with proven obstructive ASH, and even in the same patient the physical findings may be only intermittently present. For these reasons, the diagnosis usually must be documented either by echocardiography or by cardiac catheterization with angiography.

Cardiac catheterization data may appear deceptively normal, especially when ASH has not been suspected or when there is no obstruction to left ventricular ejection. Provocative measures may be required to elicit the characteristic hemodynamic abnormalities. In the presence of obstruction, the arterial pulse shows a rapid upstroke with a sharp mid-systolic fall, followed by a second "tidal" wave. Also, the intraventricular pressure tracing shows a systolic gradient from the ventricular to the aortic subvalvular area. When the cardiac catheter is further withdrawn across the aortic valve, systolic pressure remains constant, but diastolic pressure shows the normal elevation.

The subvalvular systolic pressure gradient may not be demonstrated with catheterization unless there is sympathetic stimulation such as that brought about by isoproterenol or methoxamine infusion. Another characteristic feature of ASH is a diminished arterial pulse pressure of the beats following premature ventricular contractions (PVC's). Normally, post-PVC beats exhibit an increased pulse pressure.

PATHOPHYSIOLOGY

Asymmetric septal hypertrophy is regarded at present to be a result of an autosomal dominant genetic defect with a high degree of penetrance.[3] The principal defect is hypertrophy of the interventricular septum. Histologic and electron-microscopic examination of the hypertrophied septum shows the muscle bundles to exhibit a bizarre arrangement with variations in size.[1, 11] Maron et al. found that this appearance was almost exclusively confined to the septum among patients with obstruction, but that it was also seen in the right and left ventricular free walls in patients with nonobstructive ASH.[12] Histologic confirmation of the diagnosis may be obtained by biopsy of the interventricular septum with a catheter introduced into the right ventricle.[11] Both the anterior mitral leaflet and the septal endocardium are thickened by fibrous tissue.[10]

The resultant hemodynamic derangements are dependent upon whether there is obstruction of left ventricular ejection. Echocardiographic studies of relatives of patients with proven ASH have revealed that most persons with hypertrophy of the septum do not have actual obstruction of the ventricular outflow tract.[3] Thus, the disease has a wide spectrum of severity, depending primarily on the degree of septal hypertrophy in relation to posterior wall thickness and the secondary effect on the anterior mitral leaflet position during ventricular systole.

In contrast to the "fixed" obstruction of valvular aortic stenosis, the outflow obstruction of ASH occurs mainly in mid-systole.[13] Ejection from the left ventricle in early systole is unimpeded and actually more rapid than normal. In mid-systole, obstruction occurs with a characteristic drop in the arterial systolic pressure. In late systole, left ventricular ejection again accelerates prior to aortic valve closure. The pattern of ejection–obstruction–ejection results in the bisferious, or double-peaked, pulse of obstructive ASH.

The mechanism of outflow obstruction appears to be due to the combination of septal thickening and forward displacement of the anterior mitral leaflet during ventricular systole. This is further discussed in the section on the mitral valve in this chapter.

Although in most cases of ASH with obstruction hemodynamic changes occur only on the left side of the heart, isolated right ventricular involvement occasionally occurs.[14]

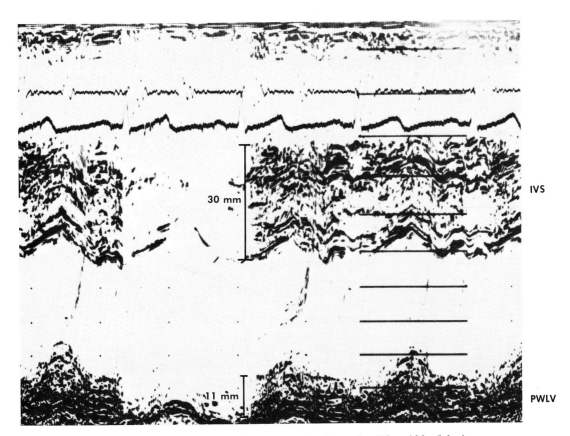

FIGURE 13–1. Asymmetric septal hypertrophy without obstruction. The width of the interventricular septum (IVS) is increased to 30 mm while the posterior left ventricular wall (PWLV) is normal in thickness (11 mm).

ECHOCARDIOGRAPHIC FEATURES

The Septum

The *sine qua non* of asymmetric septal hypertrophy with and without obstruction is disproportionate thickening of the interventricular septum relative to the posterior left ventricular wall width (Figs. 13–1 and 13–2).[15, 16] The thicknesses of the muscular septum and the posterior left ventricular wall are approximately equal in the normal heart, with the septal-to-posterior wall thickness ratio ranging from 0.9 to 1.1 (Fig. 13–3). Among persons with both nonobstructive and obstructive forms of ASH, the septum is at least 1.3 times the thickness of the posterior left ventricular wall.[15–17]

Echocardiographic assessment of the true thickness of both the septum and the posterior left ventricular wall is contingent upon optimal recording techniques. It is of paramount importance that the echo beam intersect the septum at or near a 90-degree angle and on a plane just below the mitral leaflets.[16] This angulation is important because in the presence of ASH, maximal septal thickness occurs approximately midway between the cardiac apex and the aortic valve (Fig. 13–4).[18]

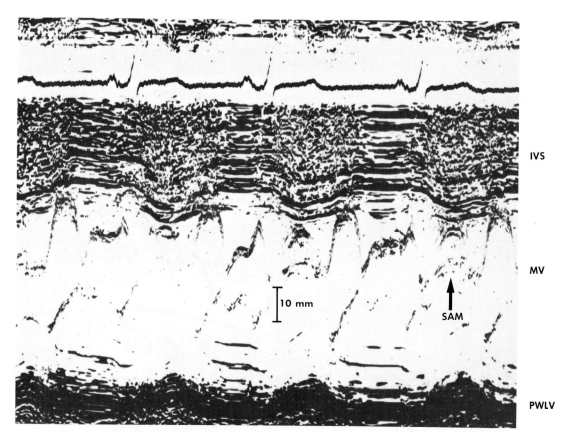

FIGURE 13–2.   Asymmetric septal hypertrophy with obstruction. The interventricular septum (IVS) is disproportionately thickened (about 30 mm) in comparison to the posterior left ventricular wall (PWLV) (about 11 mm). The septum thickens to 32 mm during ventricular systole, an increase of 7 percent. Incomplete mitral valve (MV) motion is seen, with systolic anterior motion (SAM) characteristic of obstructive ASH.

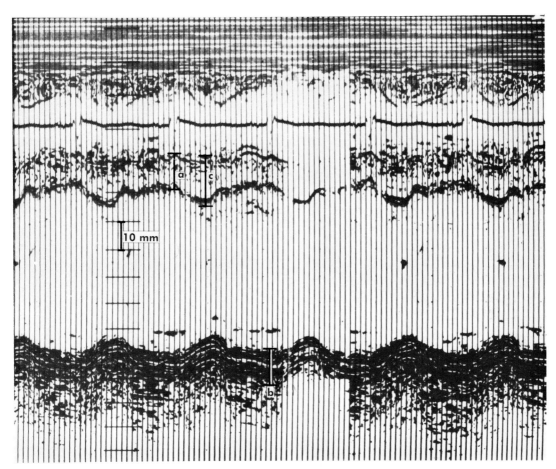

FIGURE 13-3. The normal septum and posterior wall. Both the septal width (a) and the posterior left ventricular wall width (b) measure 11 mm (ratio 1:1). Note that the septum thickens to 15 mm (36 percent increase) during ventricular systole (c).

If the echo beam strikes the septum too obliquely, factitious thickening may appear on the echocardiogram. The septal width will also be improperly measured if both the right and the left ventricular surfaces of the septum are not distinct. When the near gain control is placed too close to the right ventricular edge of the septum, septal thickness may be measured to be smaller than its actual size. This is especially likely to occur if the technologist is not forewarned of the possibility of ASH in a patient undergoing examination.

The width of the septum is measured at end-diastole, either immediately before the electrocardiographic P wave or at the initial predominant R wave or S wave of the QRS complex. (The septum has minimal motion just before atrial contraction, allowing for easier measurement, but in most cases the two points on the electrocardiogram exhibit nearly identical septal widths.)

Most patients with ASH have septal thicknesses ranging from 15 to 30 mm.[15-17] In general, the septal width is greater in patients with obstruction of left ventricular ejection than in those without resting subaortic pressure gradients.[10]

The septum may also be thickened in left ventricular hypertrophy secondary to fixed outflow obstruction (i.e., valvular aortic stenosis, membranous subvalvular stenosis, supravalvular stenosis), to systemic hypertension, or to ischem-

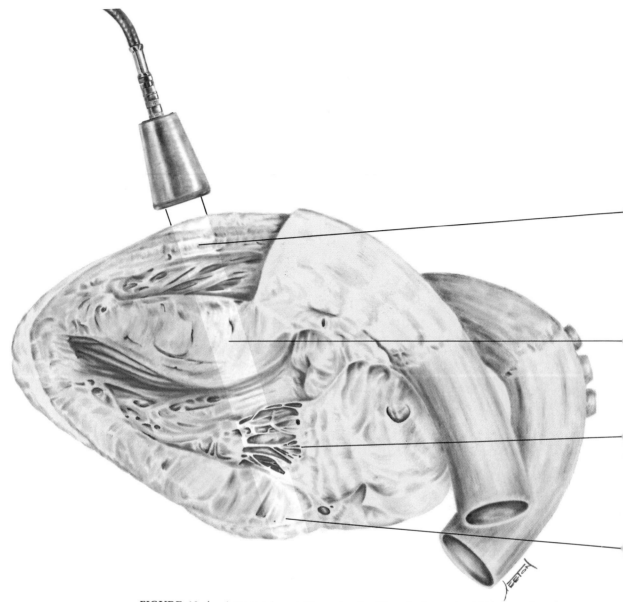

FIGURE 13-4. Asymmetric septal hypertrophy. The echo beam should intersect the septum approximately at its midportion, and the posterior left ventricular wall just below the mitral valve. Key: AWRV = Anterior wall of right ventricle. IVS = Interventricular septum. MV = Mitral valve. PWLV = Posterior wall of left ventricle.

ic heart disease. In such cases, the hypertrophy is concentric and is echo-cardiographically differentiated from ASH by the normal septum–posterior wall thickness ratio in these conditions.

Although the diastolic septal thickness is increased in ASH, the degree of systolic thickening is reduced (Fig. 13–2).[17, 19, 20] Normally the septal width increases by greater than 30 percent in systole (Fig. 13–3). Among patients with ASH, however, the septum thickens by approximately 20 percent or less. This is reflected in a reduced posterior systolic excursion as well as a decreased velocity of contraction. Therefore, the septum appears to be a hypodynamic structure in ASH, rather than a vigorously contracting structure as once believed.

AWRV

IVS

MV

PWLV

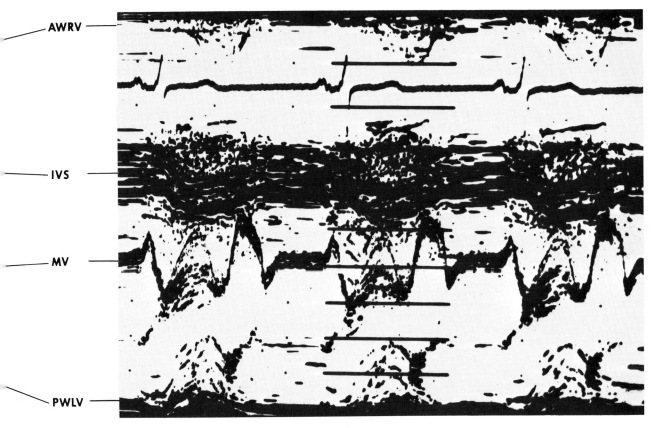

FIGURE 13-4.   Continued.

The Posterior Left Ventricular Wall

The free left ventricular wall posterior to the mitral valve is usually hypertrophied in patients with the obstructive form of ASH.[10] In most instances, the hypertrophy is less severe than the septal thickening and appears to be secondary to the outflow obstruction.[21] Among patients with nonobstructive ASH, the posterobasal wall is normal in thickness (Fig. 13–2), despite the fact that some of these patients may have primary thickening of other areas of the left ventricular wall.[10] Systolic thickening of the posterior wall is normal.[20]

The Mitral Valve

The mitral valve is often abnormal in ASH, and several echocardiographic anomalies are now well recognized.[4-6,10,15,22-28] These include (1) anterior systolic motion of the anterior leaflet, (2) reduced EF slope, (3) leaflet thickening, and (4) diastolic apposition toward the septum.

Systolic anterior motion (SAM) of the free edge of the anterior leaflet into the left ventricular outflow tract in apposition to the thickened interventricular septum appears to form the basis of the obstructive form of the disease (Figs. 13–2 and 13–5 to 13–8). This motion peaks in mid-systole and corresponds to the sudden mid-systolic drop in the intra-aortic pressure. The degree and severity of obstruction and the SAM vary from time to time in the same patient. The amount of anterior displacement of the mitral valve at the initiation of ventricular systole may determine the degree of obstruction during that cardiac cycle.[10]

Measures such as amyl nitrite inhalation and the Valsalva maneuver may provoke the SAM and outflow gradient in the patient with no apparent obstruction under basal conditions. Such intervention has the effect of increasing peripheral venous pooling with reduction in the filling pressure of the left ventricle and decreased left ventricular volume.

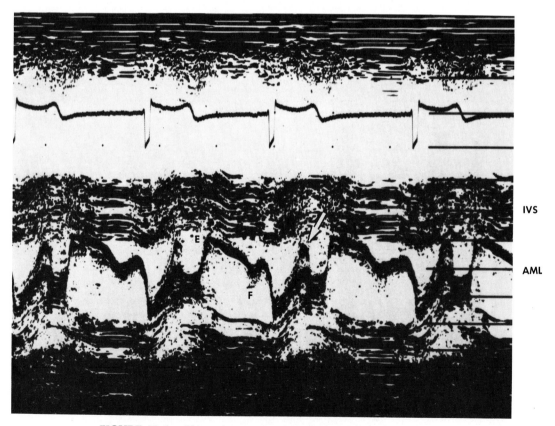

FIGURE 13–5. Obstructive asymmetric septal hypertrophy. The mitral valve anterior leaflet (AML) exhibits the characteristic systolic anterior motion (arrow). The diastolic position of the mitral leaflet (E) lies in close approximation to the septum (IVS) and the EF slope is reduced. The mitral valve leaflet appears to be slightly thickened.

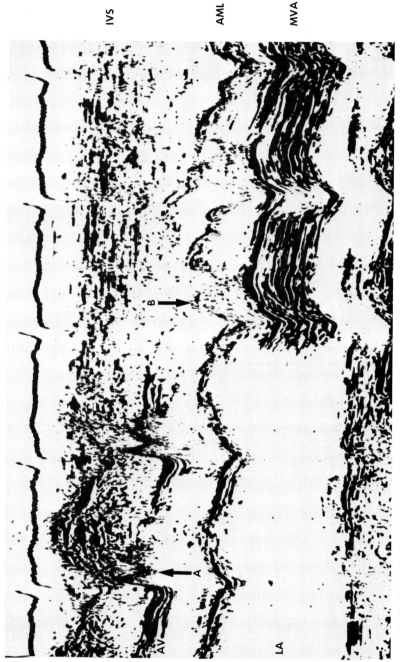

FIGURE 13–6. Sector scan in obstructive asymmetric septal hypertrophy. The aortic valve (AV) midsystolic closure (A) occurs as the anterior mitral valve leaflet (AML) shows its abnormal systolic motion (B). The mitral annulus (MVA) is markedly thickened (IVS = interventricular septum, LA = left atrium).

The alpha-sympathetic stimulators methoxamine and phenylephrine, handgrip exercises, and squatting all have the effect of increasing arterial pressure and left ventricular volume and reducing the gradient and the SAM in patients with obstructive ASH.[5, 10] Shah found the SAM to disappear in four of six patients following administration of methoxamine.[23]

Enhancement of myocardial contractility, as occurs during the administration of the beta-sympathetic stimulator isoproterenol, also increases the outflow gradient and the SAM.[22] (The effect of isoproterenol is similar to that of amyl nitrite in decreasing peripheral resistance.)

As the mitral leaflet approaches the thickened septum during systole, the effective left ventricular outflow tract is narrowed. It has been proposed that the degree and duration of this narrowing can be estimated echocardiographically and may be expressed as the "obstruction index."[5]

$$\text{Obstruction index} = \frac{\text{duration of narrowing (msec)}}{\text{average septal–mitral distance (mm)}}$$

The obstruction index has been correlated with the matched gradient across

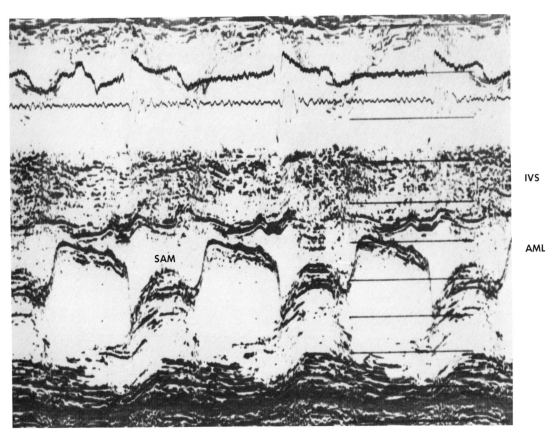

FIGURE 13–7. Asymmetric septal hypertrophy with obstruction. The interventricular septum (IVS) is thickened to 20 mm and the anterior mitral valve leaflet (AML) exhibits the SAM. The mitral diastolic closure rate is markedly reduced, without a distinct F point. The mitral valve leaflets appear thickened.

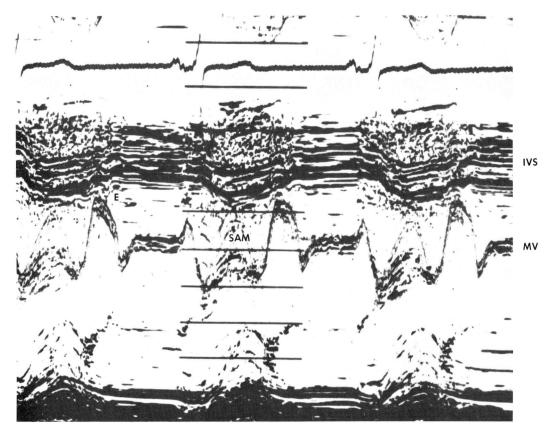

FIGURE 13–8. Asymmetric septal hypertrophy with obstruction. The mitral valve (MV) appears to contact the septum (IVS) at the time of diastolic opening (E point) and during the SAM.

the left ventricular outflow tract, and a regression equation for this has been formulated:[5]

$$\text{Gradient (mm Hg)} = (1.8 \times \text{obstruction index}) - 35$$

The degree of outflow obstruction has also been estimated by measuring only the distance from the point of maximal anterior mitral systolic displacement to the septum.[29] Expressed in millimeters, this is the minimum dimension of the left ventricular outflow tract during ventricular systole. This averaged 1.4 mm (range 0 to 5 mm) among 10 patients with obstructive ASH, with an average subvalvular gradient of 81 mm Hg (range 40 to 125 mm Hg).

Shah and associates found that the constancy of abnormal mitral systolic motion also correlated with the severity of outflow obstruction.[24] Patients in whom this abnormal motion was invariably demonstrated had an average outflow gradient of 78 mm Hg, whereas those with inconstant anterior displacement had an average peak systolic gradient of 24 mm Hg. No resting pressure gradient was measured in seven of their eight patients in whom the mitral valve motion never exhibited a SAM.

Other studies have shown, however, that marked mitral systolic motion may occur in patients with ASH but without any resting gradient.[4, 25] This phenomenon may be a result of anterior displacement of only a small portion of the anterior leaflet, insufficient to block left ventricular ejection.[4] On the other hand, the systolic anterior motion may be underestimated or even missed entirely if the apical portion of the anterior leaflet is not recorded. It is this portion that has the most abnormal motion. A false-positive diagnosis of a SAM may result if the ultrasound beam strikes the valve leaflet near its attachment to the aortic root; in such cases, the normal anterior excursion of the aortic root may be mistaken for the SAM (Fig. 13–9). When the beam is directed too far inferiorly, the posterior papillary muscle occasionally exhibits an exaggerated anterior motion in systole and may also be mistaken for a SAM (Fig. 13–10).

The mechanism of the systolic anterior mitral leaflet displacement during ventricular systole is uncertain. One explanation implicates excessive papillary muscle contraction combined with failure of the apex to move toward the base, placing abnormal traction on the chordae tendineae during systole.[30] Displacement of the anterior papillary muscle producing abnormal systolic chordal tension has also been proposed as a possible cause of displacement.[4] A more recent explanation is that the abnormal mitral systolic motion is a result of two factors acting in concert: (1) outflow narrowing at the initiation of systole and (2) hydrodynamic changes including a Venturi effect in which the mitral leaflet either is sucked forward by the rapid ejection of blood or is pushed forward from behind.[10]

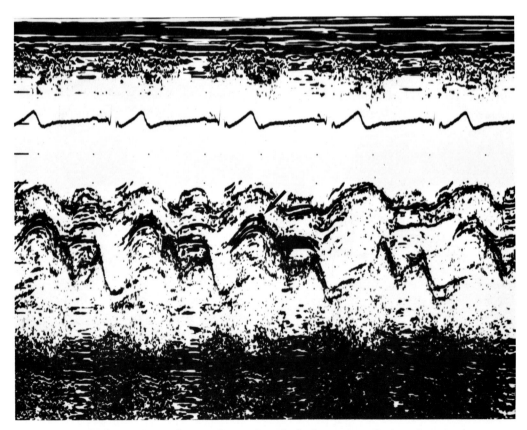

FIGURE 13–9.   "False" systolic anterior mitral valve motion. The transducer has been angled superior to the optimal mitral valve recording point, and as a result, portions of the aortic root are visible along with the mitral valve, creating the appearance of a SAM (arrow).

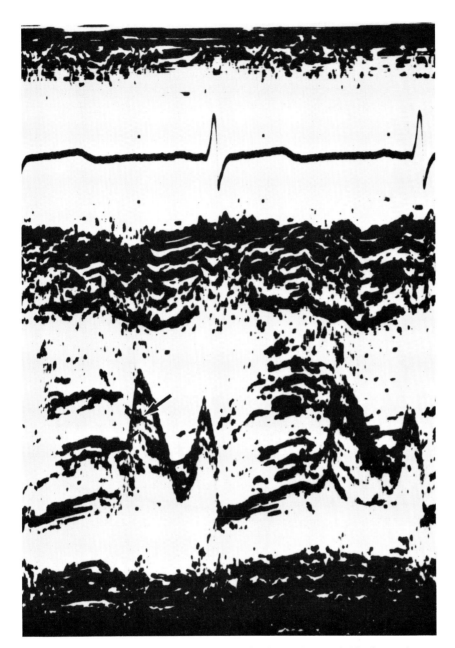

FIGURE 13-10. "False" systolic anterior mitral valve motion, probably due to the exaggerated motion of a papillary muscle. Note how these echoes (arrow) continue through the opening diastolic motion of the anterior mitral leaflet.

The anterior leaflet of the mitral valve may strike the septum during early diastolic opening (Figs. 13–5 and 13–8).[22, 25, 26] As a result, the E point may be "amputated" by the septal echo.[26] Popp et al. found mitral–septal contact in early diastole in 50 percent of cases with ASH.[22] The anterior mitral leaflet, however, may also appear to strike the septum in early diastole whenever its excursion is increased, as in chordal rupture and in Marfan's syndrome. Mitral contact with the septum may also be seen in the presence of a dilated right ventricle.[19]

The diastolic closure rate (EF slope) is frequently reduced as a result of decreased left ventricular compliance (Figs. 13–5 to 13–7).[15, 19, 22, 23, 26, 28, 29] This reduction may be quite extreme and, when coupled with the leaflet thickening, the condition resembles mitral stenosis.[28]

The anterior and posterior mitral leaflets are often thickened in both the obstructive and the nonobstructive forms of ASH (Figs. 13–5 and 13–7).[10, 28, 31] It has been speculated that this development is a result of the chronic trauma imposed on the anterior leaflet as it repeatedly strikes the septum (which also

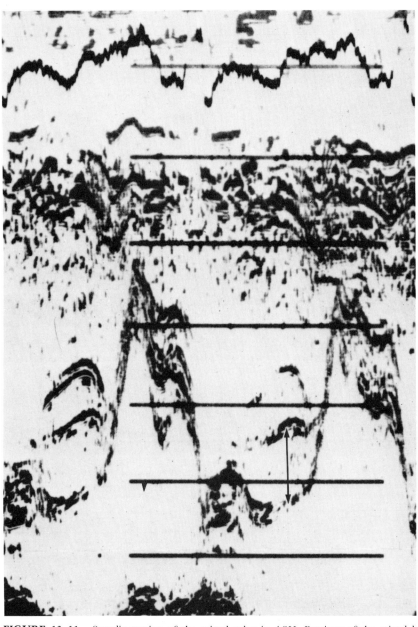

FIGURE 13–11. Systolic motion of the mitral valve in ASH. Portions of the mitral leaflets diverge (arrow) during ventricular systole, possibly accounting for the mitral regurgitation sometimes present.

exhibits endocardial fibrosis).[10] The posterior leaflet thickening could be the result of abnormal stresses caused by its anterior displacement.[10]

A large number of patients with left ventricular outflow obstruction secondary to ASH also have some degree of mitral regurgitation proved by angiography.[30, 32] While the mitral regurgitation is seldom severe, it is more pronounced in patients with high-grade left ventricular outflow obstruction. The incompetence of the mitral valve is probably caused by the displacement of the anterior leaflet during systole (Fig. 13–11). The characteristic increased diastolic opening amplitude with a rapid EF slope observed in other forms of mitral insufficiency is absent in obstructive ASH because the flow rate into the left ventricle is slowed as a result of reduced ventricular compliance. Consequently, mitral insufficiency cannot be diagnosed by echocardiography, but its presence should be suspected whenever the mitral valve exhibits abnormal systolic motion, particularly if the left atrium is markedly dilated.

The Aortic Valve

The aortic valve motion in ASH with obstruction is sometimes suggestive of this condition. The rapid early systolic ejection of blood opens the aortic

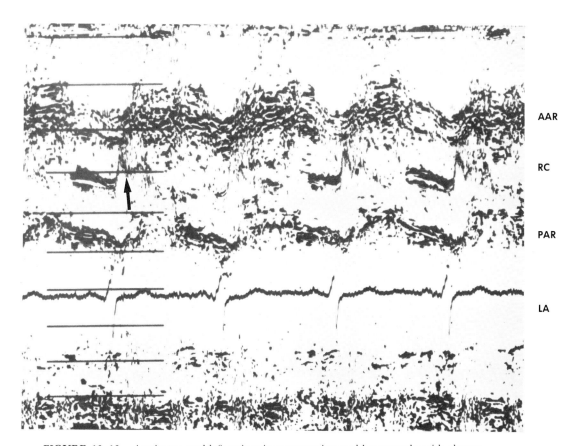

AAR

RC

PAR

LA

FIGURE 13–12. Aortic root and left atrium in asymmetric septal hypertrophy with obstruction. The aortic valve right coronary leaflet (RC) has a midsystolic closure (arrow). The left atrium (LA) is mildly dilated (5 cm) (AAR = anterior aortic root wall; PAR = posterior aortic root wall).

valve normally, but in mid-systole, the valve often exhibits total or partial closure, followed in late diastole by reopening (Figs. 13–6, 13–12, and 13–13). This motion correlates with the double-peaked pulse of obstructive ASH, the mid-systolic arterial pressure fall and aortic closure occurring simultaneously. Aortic valve motion is normal in the nonobstructive form of ASH (Fig. 13–14). (For further discussion of aortic valve motion in subaortic stenosis, see Chapter 6.)

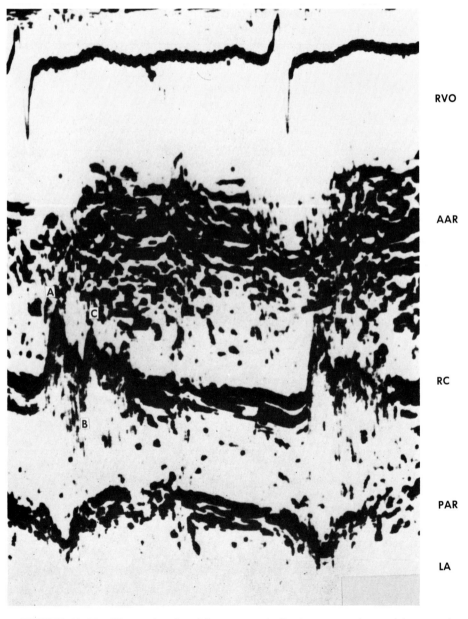

RVO

AAR

RC

PAR

LA

FIGURE 13–13. The aortic valve right coronary leaflet in asymmetric septal hypertrophy. Following early systolic opening (A), the valve closes transiently in midsystole (B), with late systolic reopening (C) (RVO = right ventricular outflow tract; AAR = anterior aortic root wall; RC = right coronary leaflet; PAR = posterior aortic root wall; LA = left atrium).

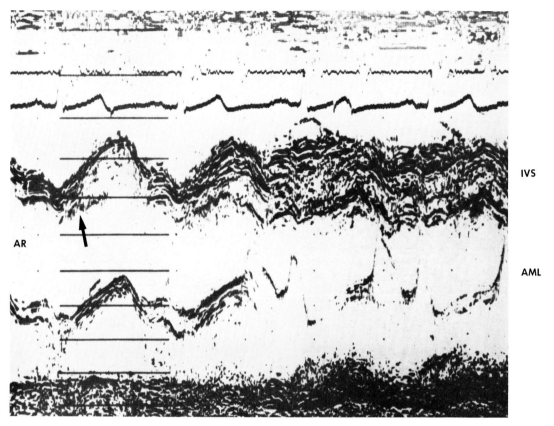

FIGURE 13–14. Nonobstructive asymmetric septal hypertrophy. Scan from the aortic root (AR) to the mitral valve shows the interventricular septum (IVS) to be thickened (20 mm), but the anterior mitral valve leaflet (AML) motion in systole is normal. There is no midsystolic closure of the aortic valve (arrow).

The Left Ventricle

In ASH, the left ventricular internal dimensions are either normal or reduced (Fig. 13–15).[10, 15] In the nonobstructive form of the disease, the echocardiographic ejection fraction is increased.[15] Fortuin et al. also found the ejection fraction and the mean velocity of circumferential fiber shortening (V_{CF}) to be increased in five patients with ASH (four with obstruction).[33]

The Left Atrium

While Roberts has observed that the left atrium in cases of ASH is almost always dilated at autopsy,[10] left atrial dilatation is less often diagnosed echocardiographically, and then is usually only mild unless left ventricular failure or significant mitral regurgitation has supervened.

Infancy

Asymmetric septal hypertrophy may occur in infants, and in severe forms it may cause death. In a series of four cases (one stillborn) in which death oc-

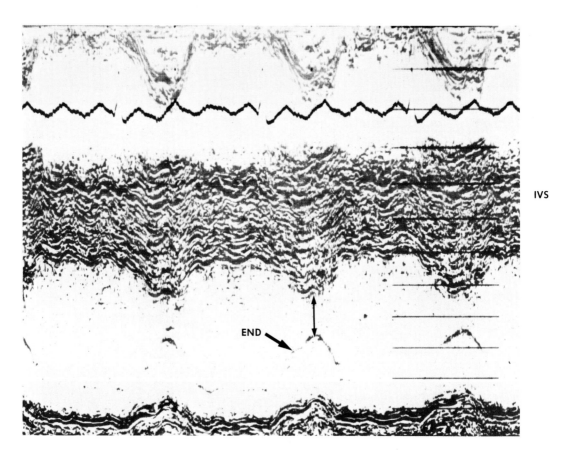

IVS

END

FIGURE 13-15. The left ventricle in nonobstrucive ASH. The interventricular septum (IVS) and the posterior left ventricular wall endocardial echo (END) closely approximate at end-systole (arrow), as the left ventricular chamber size is reduced.

curred before the age of 5 months, all had one first-degree relative with ASH.[8] The septal-to-posterior wall thickness ratios in these infants ranged from 1.8 to 2.6.

COEXISTING DISEASE

Coexisting ASH may be difficult to detect clinically in patients with other types of cardiac disease. In five of six patients with aortic valve disease (four with aortic stenosis and two with pure aortic insufficiency) and documented obstructive ASH, the ASH was not suspected clinically.[34] All six patients exhibited systolic anterior motion of the mitral valve; in the three cases in which this was only a small displacement, provocative measures failed to accentuate the motion. A single case study of combined calcific aortic valvular stenosis and ASH has been reported by Johnson et al.[35]

In a separate series of four pediatric patients with fixed left ventricular outflow obstruction, coexisting ASH was easily demonstrated, with asymmetrical septal thickening and a SAM in every case.[36] Bloom et al. found that two of twelve patients with fixed obstruction also had septal hypertrophy.[51]

Maron et al. detected disproportionate thickening of the septum in some cases of other types of congenital heart defects.[37] These have included mitral valve prolapse, interruption of the aortic arch, and ventricular septal defect. Most of these cases did not, however, exhibit the disorganized cellular structure characteristic of primary ASH.

Secondary septal thickening occurs in some cases of right ventricular hypertension as part of hypertrophy of the right ventricle.[38–40] Differentiation of right ventricular hypertrophy from primary ASH is easily made clinically.

Asymmetric septal hypertrophy also has been associated with Turner's syndrome,[41] hypertension,[42] coarctation of the aorta,[43] pulmonary artery banding,[44] aminophylline therapy,[45] and acromegaly.[46]

The frequency of atherosclerosis makes inevitable the fact that some patients will have both ASH and coronary artery disease. Clinically they are often diagnosed to have only coronary disease.[47] The ASH will be missed at cardiac catheterization as well if the evaluation consists solely of coronary arteriograms as a prelude to operative coronary revascularization. The ease with which ASH may be diagnosed echocardiographically warrants the routine performance of echocardiography in patients undergoing evaluation for ischemic heart disease. It should also be recalled that angina pectoris indistinguishable from that caused by coronary disease may be a symptom of ASH.

In the event that concomitant ASH goes undetected in the treatment of a more obvious cardiac disease state, the patient may fail to exhibit expected improvement.[36] For this reason, echocardiographic assessment for ASH is indicated in many patients who are not responding to definitive medical or surgical therapy based on a different original diagnosis.

ECHOCARDIOGRAPHIC ASSESSMENT OF THERAPY

The beta-adrenergic blocking agent propranolol forms the basis for the medical management of obstructive ASH. The mechanism of its action lies primarily in reduction of the increased fiber shortening of the left ventricular free wall during periods of stress. This reduces the amount of obstruction to the outflow of blood from the left ventricle. Elimination of the outflow gradient has been observed by Popp and associates to coincide with disappearance of the SAM during propranolol therapy in a few patients.[22] In a report of 12 patients by Shah and associates, however, there was no change in the abnormal mitral motion before and after treatment with propranolol.[48]

Septectomy is the operative treatment of choice for patients who fail to demonstrate satisfactory response to propranolol. The suggestion that mitral valve replacement may be preferable[49] has been effectively refuted by Roberts.[50] In a series of 12 patients, Bolton et al. observed the preoperative abnormal mitral motion to diminish or completely return to normal in every case following septectomy.[29] This corresponded to a change in the calculated obstruction index from a mean of 54 msec/mm before septectomy to 12 msec/mm afterwards. The left ventricular outflow tract dimension at the peak SAM increased from an average of 1.4 mm to 15 mm. Septal and posterior wall width and mitral EF slope, however, remained unchanged after operation.

References _____

1. Teare D: Asymmetrical hypertrophy of the heart in young adults. Br Heart J *20*:1–18, 1958.
2. Brock R: Functional obstruction of the left ventricle: Acquired aortic subvalvular stenosis. Guys Hosp Rep *106*:221–238, 1957.
3. Clark CE, Henry WL, and Epstein SE: Familial prevalence and genetic transmission of idiopathic hypertrophic subaortic stenosis. N Engl J Med *289*:709–714, 1973.
4. King JF, DeMaria AN, Miller RR, Hilliard GK, Zelis R, and Mason DT: Markedly abnormal mitral valve motion without simultaneous intraventricular pressure gradient due to uneven mitral-septal contact in idiopathic hypertrophic subaortic stenosis. Am J Cardiol *34*:360–366, 1974.
5. Henry WL, Clark CE, Glancy DL, and Epstein SE: Echocardiographic measurement of the left ventricular outflow gradient in idiopathic hypertrophic subaortic stenosis. N Engl J Med *288*:989–993, 1973.
6. Henry WL, Clark CE, Griffith JM, and Epstein SE: Mechanism of left ventricular outflow obstruction in patients with obstructive asymmetric septal hypertrophy (idiopathic hypertrophic subaortic stenosis). Am J Cardiol *35*:337–345, 1975.
7. Goodwin JF: ? IHSS.? HOCM.? ASH. A plea for unity (editorial). Am Heart J *89*:269–277, 1975.
8. Maron BJ, Edwards JE, Henry WL, Clark CE, Bingle GJ, and Epstein SE: Asymmetric septal hypertrophy (ASH) in infancy. Circulation *50*:809–820, 1974.
9. Adelman AG, Wigle ED, Ranganathan N, Webb GD, Kidd BSL, Bigelow WG, and Silver MD: The clinical course in muscular subaortic stenosis: A retrospective and prospective study of 60 hemodynamically proved cases. Ann Intern Med *77*:515–525, 1972.
10. Epstein SE, Henry WL, Clark CE, Roberts WC, Maron BJ, Ferrans VJ, Redwood DR, and Morrow AG: Asymmetric septal hypertrophy. Ann Intern Med *81*:650–680, 1974.
11. Alexander CS, and Gobel FL: Diagnosis of idiopathic hypertrophic subaortic stenosis by right ventricular septal biopsy. Am J Cardiol *34*:142–151, 1974.
12. Maron BJ, Ferrans VJ, Henry WL, Clark CE, Redwood DR, Roberts WC, Morrow AG, and Epstein SE: Differences in distribution of myocardial abnormalities in patients with obstructive and nonobstructive asymmetric septal hypertrophy (ASH): Light and electron microscopic findings. Circulation *50*:436–446, 1974.
13. Joyner CR, Harrison FS, and Gruber JW: Diagnosis of hypertrophic subaortic stenosis with a Doppler velocity flow detector. Ann Intern Med *74*:692–696, 1971.
14. Falcone DM, Moore D, and Lambert EC: Idiopathic hypertrophic cardiomyopathy involving the right ventricle. Am J Cardiol *19*:735–740, 1967.
15. Abbasi AS, MacAlpin RN, Eber LM, and Pearce ML: Echocardiographic diagnosis of idiopathic hypertrophic cardiomyopathy without outflow obstruction. Circulation *46*:897–904, 1972.
16. Henry WL, Clark CE, and Epstein SE: Asymmetric septal hypertrophy: Echocardiographic identification of the pathognomonic anatomic abnormality of IHSS. Circulation *47*:225–233, 1973.
17. Rossen RM, Goodman DJ, Ingham RE, and Popp RL: Ventricular systolic septal thickening and excursion in idiopathic hypertrophic subaortic stenosis. N Engl J Med *291*:1317–1319, 1974.
18. Roberts WC: Valvular, subvalvular, and supravalvular aortic stenosis: Morphologic features. Cardiovasc Clin *5*:98–126, 1973.
19. Tajik AJ, and Giuliani ER: Echocardiographic observations in idiopathic hypertrophic subaortic stenosis. Mayo Clin Proc *49*:89–97, 1974.
20. Cohen MV, Cooperman LB, and Rosenblum R: Regional myocardial function in idiopathic hypertrophic subaortic stenosis: An echocardiographic study. Circulation *52*:842–847, 1975.
21. Henry WL, Clark CE, Roberts WC, Morrow AG, and Epstein SE: Differences in distribution of myocardial abnormalities in patients with obstructive and nonobstructive asymmetric septal hypertrophy (ASH): Echocardiographic and gross anatomic findings. Circulation *50*:447–455, 1974.
22. Popp RL, and Harrison DC: Ultrasound in the diagnosis and evaluation of therapy of idiopathic hypertrophic subaortic stenosis. Circulaiton *40*:905–914, 1969.
23. Shah PM, Gramiak R, and Kramer DH: Ultrasound localization of left ventricular outflow obstruction in hypertrophic obstructive cardiomyopathy. Circulation *40*:3–11, 1969.
24. Shah PM, Gramiak R, Adelman AG, and Wigle ED: Role of echocardiography in diagnostic and hemodynamic assessment of hypertrophic subaortic stenosis. Circulation *44*:891–898, 1971.
25. Rossen RM, Goodman DJ, Ingham RE, and Popp RL: Echocardiographic criteria in the diagnosis of idiopathic hypertrophic subaortic stenosis. Circulation *50*:747–751, 1974.
26. Moreyra E, Klein JJ, Shimada H, and Segal BL: Idiopathic hypertrophic subaortic stenosis diagnosed by reflected ultrasound. Am J Cardiol *23*:32–37, 1969.

27. Wang K, Gobel FL, and Gleason DF: Bacterial endocarditis in idiopathic hypertrophic subaortic stenosis. Am Heart J *89*:359–365, 1975.

28. Smith MR, Agruss NS, Levenson NI, and Adolph RJ: Nonobstructive hypertrophic cardiomyopathy mimicking mitral stenosis: Documentation by echocardiography, phonocardiography and intracardiac pressure and sound recordings. Am J Cardiol *35*:89–96, 1975.

29. Bolton MR, King JF, Polumbo RA, Mason D, Pugh DM, Reis RL, and Dunn MI: The effects of operation on the echocardiographic features of idiopathic hypertrophic subaortic stenosis. Circulation *50*:897–900, 1974.

30. Dinsmore RE, Sanders CA, and Harthorne JW: Mitral regurgitation in idiopathic hypertrophic subaortic stenosis. N Engl J Med *275*:1225–1228, 1966.

31. Hallopeau M: Rétrécissement ventriculo-aortique. Gaz Med Paris *24*:683–684, 1969. (Cited in Epstein et al.[10])

32. Simon AL: Angiographic appearance of idiopathic hypertrophic subaortic stenosis. Circulation *46*:614–622, 1972.

33. Fortuin NJ, Hood WP, Jr., and Craige E: Evaluation of left ventricular function by echocardiography. Circulation *46*:26–35, 1972.

34. Nanda NC, Gramiak R, Shah PM, Stewart S, and DeWeese JA: Echocardiography in the diagnosis of idiopathic hypertrophic subaortic stenosis co-existing with aortic valve disease. Circulation *50*:752–757, 1974.

35. Johnson AD, Lonky SA, and Carleton RA: Combined hypertrophic subaortic stenosis and calcific aortic valvular stenosis. Am J Cardiol *35*:706–709, 1975.

36. Chung KJ, Manning JA, and Gramiak R: Echocardiography in coexisting hypertrophic subaortic stenosis and fixed left ventricular outflow obstruction. Circulation *49*:673–677, 1974.

37. Maron BJ, Edwards JF, Ferrans VJ, Clark CE, Lebowitz EA, Henry WL, and Epstein SE: Congenital heart malformations associated with disproportionate ventricular septal thickening. Circulation *52*:926–932, 1975.

38. Henry WL, Clark CE, and Epstein SE: Asymmetric septal hypertrophy (ASH): The unifying link in the IHSS disease spectrum. Circulation *47*:827–832, 1973.

39. Brown OR, Harrison DC, and Popp RL: Echocardiographic study of right ventricular hypertension producing asymmetrical septal hypertrophy (Abstr). Circulation (Suppl IV) *48*:47, 1973.

40. Goodman DJ, Harrison DC, and Popp RL: Echocardiographic features of primary pulmonary hypertension. Am J Cardiol *33*:438–443, 1974.

41. Nghiem QX, Toledo JR, Schreiber MH, Harris LC, Lockhart LL, and Tyson KRT: Congenital idiopathic hypertrophic subaortic stenosis associated with a phenotypic Turner's syndrome. Am J Cardiol *30*:683–689, 1972.

42. Hamby RI, Roberts GS, and Meron JM: Hypertension and hypertrophic subaortic stenosis. Am J Med *51*:474–480, 1971.

43. McLaughlin JS, Morrow AG, and Buckley MJ: The experimental production of hypertrophic subaortic stenosis. J Thorac Cardiovasc Surg *48*:695–703, 1964.

44. Freed MD, Rosenthal A, Plauth WH, Jr., and Nadas AS: Development of subaortic stenosis after pulmonary artery banding. Circulation (Suppl III) *47, 48*:7–10, 1973.

45. Davies H: Subaortic stenosis induced by drug therapy in a patient with an apparently normal heart. Guys Hosp Rep *119*:357–369, 1970.

46. Hearne, MJ, Sherber HS, and deLeon AC: Asymmetric septal hypertrophy in acromegaly—an echocardiographic study (Abstr). Circulation (Suppl III) *51,52*:35, 1975.

47. Whiting RB, Powell WJ, Dinsmore RE, and Sanders CA: Idiopathic hypertrophic subaortic stenosis in the elderly. N Engl J Med *285*:196–200, 1971.

48. Shah PM, Gramiak R, Adelman AG, and Wigle ED: Echocardiographic assessment of the effects of surgery and propranolol on the dynamics of outflow obstruction in hypertrophic subaortic stenosis. Circulation *45*:516–521, 1972.

49. Cooley DA, Leachman RD, and Wukasch DC: Diffuse muscular subaortic stenosis: Surgical treatment. Am J Cardiol *31*:1–6, 1973.

50. Roberts WC: Operative treatment of hypertrophic obstructive cardiomyopathy: The case against mitral valve replacement. Am J Cardiol *32*:377–381, 1973.

51. Bloom KR, Meyer RA, Bove KE, and Kaplan S: The association of fixed and dynamic left ventricular outflow obstruction. Am Heart J *89*:586–590, 1975.

14

Coronary Artery Disease

Echocardiographic recognition of some of the consequences of myocardial ischemia and infarction has been developed primarily because of the large numbers of people who are affected by coronary atherosclerosis. We can speculate that if coronary disease occurred with the incidence of, for example, asymmetric septal hypertrophy, it would be doubtful if more than a few sentences could be devoted to the subject.

The typical "coronary-prone" patient provides the ultimate challenge to the ultrasound technologist. This patient tends to be obese, to have a large chest, and all too frequently, to have obstructive lung disease as well. Unlike the bold echoes of a stenotic valve or the exaggerated septal motion of valvular insufficiency, the changes associated with coronary disease are subtle ones like dampened wall motion or small increments of change in the times of mitral opening and closure. Thus, the highest quality recording is necessary if echocardiography is to provide useful information about these patients.

The prime indication for echocardiographic examination of a patient with chest pain, whether it is typical for angina pectoris or not, is to detect a cause of ischemia other than coronary artery obstruction. For example, mitral valve prolapse and asymmetric septal hypertrophy sometimes cause chest pain. Also, even when coronary artery disease is unquestionably present, the echocardiogram is valuable in providing information about the effects of coronary obstruction on cardiac structure and function.

MYOCARDIAL ISCHEMIA

Failure to deliver adequate oxygen to viable myocardium results in alteration of its electrical and contractile properties. Several echocardiographic studies have been devoted to the detection of changes in cardiac wall motion during periods of ischemia caused by coronary artery disease.

Fogelman et al.[1] studied posterior wall motion in patients with and without coronary artery disease at rest, during exercise, and in the postexercise state. The mean and maximal systolic endocardial velocities showed a variable response, and the posterior wall excursion amplitude did not change from the resting value in coronary patients during the anginal episodes. However, these investigators observed that the patients with coronary disease had slower resting early mean diastolic endocardial velocity (DEV, 8.4 ± 0.8 cm per sec, versus 9.4 ± 1.7 cm per sec in normals) and maximal diastolic endocardial velocity (DEVM, 15.0 ± 4.0 cm per sec, versus 18.0 ± 3.0 cm per sec in normals). When the coronary patients were exercised, the DEV and DEVM remained unchanged prior to the onset of angina, but with angina, both values decreased significantly (DEV, 5.7 ± 2.2 cm per sec; DEVM, 8.2 ± 3.2 cm per sec). In contrast, the normal subjects showed a significant increase in both DEV (12.0 ± 2.0 cm per sec) and DEVM (23.0 ± 3.0 cm per sec) during exercise. The early-diastolic endocardial velocity is a manifestation of myocardial relaxation. Because this is an active process, it may be affected by inadequate oxygenation, which may account for the changes observed during episodes of ischemia. The slightly slower DEV and DEVM at rest in the coronary patients may be due either to chronic ischemia or, as these investigators point out, to decreased isovolumetric relaxation associated with age.

Kerber and associates[2] have shown in experimental studies that there is a good correlation between the endocardial systolic wall velocity and the degree of reduction of coronary perfusion. Decreased perfusion also correlated with the development of aneurysmal bulging during the period of isometric contraction.

Ludbrook and coworkers,[3] however, have pointed out the difficulties in reproducing posterior wall velocities and in correlating these indices with other parameters of left ventricular function in patients with coronary artery disease. While it is reasonable to assume that changes occur in the motion of ischemic segments of myocardium, more studies are warranted before the true value and limitations of the echo detection of these changes are known with certainty.

MYOCARDIAL INFARCTION: ACUTE STAGE

Echocardiographic examination of the patient during the acute phase of myocardial infarction ranks second only to that of the immediate postoperative patient in the challenge it presents to the technologist. Except in specific circumstances, the examination probably should not be attempted as long as the patient is experiencing the initial chest pain. Assessment of an unexplained murmur, possible acute tamponade, and unexplained shock would be among exceptional indications for clinical echocardiography during the first hours following infarction. Even in these instances, however, the examination should be limited to the diagnosis or exclusion of specific problems. An additional electronic device may serve to heighten the patient's anxiety at a time when maximal effort should be directed toward sedation and the relief of his discomfort. Furthermore, the echocardiographic examination of the patient experiencing severe chest pain is frequently of suboptimal quality. In one study,[4] suitable echocardiograms were obtainable in only 60 percent of patients sustaining acute infarction, although Corya et al.[5] reported satisfactory examinations on more than 90 percent of such patients.

The ultimate prognosis for the patient with an acute myocardial infarction is dependent on two interrelated factors, and extensive research with ultrasound, as well as other techniques, is now being directed to both: (1) the amount of affected muscle mass and (2) complications such as septal perforation and papillary muscle disruption.

Altered Wall Motion

Experimental infarction of the posterior left ventricular wall in dogs has been found to result in changes in the motion of the endocardium in the affected area within 15 minutes after coronary embolism.[6] The most characteristic change in this experimental series was a reduction in the amplitude of endocardial excursion by a mean of 36 percent. The mean and maximal systolic velocities of excursion were also significantly reduced by over 30 percent. These changes were accounted for by reduced myocardial contractility as a result of the infarction.

Another study on dogs undergoing experimental acute myocardial infarction demonstrated that infarction of the posterior wall profoundly altered the motion of that wall, with marked diminution in the mean posterior wall velocity and the amplitude of excursion.[7] In addition, there was a striking alteration in the contour of the wall motion within the infarcted area as the posterior displacement of the wall during the isovolumetric contraction period became markedly accentuated. This was followed by a slow anterior excursion during ventricular ejection and rapid anterior movement during the isovolumetric relaxation period. These paradoxical movements were attributed to recording the actual dyskinetic area of infarction. When the infarction involved the apical myocardium, however, there were no significant changes in the posterior wall motion.

Inoue et al.[8] have described aberrations in the posterior wall motion in 10 of 11 patients during the acute phases of myocardial infarction. Specifically, these investigators noted anterior bulges of the endocardium during both ventricular systole and diastole, but their significance in this study is unclear. In addition, the mean posterior wall velocities and amplitudes of excursion were observed to be reduced. Smithen and associates[9] found a 26 percent decrease in the maximal posterior wall systolic velocity and a 46 percent reduction in the systolic anterior excursion during the first 36 hours following acute anterior wall infarction in eight patients.

In a study of 10 patients with acute myocardial infarction, Ratshin and associates[10] found the mean (2.76 ± 0.30 cm per sec) and maximum (4.97 ± 0.64 cm per sec) posterior wall velocities in patients with inferior wall infarctions to be slower than those in patients with anterior myocardial infarctions (3.19 ± 0.48 cm per sec and 5.89 ± 0.80 cm per sec). In a separate report of 22 patients with acute posterior myocardial infarction, Chapelle et al.[11] found that within 24 hours of infarction the maximal velocity of posterior wall excursion was significantly reduced.

Heikkilä and Nieminen[12] studied 30 patients with acute myocardial infarction within twelve hours after admission to the coronary care unit. In all patients the asynergistic area of infarcted myocardium could be detected echocardiographically. The anterior and anteroseptal infarctions were consistently associated with paradoxical septal motion of up to 5 mm anteriorly during ventricular systole. Diminished or absent posterior wall motion was seen in all patients with inferior or posterior wall infarctions. The noninfarcted areas of myocardium often exhibited increased amplitude of motion. The echocardiographic localization of infarction directly correlated with the electrocardiographic data.

Corya et al.[13] found that 25 of 26 patients with acute myocardial infarction showed abnormal anterior left ventricular wall motion on the echocardiogram and anterior or lateral wall electrocardiographic changes consistent with transmural or subendocardial infarction. Of 34 patients with anterior or lateral wall electrocardiographic changes of infarction, 25 had abnormal echocardiographic anterior wall motion. Conversely, only one of 16 patients with acute inferior infarction showed altered echocardiographic anterior wall motion.

Therefore, while more studies are obviously needed, the echocardiographic findings in acute infarction appear to be principally dependent on the position of the infarcted area relative to the echo beam. When the area of acute infarction itself is analyzed, systolic changes of the wall motion are dramatic. However, if the acutely infarcted area of the ventricle is remote from the portion recorded, the findings are nonspecific and are related primarily to depressed myocardial contraction or to compensatory increases in wall motion.

Left Ventricular Dimensions and Function

Henning and associates[14] have studied patients with transmural myocardial infarction and have compared the ejection fraction as determined by echocardiogram and by radionuclide angiography. In their report they pointed out a tendency of the echocardiogram to overestimate left ventricular function in the presence of a previous infarction. Pombo et al.,[4] however, compared stroke volume and cardiac output determinations obtained by ultrasound to the dye-dilution measurements in a group of nine patients with acute myocardial infarction. They found close correlation between the two methods in determining both stroke volume and cardiac output, although larger stroke volumes were estimated by echocardiography in patients with inferior wall myocardial infarctions. Smith et al.[15] found a closer correlation between the left ventricular end-diastolic volume determined echocardiographically and cineangiographically than between the end-systolic determinations. The discrepancy between the accuracy of end-systolic and end-diastolic determinations may be explained by geometric distortions of the myocardium that occur during ventricular systole in the presence of infarction. The echo beam may then intersect a hypermobile noninfarcted segment or a hypomobile infarcted segment of myocardium, and in either instance, the end-systolic dimension does not reflect the changes in the volume of the ventricle as a whole. Therefore, if the recording is made across noninfarcted segments of the left ventricle, end-systolic volume will be calculated as smaller than the true volume, and the stroke volume will be calculated as larger than is truly the case. Sweet et al.[16] have proposed that the difference between the stroke volume determined by echocardiography and by invasive methods provides a means for estimating the size of the abnormally contracting segment of myocardium.

Broder and Cohn[17] studied 12 patients with acute myocardial infarction and found the echocardiographic end-diastolic dimension to be normal in the presence of elevated left ventricular end-diastolic pressure determined by simultaneous left ventricular catheterization. This implies a reduction in myocardial compliance in these circumstances. A report by Corya et al.[5] showed that an increased echocardiographic left ventricular internal end-diastolic dimension (LVID$_d$) correlated with the clinical diagnosis of heart failure. Subsequent hospital mortality could be predicted by relating the LVID$_d$ to the period of mitral valve closure, which is a reflection of the left ventricular end-diastolic pressure (PR-AC interval). Six of eight patients with LVID$_d$/PR-AC ratios greater than 65 died, whereas only one of 27 patients with a ratio less than 65 expired.

The mitral valve EF slope was serially determined by Bergeron and associates[18] during the hospitalization of patients with acute myocardial infarction. On echocardiograms recorded within 5 hours of admission, they found the EF slope to be slightly reduced (mean 79 ± 6 mm per sec) in comparison to a repeat study performed 13 to 30 days after the infarction (mean 102 ± 2.5 mm per sec). This is probably a result of reduced ventricular compliance during the acute infarction period and increasing compliance with healing. Alterations in ventricular geometry also may have an effect on the pressure–volume relationship of the left ventricle and thus contribute to changes in the mitral diastolic closure velocity. The mitral valve amplitude of excursion was also measured in this study, and this parameter showed no significant change from the initial recording until discharge.

Further echocardiographic studies on left ventricular function in patients with acute myocardial infarction may provide the clinician with better objective criteria for specific therapeutic intervention. For example, serial echocardiograms may prove to be useful in detecting an extension of infarction and may be valuable in alerting the physician to earlier evidence of left ventricular failure than current standard practices provide.

Mitral Regurgitation

As a complication of acute myocardial infarction, mitral regurgitation may occur either as a consequence of combined papillary dysfunction and left ventricular dyskinesia or dilatation[19] or from acute papillary muscle disruption. The former may be intermittent[20] and often is not associated with a murmur.[21] Its echocardiographic features are those of a low-flow mitral motion in left heart failure, which is discussed in Chapter 8.

Papillary muscle rupture, which may result in acute mitral regurgitation during the first few days after a myocardial infarction, is usually heralded by the sudden development of pulmonary edema and a loud holosystolic murmur.[22] Cardiac decompensation may ensue rapidly, and death usually occurs unless there is operative intervention.[23, 24] Acute papillary muscle transection is similar to acute chordal rupture (Chapter 4). The valve leaflets are usually thin, with no evidence of prior disease, and they exhibit marked excursion which, combined with the accompanying tachycardia, may be difficult to record completely

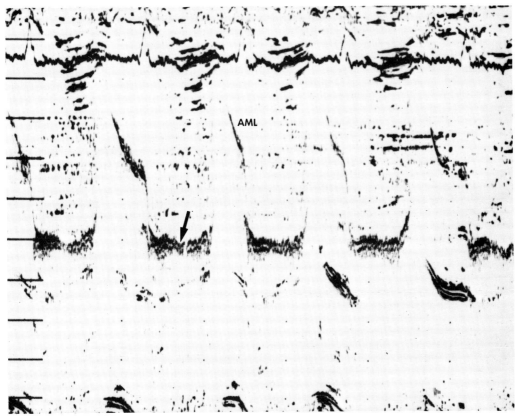

FIGURE 14-1. Transected posteromedial papillary muscle in acute inferior wall myocardial infarction. The mitral valve has a rapid fluttering motion during ventricular systole (arrow). The increased rate of diastolic opening of the anterior leaflet (AML) makes this portion of its motion difficult to record.

on the echocardiogram (Fig. 14–1). The anterior leaflet echo is often "lost" in the echo from the interventricular septum. A fluttering motion of the leaflets during ventricular systole is highly characteristic when observed. The leaflets may also prolapse into the left atrium, where they sometimes appear as one or more faint echoes with slight anterior motion during ventricular systole (Fig. 14–2). In the very acute stage of mitral insufficiency, the left atrium will be normal in size or only slightly dilated. The left ventricle may also have normal dimensions. The interventricular septum may show exaggerated systolic posterior motion[25] unless it has been involved in the infarction, in which case it will appear paradoxical.

Rupture of the Interventricular Septum

Septal rupture occurs suddenly, with clinical signs resembling those of acute mitral regurgitation. Chandraratna and associates[25] studied three patients with anatomically proven septal rupture and found the echocardiographic features to be nonspecific. Right ventricular dilatation was present in all three of these cases, whereas four patients with acute mitral regurgitation had normal

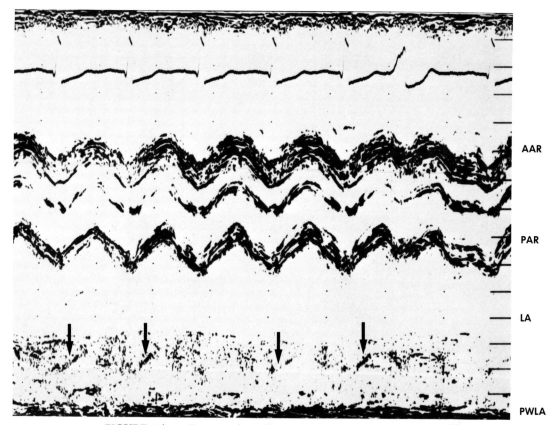

FIGURE 14-2. Transected papillary muscle in acute inferior wall myocardial infarction. In this view through the left atrium (LA) a portion of the posterior mitral leaflet appears during ventricular systole (arrows). The left atrium is dilated. On postmortem examination, the posterior leaflet was totally flail and was lying in the left atrium (AAR = anterior aortic root wall; PAR = posterior aortic root wall; PWLA = posterior wall of left atrium).

right ventricular dimensions. Also, the septum had a normal systolic amplitude of motion, which is not the case in mitral regurgitation. In a single case study by DeJoseph et al.,[26] the septum was observed to exhibit little motion prior to rupture. After rupture, however, the upper portion of the septum moved anteriorly with an exaggerated motion, accompanied by a marked posterior excursion at the onset of ventricular diastole. The lower septum remained akinetic. Mitral valve motion may be normal or exaggerated, depending on the volume of the flow through the septal defect.

The differentiation of acute mitral regurgitation from septal perforation at present is made on clinical grounds, utilizing all the information of the event, type of infarction, characteristics of the murmur, etc. The echocardiographic features are of limited value because data from large series of each of these complications are not yet available for analysis. The mitral valve motion is similar in that both lesions result in increased flow across the valve, but systolic fluttering and systolic prolapse into the left atrium are features only of acute mitral insufficiency. Right ventricular dilatation, however, is characteristic of a perforated interventricular septum but not of acute mitral regurgitation.

MYOCARDIAL INFARCTION: CHRONIC CHANGES

Myocardial infarction causes a functional loss of a segment of the myocardium that ceases to participate in the contractile process of the heart. As a consequence, the infarcted area may exhibit (1) normal direction but diminished amplitude of motion, (2) absent (akinetic) motion, or (3) reversed (dyskinetic) motion. In addition, the character of the echoes from the infarcted area may be altered, and the wall thickness may become reduced when myocardium is replaced by scar tissue. Noninfarcted areas, on the other hand, may hypertrophy and have hyperdynamic contractile motion. Echocardiographic detection of these changes is dependent on the location and extent of the infarction. It must be emphasized that, because coronary disease affects only segments of the myocardium, multiple areas of septum and free wall must be recorded before the echocardiographic evaluation can be considered adequate. Even then, sizable infarcted areas (especially anterolateral and apical) may be overlooked.

Interventricular Septum

The septum has a dual blood supply, generally with its anterior two thirds supplied by perforating branches of the left anterior descending coronary ar-

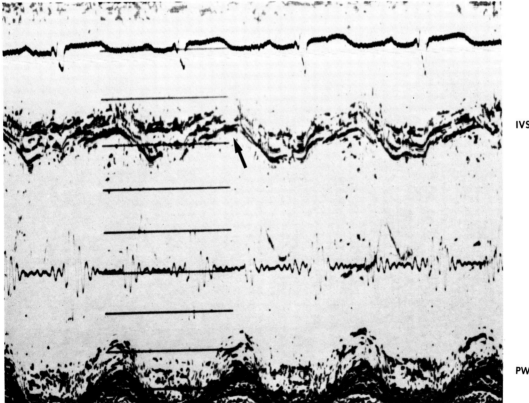

FIGURE 14-3. Infarction of the interventricular septum (IVS). The septum moves paradoxically (arrow) during ventricular systole, without systolic thickening. The posterior left ventricular wall (PWLV) shows normal motion.

tery and its posterior one third served by the posterior circulation. Its supply, however, is variable, and in atherosclerotic disease, either of these coronary arteries can assume a more important role in supplying blood to the septum. For these reasons, septal infarction can vary so much in extent and location that echocardiographic changes can be prominent, subtle, or totally absent.

Either absent (type B) motion or truly paradoxical (type A) (Fig. 14–3) motion is observed in the majority of cases.[27, 28] In either instance, the area of septum exhibiting the abnormal pattern has become a passive structure. Anterior motion during ventricular systole is a result of (1) the normal anterior displacement of the entire heart during ventricular systole, and (2) the pressure within the left ventricle during systole, which is higher than that in the right ventricle and which "pushes" the noncontractile area of the septum anteriorly into the right ventricle.

Displacement of the infarcted septum to a more anterior position can be appreciated on a scan from the aorta to the left ventricle. Under normal circumstances, the septum lies at approximately the same depth as the anterior wall of the aortic root, but in the presence of septal infarction, the septum is often distinctly closer to the anterior chest wall.

A study of 38 coronary patients in which the coronary and left ventricular angiograms were correlated with the echocardiograms revealed that 30 had abnormal septal motion.[28] These 30 all had 75 percent or greater blockage of the

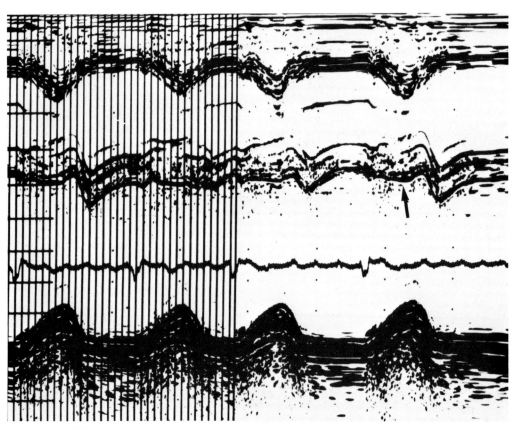

FIGURE 14–4. Anteroseptal myocardial infarction. The posterior systolic amplitude of motion of the interventricular septum is markedly diminished (arrow).

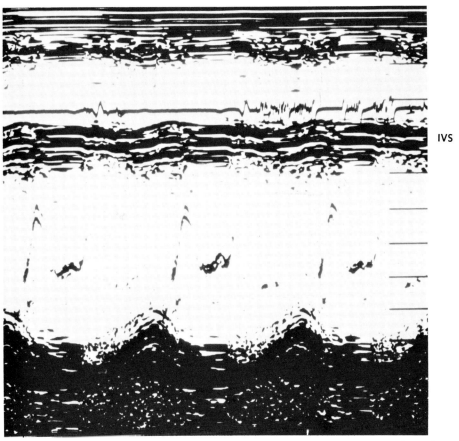

IVS

FIGURE 14-5. Infarction of the interventricular septum (IVS). The infarcted area is composed of heavy, distinct parallel echoes that move slightly anteriorly during ventricular systole.

left anterior descending coronary vessel. Of the eight with normal septal motion and greater than 75 percent blockage of the anterior descending artery, only one had evidence of a transmural infarction on the resting electrocardiogram. Among an additional 10 patients without significant obstruction of the anterior descending coronary artery, none had abnormal septal motion. In analyzing both septal and posterior wall motion, no patient with electrocardiographic documentation of a transmural infarction had completely normal wall motion on the echocardiogram. This study also suggests that the echocardiogram is more sensitive than the left ventricular angiogram in detecting myocardial asynergy associated with blockage of the left anterior descending coronary vessel. Whether septal wall motion will appear altered on the echocardiogram will depend on the amount of infarction as well as on its location relative to the ultrasound beam. Certainly, even if the beam transects an area of infarction that is very small, it is conceivable that this segment of the septum may be pulled posteriorly by adjacent viable septal myocardium. It is also possible to miss an area of septal infarction, especially if it involves the lower one third or posterior aspect of the septum. To minimize the possibility of obtaining such false impressions, scans of as much of the septum as possible should be considered routine in every case of coronary disease.[29]

In some instances of previous infarction, the septum maintains its normal posterior direction of excursion during ventricular systole, but the amplitude is reduced — less than 3 mm from end-diastole to normal posterior position of the left ventricular endocardial edge (Fig. 14–4).[28] The septal width in these instances may show minimal systolic increase with a decreased rate of posterior motion as well. This type of reduced motion is also observed in patients with congestive cardiomyopathy.

Burch et al.[30] reported a case of paradoxical septal motion in ischemic cardiomyopathy. At postmortem examination, the septum was observed to be hypertrophied, with extensive fibrosis but without discrete infarction or aneurysm.

Finally, the septum sometimes appears as a thin band of parallel-moving echoes of increased intensity, presumably due to fibrosis in the area of infarction (Fig. 14–5).

It must be reiterated that conclusions about septal motion presume that the echo beam is traversing the muscular (not membranous) septum and that the beam is close to intercepting the septum at 90 degrees. Failure to satisfy either of these technical requirements may lead to false findings.

Left Ventricular Free Wall

Infarction of the posterior left ventricular wall is either restricted to that area of the myocardium or may actually be an extension of a diaphragmatic or a lateral wall infarction. In practice, it can be difficult to determine precisely what anatomical portion of the left ventricular free wall one is recording in a single patient. Because the electrocardiographic precision in location of myocardial infarction is far from perfect, failure to record an abnormal posterior wall in the presence of a posterior infarction by electrocardiogram should not be overly distressing. (The echocardiogram may actually be a far more sensitive means for the detection and location of an infarction than the electrocardiogram, particularly when the infarction is not transmural. The superiority of the electrocardiogram lies primarily in the fact that it is relatively thorough in its coverage of the major areas of the left ventricular myocardium. The echocardiogram cannot, with present techniques, "see" all areas, but there is reason to be optimistic about the possibility for improvements that will permit more complete recording of the left ventricular walls.)

The posterior wall echo may show reduced amplitude of systolic excursion, or it may actually appear flat (Fig. 14–6). Eight of the 38 patients studied by Jacobs[28] had abnormal posterior wall motion, which he defines as less than 0.8 cm of systolic anterior excursion. Reduced or absent systolic thickening may also be observed.

Compensatory Changes

When infarction has occurred, noninfarcted areas of the left ventricular myocardium may exhibit compensatory changes. Hypertrophy of the remaining myocardium appears to occur as a result of the dysynergy and dilatation of the

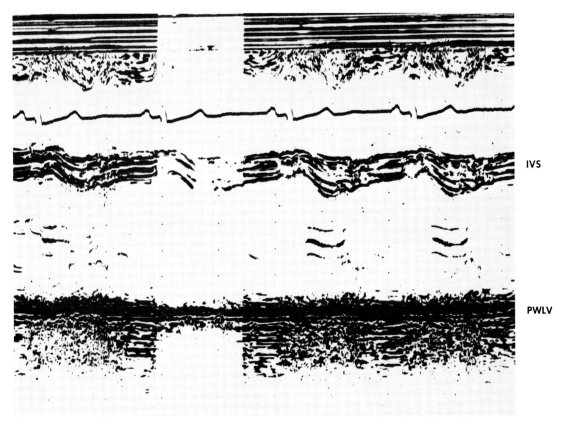

FIGURE 14-6. Posterior left ventricular wall myocardial infarction. There is no discernible posterior wall (PWLV) motion during ventricular systole. The septum (IVS) shows normal motion.

left ventricle, which increase the amount of energy expended by these noninfarcted areas.[31] Rackley et al.[32] found that the extent of left ventricular hypertrophy was related to the degree of dilatation. It must be recalled that patients with coronary disease also may have a concentric form of hypertrophy on the basis of systemic hypertension, as well as nonrelated disease processes such as aortic stenosis.

A more dramatic compensatory change observed on the echocardiogram is the increase in either septal or posterior wall amplitude of excursion when infarction occurs elsewhere. In the coronary patient, septal excursion exceeding 8 mm raises the possibility of infarction of another area of the myocardium[28] (valvular insufficiency, especially mitral regurgitation, must be excluded) (Fig. 14-7). Posterior wall endocardial anterior movement exceeding 16 mm also should be considered an abnormal change suggesting infarction of another region of the myocardium.

Ventricular Aneurysm

An important and common sequela of transmural myocardial infarction is ventricular aneurysm. Aneurysm of the ventricular wall is most often detected

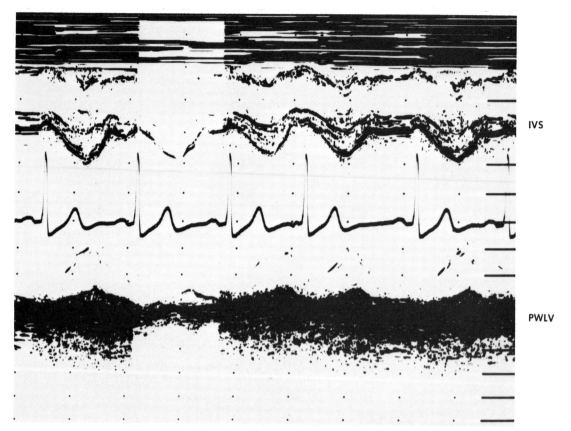

IVS

PWLV

FIGURE 14–7.   Posterior left ventricular wall infarction. There is a marked decrease in motion of the posterior left ventricular wall (PWLV), but the amplitude of the systolic motion of the interventricular septum (IVS) is increased.

echocardiographically when it involves the posterior left ventricular myocardium. As the beam is directed into a posterior wall aneurysm, the wall has absent systolic anterior excursion. The septal-to-posterior wall dimension at that level is increased. As the beam is scanned out of the aneurysm, this dimension abruptly diminishes as the posterior wall becomes positioned farther anteriorly.[33] The adjacent unaffected myocardium may possess normal, diminished, or even exaggerated (compensatory) anterior systolic contractile motion. Abnormal anterior wall motion has been described in cases of anterior aneurysm when the transducer is placed over the precordial impulse.[34]

"Pseudoaneurysm" of the left ventricle also may occur after a myocardial infarction. The echocardiographic features of one case have been described by Roelandt et al.,[35] who found the pseudoaneurysm to resemble a very large, loculated pericardial effusion. The chief value of the echocardiogram in this case was in differentiating the pseudoaneurysm from a true ventricular aneurysm.

Ventricular Thrombus

Thrombus formation may occur adjacent to an infarction of the endocardium and is also frequent within an aneurysm (Fig. 14–8). While the echocar-

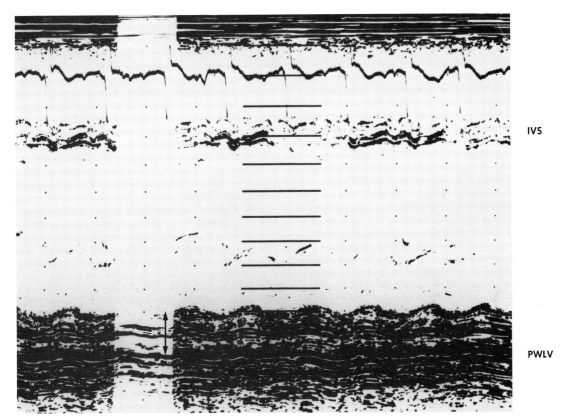

IVS

PWLV

FIGURE 14-8. Ventricular aneurysm with thrombus formation. The left ventricular internal dimension is markedly increased, with diminished posterior wall (PWLV) excursion and paradoxical septal (IVS) motion. Post mortem, the apparent disproportionate thickness of the posterior wall (arrow) was found to be part of a large calcified thrombus.

diographic detection of a thrombus within the left ventricle is unusual, if the thrombus becomes calcified, it may be observed as a dense, multiple-layered echo lying adjacent to the cardiac wall.

Anomalous Origin of the Left Coronary Artery

In isolated instances, the left coronary artery may arise from the pulmonary artery, in which case the portion of the left ventricular myocardium it supplies becomes thinned and scarred, with chamber dilatation. The remaining myocardium, which is supplied by the right coronary arterial system, becomes hypertrophied.[36]

A study of four patients with anomalous origin of the left coronary artery showed the following echocardiographic characteristics: (1) a large right coronary aortic valve cusp; (2) posterior dislocation of the aortic valve apparatus; (3) a dilated left ventricle with a poorly contractile posterior wall; (4) abnormal septal motion (when the anterior descending coronary artery was anomalous); and (5) intermittent papillary muscle dysfunction.[37]

References

1. Fogelman AM, Abbasi AS, Pearce ML, and Kattus AA: Echocardiographic study of the abnormal motion of the posterior left ventricular wall during angina pectoris. Circulation 46:905–913, 1972.

2. Kerber RE, Marcus ML, Ehrhardt J, Wilson R, and Abboud FM: Correlation between echocardiographically demonstrated segmental dyskinesis and regional myocardial perfusion. Circulation 52:1097–1104, 1975.

3. Ludbrook P, Karliner JS, London A, Peterson KL, Leopold GR, and O'Rourke RA: Posterior wall velocity: An unreliable index of total left ventricular performance in patients with coronary artery disease. Am J Cardiol 33:475–482, 1974.

4. Pombo JF, Russell RO, Rackley CE, and Foster GL: Comparison of stroke volume and cardiac output determination by ultrasound and dye dilution in acute myocardial infarction. Am J Cardiol 27:630–635, 1971.

5. Corya BC, Rasmussen S, Knoebel SB, and Feigenbaum H: Echocardiography in acute myocardial infarction. Am J Cardiol 36:1–10, 1975.

6. Stefan G, and Bing RJ: Echocardiographic findings in experimental myocardial infarction of the posterior left ventricular wall. Am J Cardiol 30:629–639, 1972.

7. Kerber RE, and Abboud FM: Echocardiographic detection of regional myocardial infarction: An experimental study. Circulation 48:997–1005, 1973.

8. Inoue K, Smulyan H, Mookherjee S, and Eich RH: Ultrasonic measurement of left ventricular wall motion in acute myocardial infarction. Circulation 43:778–785, 1971.

9. Smithen C, Wharton C, and Sowton E: Changes in left ventricular wall movement following exercise, atrial pacing and acute myocardial infarction measured by reflected ultrasound (Abstr). Am J Cardiol 29:293, 1972.

10. Ratshin RA, Rackley CE, and Russell RO: Serial evaluation of left ventricular volumes and posterior wall movement in the acute phase of myocardial infarction using diagnostic ultrasound (Abstr). Am J Cardiol 29:286, 1972.

11. Chapelle M, Senekies A, Benaim R, and Chiche P: Evaluation of left ventricular function by echocardiography in acute myocardial infarction (Abstr). Proc Second World Congress on Ultrasonics in Medicine, Rotterdam, 1973.

12. Heikkilä J, and Nieminen M: Echoventriculographic detection, localization, and quantification of left ventricular asynergy in acute myocardial infarction. Br Heart J 37:46–59, 1975.

13. Corya BC, Feigenbaum H, Rasmussen S, and Black MJ: Anterior left ventricular wall echoes in coronary artery disease: Linear scanning with a single element transducer. Am J Cardiol 34:652–657, 1974.

14. Henning H, Schelbert H, Crawford MH, Karliner JS, Ashburn W, and O'Rourke RA: Left ventricular performance assessed by radionuclide angiocardiography and echocardiography in patients with previous myocardial infarction. Circulation 52:1069–1075, 1975.

15. Smith McK, Ratshin RA, Harrell FE, Jr, Russell RO, and Rackley CE: Early sequential changes in left ventricular dimensions and filling pressure in patients after myocardial infarction. Am J Cardiol 33:363–369, 1974.

16. Sweet L, Moraski RE, Russell RO, and Rackley CE: Relationship between echocardiography, cardiac output, and abnormally contracting segments in patients with ischemic heart disease. Circulation 52:634–641, 1975.

17. Broder MI, and Cohn JN: Evaluation of abnormalities in left ventricular function after acute myocardial infarction. Circulation 46:731–743, 1972.

18. Bergeron GA, Cohen MV, Teichholz LE, and Gorlin R: Echocardiographic analysis of mitral valve motion after acute myocardial infarction. Circulation 51:82–87, 1975.

19. Mittal AK, Langston M, Cohn KE, Selzer A, and Kerth WJ: Combined papillary muscle and left ventricular wall dysfunction as a cause of mitral regurgitation: An experimental study. Circulation 44:174–180, 1971.

20. Lipp H, Gambetta M, Schwartz J, de la Fuente D, and Resnekov L: Intermittent pansystolic murmur and presumed mitral regurgitation after acute myocardial infarction. Am J Cardiol 30:690–694, 1972.

21. Forrester JS, Diamond G, Freedman S, Allen HN, Parmley WW, Matloff J, and Swan HJC: Silent mitral insufficiency in acute myocardial infarction. Circulation 44:877–883, 1971.

22. Dugall JC, Pryor R, and Blount SG, Jr: Systolic murmur following myocardial infarction. Am Heart J 87:577–583, 1974.

23. De Busk RF, and Harrison DC: The clinical spectrum of papillary-muscle disease. N Engl J Med 281:1458–1467, 1969.

24. Austen WG, Sokol DM, DeSanctis RW, and Sanders CA: Surgical treatment of papillary-muscle rupture complicating myocardial infarction. N Engl J Med 278:1137–1141, 1968.

25. Chandraratna PAN, Balachandran PK, Shah PM, and Hodges M: Echocardiographic observations on ventricular septal rupture complicating acute myocardial infarction. Circulation 51:506–510, 1975.

26. DeJoseph RL, Seides SF, Lindner A, and Damato AN: Echocardiographic findings of ventricular septal rupture in acute myocardial infarction. Am J Cardiol 36:346–348, 1975.
27. Diamond MA, Dillon JC, Haine CL, Chang S, and Feigenbaum H: Echocardiographic features of atrial septal defect. Circulation 43:129–135, 1971.
28. Jacobs JJ, Feigenbaum H, Corya BC, and Phillips JF: Detection of left ventricular asynergy by echocardiography. Circulation 48:263–271, 1973.
29. Winters WL, Jr, and Chapman R: Variations in ventricular septal motion defined by echocardiography (Abstr). Circulation 48:231, 1973.
30. Burch GE, Giles TD, and Martinez E: Echocardiographic detection of abnormal motion of the interventricular septum in ischemic cardiomyopathy. Am J Med 57:293–297, 1974.
31. Badeer HS: Pathogenesis of cardiac hypertrophy in coronary atherosclerosis and myocardial infarction. Am Heart J 84:256–264, 1972.
32. Rackley CE, Dear HD, Baxley WA, Jones WB, and Dodge HT: Left ventricular chamber volume, mass, and function in severe coronary artery disease. Circulation 41:605–613, 1970.
33. Kreamer R, Kerber RE, and Abboud F: Ventricular aneurysm: Use of echocardiography. J Clin Ultrasound 1:60–63, 1971.
34. Yoshikawa J, Owaki T, Kato H, and Tanaka K: Ultrasonic diagnosis of ventricular aneurysm (Abstr). Circulation (Suppl III) 49, 50:30, 1974.
35. Roelandt J, van den Brand M, Vletter WB, Nauta J, and Hugenholtz PG: Echocardiographic diagnosis of pseudoaneurysm of the left ventricle. Circulation 52:466–472, 1975.
36. Perloff JK: The Clinical Recognition of Congenital Heart Disease. Philadelphia, W. B. Saunders Company, 1970.
37. Glaser J, Bharati S, Whitman V, and Liebman J: Echocardiographic (EG) findings in patients (pts) with anomalous origin of the left coronary artery (ALCA) (Abstr). Circulation (Suppl IV) 7, 8:63, 1973.

15

Cardiac Valve Surgery

Since the development of prosthetic replacements for diseased cardiac valves, physicians have been challenged to develop reliable means for assessing the function of valve replacements without introducing additional risks to the patient. The difficulties inherent in this task have been compounded by the development of numerous types of prosthetic valves, each with its own unique structural characteristics. For the most part, evaluation has focused on analysis of the sounds generated by prosthetic valve motion to provide clues of valve function. Hence auscultation and, for objective definition of these sounds, phonocardiography have been the principal means for assessing patients with prosthetic valves.

The echocardiogram ultimately may provide the best clinical data in detecting prosthetic valve malfunction. To date, reports detailing the echocardiographic features are for the most part confined to isolated instances of valve failure. Much more information on the ultrasound characteristics of normal function as well as failure is required before the full value of echocardiographic evaluation of prosthetic valves will be known.

GENERAL PRINCIPLES OF RECORDING AND INTERPRETATION

Knowledge of the construction of the prosthetic valves that may be encountered is imperative to an understanding of their appearance on the echocardiogram. There are three basic types of prosthetic valve: the ball valve, the disc valve, and the tilting disc valve.[1] Any of these three types of prosthetic valve may be used in all of the cardiac valve positions. In a later section, the value of echocardiography in valve selection is discussed in some detail.

Practically all prosthetic valves consist of three basic components: the sewing ring, the struts, and the poppet (ball or disc). (An exception is the Wada-Cutter valve which does not have struts.) When a valve is in the mitral position, each of these parts can usually be identified on the echocardiogram, although often it is possible to record the poppet motion without visualizing the struts (Figs. 15–1 to 15–5). The parts of the prosthetic aortic valve, except the poppet, generally are less easily identified.

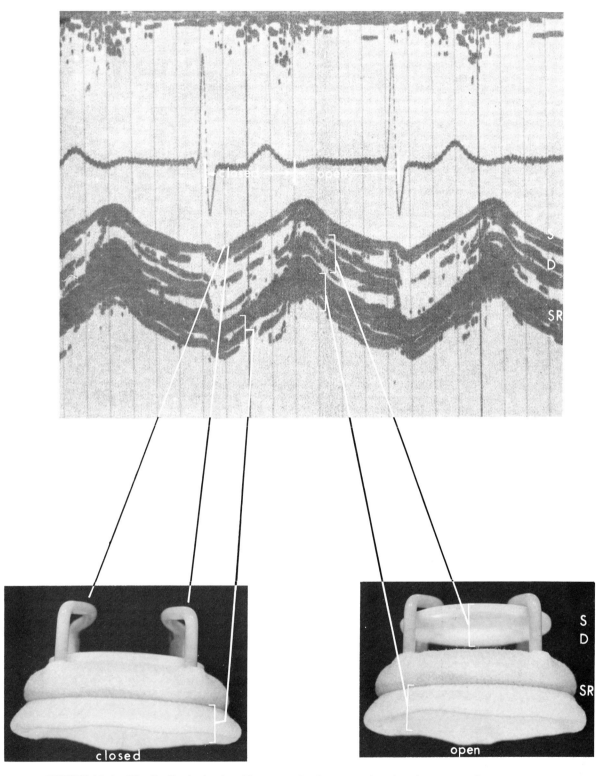

FIGURE 15–1. The Beall mitral valve. The struts (S), disc (D), and sewing ring (SR) can be identified on the echocardiogram.

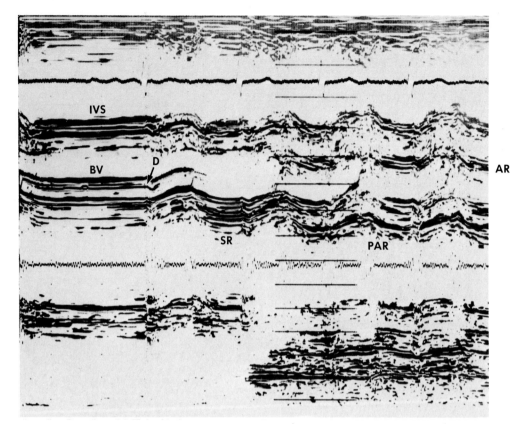

FIGURE 15–2. Sector scan from the Beall mitral valve (BV) to the aortic root (AR) demonstrates the contiguity from the sewing ring (SR) to the posterior aortic root wall (PAR) (D = disc; IVS = interventricular septum).

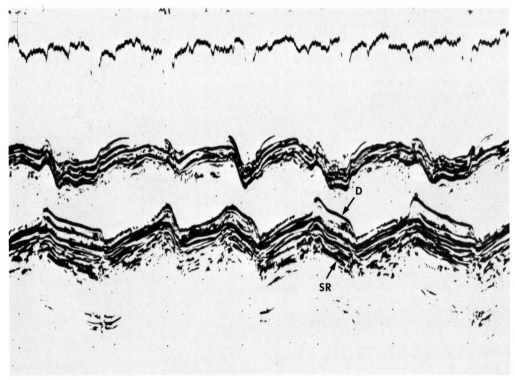

FIGURE 15–3. In this recording of a Beall mitral valve, only the disc (D) and sewing ring (SR) are recorded.

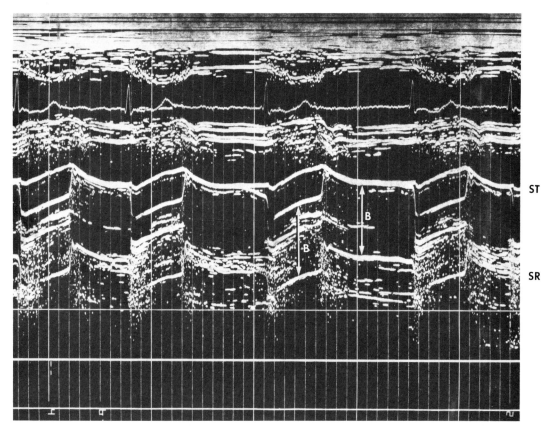

FIGURE 15-4. Starr-Edwards mitral ball valve. The struts (ST), sewing ring (SR), and leading and trailing edges of the ball (B) are recorded.

Because of the strong acoustical interface between the artificial valve and the surrounding blood and cardiac tissue, its echoes are very intense and deceptively easy to record. Therefore, without close attention, only the supporting structures may be recorded, without discernible ball or disc motion (Fig. 15–6). The same attention to transducer angle and fine controls necessary for recording any of the cardiac structures is equally necessary for satisfactory recordings of prosthetic valves. As a general rule, the best recording is the one that clearly defines the time of valve opening and closure and, in the mitral position, most closely approximates the normal excursion amplitude of the poppet. Therefore, the exact model and size of prosthetic valve should be known to the technologist before any attempt is made to record the valve. Unfortunately, this information is not always available.

The motion of a prosthetic valve is determined not only by the valve characteristics themselves, but also by the motion of the entire cardiac structure and by the hemodynamics on either side of the valve. Each of these variables should be taken into account when studying prosthetic valve echocardiograms, although present knowledge is inadequate for quantifying their exact effects.

It has been established that the transducer angle relative to the position of the valve is critical for measurements of the amplitude of excursion of the poppet. Unless the beam parallels the axis of the opening and closing movements, measurements of amplitude are not of value, except when the relative position

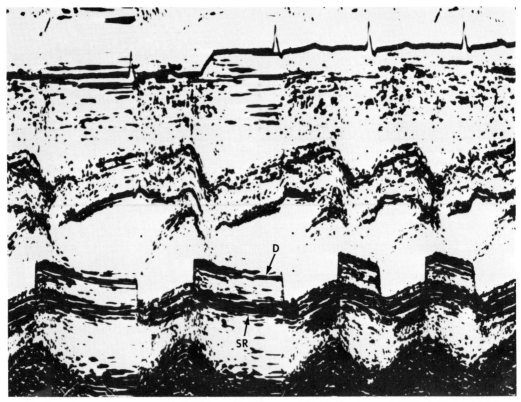

FIGURE 15-5. The Bjork-Shiley mitral valve. The disc (D) and sewing ring (SR) are recorded, without the struts.

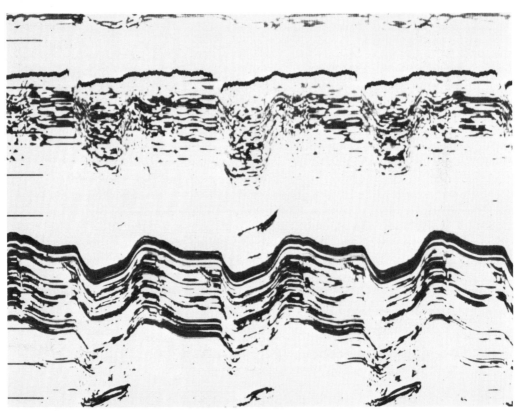

FIGURE 15-6. In this recording of a Beall mitral valve, the disc motion is not discernible. Only multiple parallel echoes from the struts are seen.

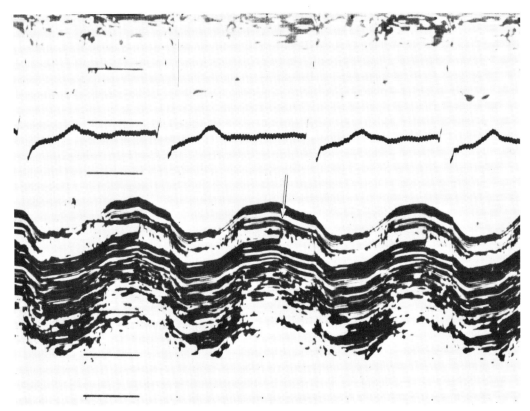

FIGURE 15-7. Echocardiogram of a Beall mitral valve two hours after implantation. The disc is opening extremely late in diastole (arrow). The patient was found to be hypovolemic, and following fluid restoration the disc opening occurred normally (see Fig. 15-8).

of the beam to the valve remains absolutely fixed and the amplitude definitely changes from beat to beat. Valve excursion in the aortic position, however, is very rarely parallel to the beam and therefore is usually not a useful echocardiographic measurement.

Although long-term supporting data are not yet available, the optimal application of echocardiography in prosthetic valve assessment may be serial evaluations, with a control recording made after the immediate postoperative period. Studies obtained during the recovery period thus far appear to be useful only in the detection of gross abnormalities of valve function, and must be interpreted with exceptional caution (Figs. 15-7 and 15-8). Such subtle parameters of valve function as opening and closing intervals change as the heart and the pulmonary and systemic circulatory systems adjust to both the valve itself and to the effects of surgery during the first weeks following operation. Beyond the early recovery period, however, fine changes in valve motion probably assume great significance.

MITRAL PROSTHETIC VALVE

Normal Function

Prosthetic valves in the mitral position are easy to record because the ultrasound beam and the axis of the poppet motion are approximately parallel.

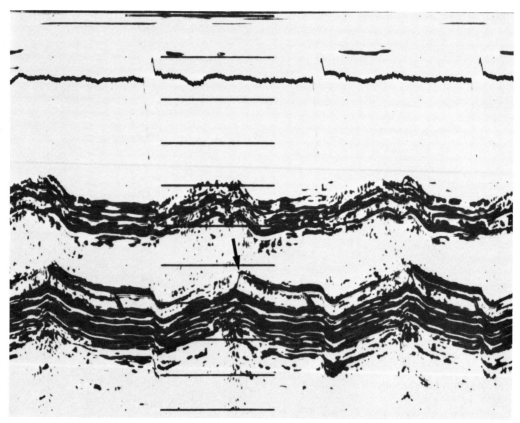

FIGURE 15–8.   Twenty-four hours after the recording seen in Figure 15–7, the patient has been rehydrated, and the time of valve opening has normalized (arrow).

Consequently, the true amplitude of opening and closing is recorded, as the ball or disc remains within the ultrasound beam path throughout the cardiac cycle.

Whereas only the motion of the ball or disc is pertinent to valve function, the passive movements of the valve apparatus as a whole must be taken into account in amplitude measurements. The movements of the apparatus are due to both the normal anteroposterior motion of the heart and to the filling and emptying of the left ventricle and the left atrium throughout each cardiac cycle (i.e., as the left ventricle fills during ventricular diastole, the valve apparatus "floats" toward the emptying left atrium, moving superiorly and posteriorly; the reverse occurs during ventricular ejection) (Fig. 15–9). The time of opening and closure is mainly a function of the relative pressures in the left atrium and the left ventricle. Gravity also appears to play a role in that the opening speed is slower against gravity (supine) than when opening is in the same direction (prone).[2]

The position of the poppet relative to the other components of the valve is twofold, i.e., either open or closed. The valve does not normally have periods of only partial opening analogous to the mid-diastolic position of the normal mitral leaflets. Siggers et al. have proposed that there is no mid-diastolic closure of the prosthetic valve because the vortex mechanism that may be in part responsible for normal mid-diastolic leaflet closure does not occur in association with the prosthetic valve.[2] Movements of the poppet during diastole are associated with motion of the entire apparatus, such as a slight anterior displacement sometimes observed during atrial systole. Alderman et al. have noted that the poppet may show some low-amplitude oscillations in the presence of atrial flutter.[3]

Valve opening occurs when the left atrial pressure exceeds the intraventricular pressure, with an insignificant delay to overcome both the inertia of the closed valve and the force of gravity when the patient is in the supine position. The opening velocity of the ball and disc prosthetic mitral valves is in the range of 200 to 500 mm per sec.[2,4–7] Closure rates are usually faster, except in instances of long diastolic cycles when the valve may slowly float shut prior to the onset of the next ventricular systole (Fig. 15–9). Johnson et al. have pointed out that opening and closing velocities normally have great variability even in the same patient, and therefore these measurements are of dubious value.[6]

At the time of opening, the poppet is frequently observed to reverberate for one or two very short cycles and then remain adjacent to the apex of the valve for the duration of ventricular diastole.[4]

The time of mitral valve opening relative to the time of aortic valve closure is an important manifestation of the function of the prosthetic mitral valve and

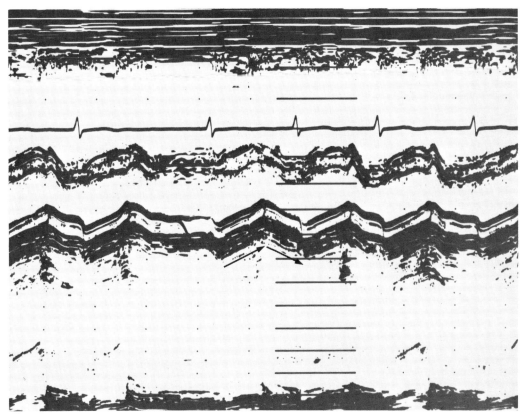

FIGURE 15-9. Normal disc mitral valve. The normal anterior direction of the entire valve apparatus during ventricular systole and posterior excursion during diastole are observed (arrows). Notice that during the second diastolic cycle, which is longer than the others, the valve closes prior to the onset of the next QRS complex.

of the left ventricle. The interval from aortic closure to mitral opening (A_2–MVO) can be measured by recording a simultaneous phonocardiogram in which the aortic component of the second heart sound (A_2) is displayed with the echocardiogram of the prosthetic valve (Fig. 15–10). An alternative method is to measure the time of echocardiographic aortic closure after the QRS complex of the electrocardiogram and to take the same measurement of mitral

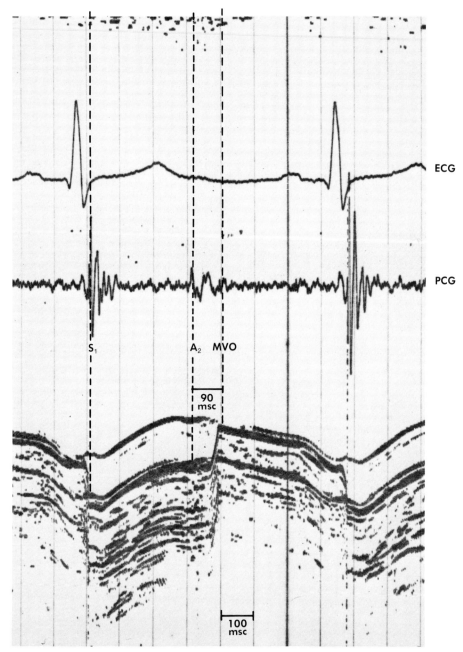

FIGURE 15-10.   Mitral disc opening (MVO) occurs about 90 msec after the aortic component of the second heart sound (A_2) (ECG = electrocardiogram; PCG = phonocardiogram; S_1 = first heart sound).

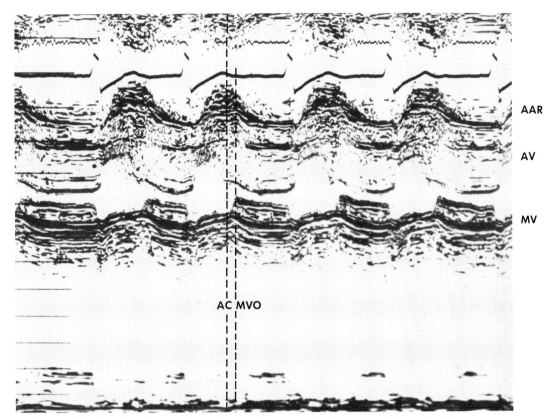

FIGURE 15-11. In this recording of a Starr-Edwards mitral valve (MV), its motion is seen along with one leaflet of the aortic valve (AV). The time from aortic valve closure (AC) to the mitral prosthetic opening (MVO) can be measured directly (AAR = anterior aortic root wall).

opening. The third, and most precise, method, although usually not technically possible, is to record both the aortic and the prosthetic mitral valve simultaneously (Fig. 15-11). The A_2–MVO interval is determined principally by the isovolumetric relaxation of the left ventricle, which is a function of the end-systolic aortic pressure, the left atrial pressure at the time of mitral valve opening, and the rate of fall of left ventricular pressure.[8] For example, an increase in the left atrial pressure with constant aortic and left ventricular pressure causes earlier opening of the mitral valve and shortening of the A_2–MVO interval.

The time of prosthetic mitral valve closure begins when the pressure within the ventricle rises during isovolumetric contraction, after the initial inscription of the QRS complex. Closure sometimes occurs earlier during long periods of diastole (see Fig. 15-9).

The normal true amplitude of poppet excursion is a function only of the valve construction, but the recorded amplitude is affected by beam angle as well. When the ultrasound beam is exactly parallel to the axis of the ball or disc motion, then the true excursion is measured.[9] However, with lesser angles, the apparent excursion becomes reduced. *In-vitro* studies showed that transducer angles greater than 30 degrees from the optimal parallel transducer-poppet position rendered this measurement very difficult.[10] Johnson et al. nevertheless showed that the actual excursion of prosthetic mitral valves, compared with manufacturer's specifications, can be calculated echocardiographically.[6] Even when optimal angulation cannot be achieved, serial studies showing changes in measured excursion may prove to be of value as long as the transducer position is the same with each test.

Prosthetic Mitral Valve Malfunction

Malfunction of artificial cardiac valves may occur from any of a variety of causes, depending on the type and age of the valve.[1, 11-26] Many of the complications of prosthetic valve implacement, both in the intraoperative and remote postoperative periods, are not due to actual malfunction of the valve. When this is the case, echocardiography cannot be relied upon to delineate the problem. Furthermore, thrombus or pannus formation in many instances cannot be detected echocardiographically unless there is actual alteration in poppet motion.

Change in the A_2–MVO interval, either by shortening or by prolongation, is one of the most important echocardiographic features of the abnormally functioning mitral valve. When thrombus or pannus impedes the poppet motion, an intermittent delay in valve opening may occur, or there may be no opening during some cardiac cycles.[14, 24, 27] In the case of the disc valve, because only part of the disc may exhibit this type of abnormal motion, with the remainder unaffected, it is necessary to record multiple views at varying transducer angles. Delayed opening is also sometimes associated with decreased amplitude of excursion of the poppet.[14]

Early valve opening with shortening of the A_2–MVO interval also may occur (Fig. 15–12).[7, 8, 13] This too may be a result of thrombus formation, as well as paravalvular or intravalvular regurgitation. A decreased A_2–MVO interval is most often due to increased left atrial volume in valvular regurgitation. Thrombus formation may cause early valve opening by increased left atrial pressure.[8]

A shortened or prolonged A_2–MVO interval is not diagnostic of valvular malfunction,[8] as other causes of altered left heart hemodynamics can have similar effects. For example, decreased left atrial filling pressure, as in circulatory hypovolemia, can result in delayed mitral opening (see Fig. 15–7). Left ventricular dysfunction can either shorten or prolong the A_2–MVO interval.[8]

Reduced amplitude of poppet excursion is also an important sign of valve malfunction. It may be a result of thrombus or pannus formation, or of interference by the walls of a ventricle that is too small for the implanted valve. The decreased amplitude may be gross or subtle, and it may be constant or intermittent. Oliva et al.[19] and Johnson et al.[6] have reported the significance of decreased excursion of the Beall valve and of the Kay-Shiley disc valve in patients with confirmed thrombus formation. Belenkie et al. reported a single case of Cutter-Smellof ball valve malfunction due to fibrous overgrowth in which intermittent partial opening of the valve occurred.[24]

In some instances of valvular malfunction, the actual thickness of the valve poppet may increase due to lipid absorption (termed *variance*) resulting in either obstruction or regurgitation. This occurs primarily in the older types of valves. The diameter of the ball can be measured echocardiographically as

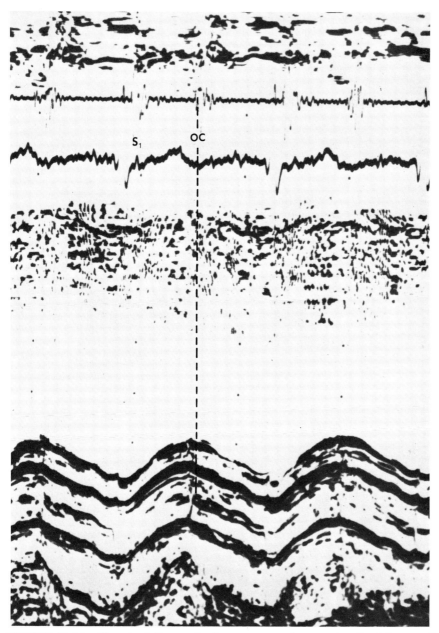

FIGURE 15–12. The mitral disc opening is premature and occurs virtually at the same time as the aortic component of the second heart sound, which is obscured by the opening click (OC) of the prosthetic valve. The patient had severe paraprosthetic valve regurgitation (S_1 = first heart sound).

described by Johnson et al. (Fig. 15–13).[5] Sound travels more slowly through prosthetic valves than through the body tissue; hence the apparent ultrasonic dimension through the poppet is greater than the actual diameter, and a correction factor depending on the composition of the prosthetic valve must be employed in the calculation. For silicone rubber, as used in the Starr-Edwards valve, the correction factor is 0.64. Therefore the diameter of the Starr-Edwards ball is determined by multiplying the echocardiographic dimension by

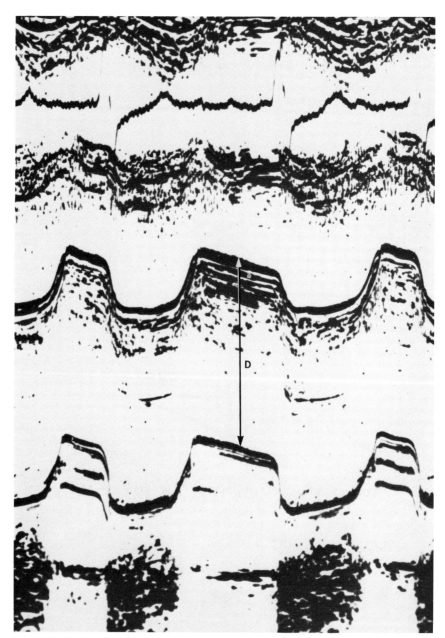

FIGURE 15–13.   The diameter (D) of the ball (mitral Starr-Edwards model No. 6000) can be measured directly from the echocardiogram. The measured dimension (3.9 cm) is corrected by the factor 0.64 to give a true diameter of 2.5 cm.

0.64. Further *in-vitro* studies of poppet size are needed before the value of this parameter can be realized, but studies to date indicate that this is a very sensitive method.[28]

Thrombus formation itself is seldom recorded by echocardiography, although pannus ingrowth may be easier to detect if it is sufficiently thick. From a practical standpoint, the echoes from the various components of the valve are generally so intense that superimposed echoes from clot or fibrous tissue are difficult to discern, unless one has the benefit of prior recordings for comparison.

The ultrasonic features of the cardiac structures other than the prosthetic valve are useful and should always be included in the examination. Disease of the other cardiac valves, especially the aortic valve, as well as the functional abnormalities imposed by disease of the replaced valve prior to surgery are frequently observed. Differentiation of progressive left ventricular dysfunction from prosthetic mitral valve malfunction is aided by the echocardiogram. For example, the cause of shortening of the A_2–MVO interval is probably paravalvular regurgitation when hyperdynamic systolic motion of the interventricular septum is recorded.[8] When the valve is obstructed, the left ventricular internal dimension does not increase in comparison to prior recordings, whereas left ventricular dysfunction and paravalvular regurgitation are associated with increasing ventricular dimensions.

AORTIC PROSTHETIC VALVE

Echocardiographic assessment of the prosthetic aortic valve is not as rewarding as that of the mitral valve, principally because, from standard

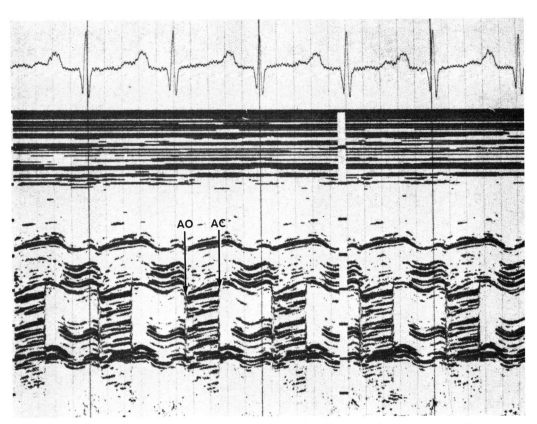

FIGURE 15–14. Starr-Edwards valve in the aortic position. The time of valve opening (AO) and closure (AC) is easily identified, as the ball appears as a mass of echoes within the aortic root during ventricular ejection. The ball diameter and amplitude of excursion, however, cannot be determined in this type of recording.

recording positions, the axis of the poppet motion is perpendicular to the echo beam. Consequently, it is often difficult to observe both the open and closed positions of the valve in the same view. For the same reason, one cannot be certain of the significance of deviations in echocardiographic measurements of poppet excursion. An exception to this is the tilting disc valve in which the direction of opening motion of the disc may be toward the ultrasound beam, depending on the placement of the valve within the aorta.[15]

The echocardiographic recording of the prosthetic aortic valve, most commonly the ball type, is marked by the appearance of the ball within the aortic root either in its open position during ventricular ejection or closed during diastole (Figs. 15–14 and 15–15). This pattern is caused by movement of the ball into and out of the beam target area. The poppet can often be observed to oscillate at the time of initial opening, an appearance that has also been observed fluoroscopically (Fig. 15–16).[29]

Two measurements that are of potential but unproven value in assessing aortic prosthetic valve function are the interval from the beginning of electromechanical systole to valve opening, and the duration of valve opening. The obvious advantage of these two parameters is the ease with which they can be determined echocardiographically, as they are not dependent on aligning the beam with the poppet axis. The main difficulty in using these intervals is that they are probably much more often altered by changes in left ventricular func-

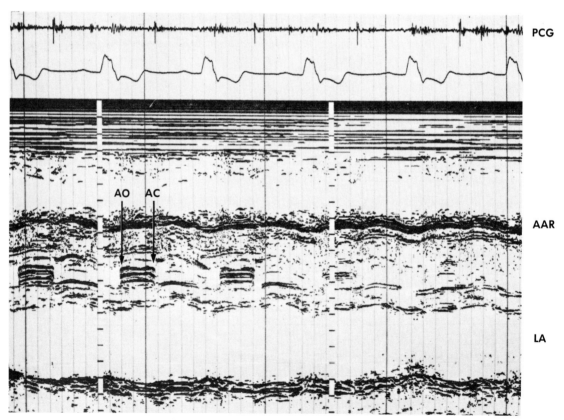

FIGURE 15–15. Bjork-Shiley aortic prosthetic valve. The tilting disc in this case is opening toward the transducer, and the time of opening (AO) and closure (AC) is evident. Note the corresponding prosthetic sounds recorded on the phonocardiogram (PCG) (AAR = anterior aortic root wall; LA = left atrium).

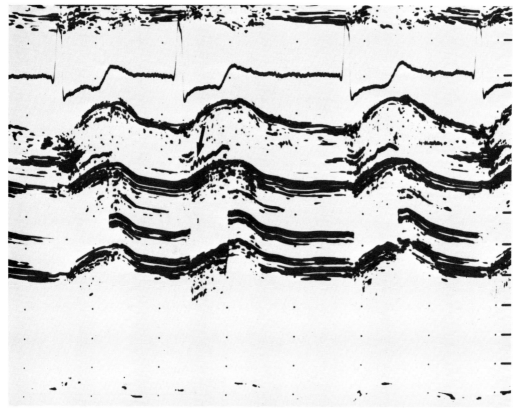

FIGURE 15-16. In this recording of an aortic ball (Smeloff-Cutter) valve, note the oscillations (arrow) which occur at the time of valve opening.

tion than by changes in the valve itself. Until serial studies of these measurements are carried out in patients with prosthetic aortic valves, their precise value to the clinician will not be known. For example, it would be expected that marked beat-to-beat variation in the time of opening and closing will occur if the poppet intermittently lodges in the base or apex of the valve.

Ben-Zvi et al. have reported the echocardiographic features of two instances of thrombosis on Björk-Shiley aortic prostheses.[15] In neither case was there detectable disc motion, and the valve area was filled in with dense echoes. After thrombectomy and débridement, however, disc motion was discernible and the root was no longer filled in with dense echoes.

The mitral valve recording also may provide important clues to aortic valve malfunction. It must be realized, however, that all types of normally functioning prosthetic aortic valves, especially the tilting disc types, are associated with a small amount of regurgitation in some cases.[30] Consequently, secondary mitral valve fluttering is not regarded as a definite sign of valve malfunction unless it occurs as a new finding in a patient with previous post-replacement echocardiograms. Premature mitral valve closure may result from acute aortic regurgitation.

Left ventricular measurements may also provide evidence for prosthetic valve malfunction. For example, increase in the internal dimension at end-diastole and exaggerated septal and posterior wall motion can signify aortic regurgitation. Burrgraf and Craige revealed that successful valve replacement for aortic regurgitation resulted in significant decrease in the left ventricular end-diastolic dimension and septal excursion.[31] Interpretation of left ventricular recordings, however, is tempered by the fact that 90 percent of patients undergoing prosthetic aortic valve replacement had postoperative hypokinetic or paradoxical septal motion, a finding that in time disappeared in most such patients. Yoshikawa also documented abnormal septal motion following prosthetic aortic valve replacement.[32]

PREOPERATIVE EVALUATION

Roberts et al. found that the most common cause of death among 45 patients who died within 2 months of mitral or aortic prosthetic valve replacement was a disproportionately large valve for the size of the aorta or left ventricle into which it was inserted.[25] Selection of the appropriate type of prosthetic valve may be assisted by the preoperative echocardiographic findings.

Nanda et al. measured the size of the left ventricular outflow tract in patients with mitral stenosis prior to valve replacement.[33] They defined the outflow tract width as the distance between the anterior mitral valve leaflet and the left ventricular edge at the beginning of ventricular systole (C point) (Fig. 15–17). Five of seven patients who received Starr-Edwards valves and had left ventricular outflow widths smaller than 20 mm expired, and four of the five had low cardiac output syndrome. By contrast, only one of seven patients who received low-profile Cross-Jones disc valves and had an outflow tract of less than 20 mm died. Although this is a small series, the implication is that echocardiographic determination of the left ventricular outflow tract size should be a factor in selecting the type of valve used for implantation in the mitral position.

Massive mitral annulus calcification has been reported as an important predisposing factor to the development of valve dehiscence.[18] Therefore, echocardiographic recognition of a markedly thickened annulus should be reported to the surgeon prior to operation for valve replacement.

The presence of calcium in the stenotic mitral valve is an important contraindication to the commissurotomy procedure. Nanda et al. reported that preoperative echocardiographic assessment for valvular calcification is generally a reliable means for determining whether commissurotomy or valve replacement is indicated.[34] In their study, multiple conglomerate echoes usually indicated the presence of calcium, but in most instances much of the increase in echo density was due to fibrous tissue. Therefore, although it is tempting to conclude that a greatly thickened valve is calcified, total reliance on the echodardiogram for the detection of calcium is not justified, especially without gray scale recordings. These authors also found that cusp mobility, or amplitude of opening (defined as the C-E distance) was also a good basis for determining the type of procedure to be carried out. In all cases in which the opening amplitude of the anterior leaflet was less than 15 mm, the valve was replaced, whereas in 23 of 28 patients with C-E amplitudes of 20 mm or greater, commissurotomy was the treatment of choice.

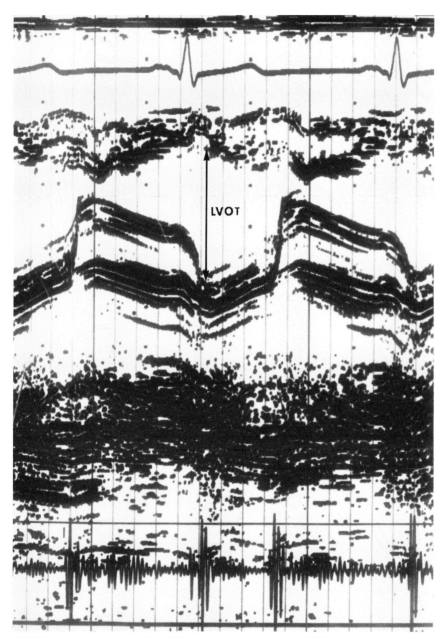

FIGURE 15–17.   The size of the left ventricular outflow tract (LVOT) is measured from the C point of the mitral valve to the interventricular septum.

The aortic root may be too narrow to accommodate a prosthetic valve, in which case implantation will result in prosthetic valve stenosis.[35–37] This is particularly serious in the patient with concomitant mitral regurgitation, which is worsened by the new outflow obstruction when prior pure aortic regurgitation was present.[25] Echocardiographic studies of aortic root size are needed to determine the usefulness of this technique in the selection of the type and size of prosthetic valve to be inserted.

MITRAL COMMISSUROTOMY

Mitral commissurotomy was among the earliest forms of cardiac surgery, and it remains the procedure of choice in patients with pure, non-calcific mitral stenosis. The echocardiogram, in addition to its use in the preoperative evaluation, is an important means for determining the immediate result of the commissurotomy and serves also as a valuable means for long-term follow-up (Figs. 15–18 and 15–19).

Johnson et al. first described the feasibility of recording the mitral valve by echocardiography at the time of operation with placement of the gas-sterilized transducer directly on the exposed heart. In their study they showed an excellent correlation between the intraoperative mitral EF slope and the same measurements obtained before and after mitral commissurotomy.[38] In a similar study of six cases, we found that the intraoperative EF slope increased an average of 28 mm per sec. (Table 15–1). Subsequent examinations for periods of up to 3 years showed no significant change in the EF slopes of these patients, all of whom remained clinically improved.

Effert found the average EF slope to increase by 25 mm per sec after commissurotomy in a series of 279 patients.[39] Most showed an increase from 10 to 30 mm per sec and some had increases exceeding 70 mm per sec. There was,

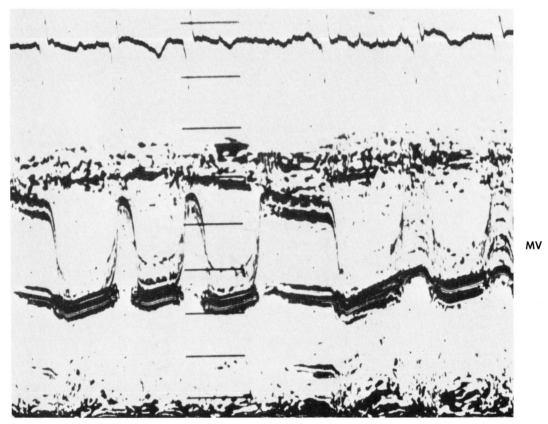

MV

FIGURE 15–18.   Intraoperative recording of a stenotic mitral valve (MV) with transducer placed directly on the heart. The diastolic closure rate is 10 mm per sec. (See Figure 15–19 for postcommissurotomy recording).

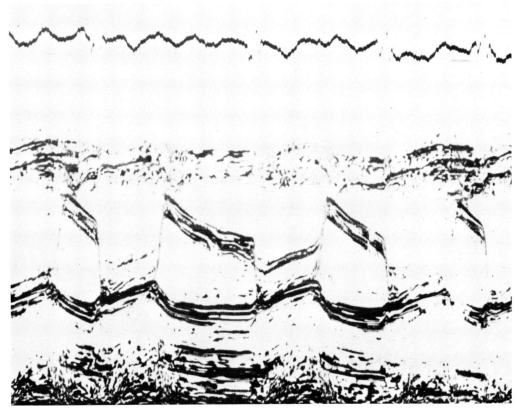

FIGURE 15-19. Intraoperative recording following mitral commissurotomy. Note the improvement in the rate of diastolic closure, which now measures 44 mm per sec, compared to Figure 15-18.

however, no correlation between the preoperative slope and the degree of improvement of this measurement. Silver et al. reported the single case of a 13-year-old boy with mitral stenosis in whom there was a similar increase in the EF slope following commissurotomy.[40]

The intraoperative study may also be of value in detecting surgical inducement of mitral regurgitation. In one case, we recorded a marked increase in the amplitude of the anterior leaflet excursion following commissurotomy, and the patient then developed significant mitral regurgitation in the postoperative period. Further studies are needed to define the intraoperative echocardiographic criteria for mitral regurgitation caused by commissurotomy. Specific intraoperative parameters for detection of this complication could help to prevent reoperation for valve replacement.

MITRAL VALVULOPLASTY

Mary et al. studied 15 patients at varying intervals following reconstructive mitral valve surgery.[41] This study suggests that the echocardiogram may be of value in following such patients for evidence of stenosis. However, one patient developed significant mitral regurgitation without change in the opening

TABLE 15-1 PRE- AND POSTCOMMISSUROTOMY MITRAL VALVE EF SLOPES
MEASURED IN SIX PATIENTS

CASE	PRE-COMMISSUROTOMY*	IMMED. POST-COMMISSUROTOMY*	1–3 MONTHS	1 YEAR	2 YEARS	3 YEARS
1	5 mm/sec	36 mm/sec	36	36	—	36
2	8 mm/sec	42 mm/sec	—	48	56	—
3	14 mm/sec	48 mm/sec	56	—	56	—
4	5 mm/sec	36 mm/sec	44	—	50	44
5	16 mm/sec	40 mm/sec	—	—	38	—
6	14 mm/sec	32 mm/sec	—	44	38	44
Mean	11 mm/sec	39 mm/sec	45	43	48	41

*Intraoperative measurements.

amplitude or diastolic closure rate. Comparison with preoperative studies was not reported.

MITRAL FASCIA LATA GRAFTS

Studies on 19 patients with stented fascia lata mitral grafts were carried out at varying periods averaging 3 years after surgery.[42] The mitral EF slope showed a good correlation with calculations of the effective graft area derived from cardiac catheterization data. The EF slope and mitral amplitude, however, were not useful in detecting mitral regurgitation in this series.

HOMOGRAFT AORTIC VALVE

Ratshin et al. have reported that homograft aortic valve leaflets typically exhibit coarse systolic vibrations when a systolic murmur is present and that the intensity of the murmur appears to correlate with the amplitude of the vibrations.[43] It should be added that the echocardiographic recording of the homograft leaflets is sometimes obscured by redundant echoes within the aortic root, which may represent scar tissue around the valve. We have observed one case of acute aortic regurgitation of a homograft valve in which the typical premature mitral valve closure was apparent.

References

1. Pluth JR, and McGoon DC: Current status of heart valve replacement. Mod Con Cardiovasc Dis 43:65–70, 1974.
2. Siggers DC, Srivongse SA, and Deuchar D: Analysis of dynamics of mitral Starr-Edwards valve prosthesis using reflected ultrasound. Br Heart J 33:401–408, 1971.
3. Alderman EL, Rytand DA, Crow RS, Finegan RE, and Harrison DC: Normal and prosthetic atrioventricular valve motion in atrial flutter. Circulation 45:1206–1215, 1972.
4. Winters WL, Gimenez J, and Soloff LA: Clinical application of ultrasound in the analysis of prosthetic ball valve function. Am J Cardiol 19:97–106, 1967.
5. Johnson ML, Paton BC, and Holmes JH: Ultrasonic evaluation of prosthetic valve motion. Circulation (Suppl II) 41,42:3–9, 1970.
6. Johnson ML, Holmes JH, and Paton BC: Echocardiographic determination of mitral disc valve excursion. Circulation 47:1274–1280, 1973.
7. Gibson TC, Starek PJK, Moos S, and Craige E: Echocardiographic and phonocardiographic characteristics of the Lillehei-Kaster mitral valve prosthesis. Circulation 49:434–440, 1974.
8. Brodie BR, Grossman W, McLaurin L, Starek PJK, and Craige E: Diagnosis of prosthetic mitral valve malfunction with combined echo-phonocardiography. Circulation 53:93–100, 1976.
9. Douglas JE, and Williams GD: Echocardiographic evaluation of the Bjork-Shiley prosthetic valve. Circulation 50:52–57, 1974.
10. Friedewald VE, Jr., Futral JE, Diethrich EB, and Phillips B: In vitro prosthetic valve studies utilizing echocardiography (Abstr). *In* White D (Ed.): Ultrasound in Medicine. New York, Plenum Press, 1975, p. 103.
11. Morrow AG, Oldham HN, Elkins RC, and Braunwald E: Prosthetic replacement of the mitral valve. Circulation 35:962–979, 1967.
12. Levine FH, Copeland JG, and Morrow AG: Prosthetic replacement of the mitral valve. Circulation 47:518–526, 1973.
13. Willerson JT, Kastor JA, Dinsmore RE, Mundth E, Buckley MJ, Austen WG, and Saunders CA: Non-invasive assessment of prosthetic mitral paravalvular and intravalvular regurgitation. Br Heart J 34:561–568, 1972.
14. Pfeifer J, Goldschlager N, Sweatman T, Gerbode F, and Selzer A: Malfunction of mitral ball valve prosthesis due to thrombus. Am J Cardiol 29:95–99, 1972.

15. Ben-Zvi J, Hildner FJ, Chandraratna PA, and Samet P: Thrombosis on Bjork-Shiley aortic valve prosthesis. Am J Cardiol *34*:538–544, 1974.

16. Gold H, and Hertz L: Death caused by fracture of Beall mitral prosthesis. Am J Cardiol *34*:371–375, 1974.

17. Roberts WC, Levinson GE, and Morrow AG: Lethal ball variance in the Starr-Edwards prosthetic *mitral* valve. Arch Intern Med *126*:517–521, 1970.

18. Leachman RD, and Cokkinos DVP: Absence of opening click in dehiscence of mitral-valve prosthesis. N Engl J Med *281*:461–464, 1969.

19. Oliva PB, Johnson ML, Pomerantz M, and Levene A: Dysfunction of the Beall mitral prosthesis and its detection by cinefluoroscopy and echocardiography. Am J Cardiol *31*:393–396, 1973.

20. Hylen JC: Mechanical malfunction and thrombosis of prosthetic heart valves. Am J Cardiol *30*:396–404, 1972.

21. Hylen JC: Durability of prosthetic heart valves (Editorial). Am Heart J *81*:299–303, 1971.

22. Horsley HT, Rappoport WJ, Vigoda PS, and Vogel JHK:Fatal malfunction of Edwards low-profile mitral valves. Circulation (Suppl II) *41,42*:39–42, 1970.

23. Hodam R, Starr A, Raible D, and Griswold H: Totally cloth-covered prosthesis: A review of two years' clinical experience. Circulation (Suppl II) *41,42*:33–38, 1970.

24. Belenkie I, Carr M, Schlant RC, Nutter DO, and Symbas PN: Malfunction of a Cutter-Smeloff mitral ball valve prosthesis: Diagnosis by phonocardiography and echocardiography. Am Heart J *86*:399–403, 1973.

25. Roberts WC, Fishbein MC, and Golden A: Cardiac pathology after valve replacement by disc prosthesis. Am J Cardiol *35*:740–760, 1975.

26. Barnhorst DA, Oxman HA, Connolly DC, Pluth JR, Danielson GK, Wallace RB, and McGoon DC: Long-term follow-up of isolated replacement of the aortic or mitral valve with the Starr-Edwards prosthesis. Am J Cardiol *35*:228–233, 1975.

27. Craige E, Hutchin P, and Sutton R: Impaired function of cloth-covered Starr-Edwards mitral valve prosthesis. Circulation *41*:141–148, 1970.

28. Johnson ML: Echocardiographic evaluation of prosthetic heart valves. *In* Gramiak R, and Waag RC (Eds.): Cardiac Ultrasound. St. Louis, The C. V. Mosby Company, 1975, pp. 149–184.

29. Hamby RI, Lee RL, Aaitablian A, Wisloff BG, and Hartstein ML: Cinefluorographic study of the aortic ball-cage prosthetic valve. Am J Cardiol *34*:276–283, 1974.

30. Bjork VO, and Olin CA: A hydrodynamic comparison between the new tilting disc aortic valve prosthesis (Bjork-Shiley) and the corresponding prostheses of Starr-Edwards, Kay-Shiley, Smelloff-Cutter and Wada-Cutter in the pulse duplicator. Scand J Thorac Cardiovasc Surg *4*:31, 1970.

31. Burgraff GW, and Craige E: Echocardiographic studies of left ventricular wall motion and dimensions after valvular heart surgery. Am J Cardiol *35*:473–480, 1975.

32. Yoshikawa J, Owaki T, Kato H, Tanaka K: Abnormal motion of interventricular septum of patients with prosthetic valve. *In* White D (Ed.): Ultrasound in Medicine. New York, Plenum Press, 1975, p. 1.

33. Nanda NC, Gramiak R, Shah PM, DeWeese JA, and Mahoney EB: Echocardiographic assessment of left ventricular outflow width in the selection of mitral valve prosthesis. Circulation *48*:1208–1213, 1973.

34. Nanda NC, Gramiak R, Shah PM, and DeWeese JA: Mitral commissurotomy versus replacement: Preoperative evaluation by echocardiography. Circulation *51*:263–267, 1975.

35. Quattlebaum FW, Kalke B, Edwards TE, et al.: Obstruction of the aorta by prosthetic aortic valve. J Thorac Cardiovasc Surg *55*:231–237, 1968.

36. Najafi H, and DeWall RA: Fatal obstruction of the aortic root by Starr-Edwards aortic ball valve prosthesis. J Thorac Cardiovasc Surg *51*:180–184, 1966.

37. Najafi H, Ostermiller WE, Javid H, et al.: Narrow aortic root complicating aortic valve replacement. Arch Surg *99*:690–694, 1969.

38. Johnson ML, Holmes JH, Spangler RD, and Paton BC: Usefulness of echocardiography in patients undergoing mitral valve surgery. J Thorac Cardiovasc Surg *64*:922–934, 1972.

39. Effert S: Pre- and postoperative evaluation of mitral stenosis by ultrasound. Am J Cardiol *19*:59–65, 1967.

40. Silver W, Rodriguez-Torres R, and Newfeld E: The echocardiogram in a case of mitral stenosis before and after surgery. Am Heart J *78*:811–815, 1969.

41. Mary DAS, Pakrashi BC, Wooler GH, and Ionescu MI: Study with reflected ultrasound of patients with mitral valve repair. Br Heart J *35*:480–487, 1973.

42. Mary DAS, Pakrashi BC, Catchpole RW, and Ionescu MJ: Echocardiographic studies of stented fascia lata grafts in the mitral position. Circulation *49*:237–245, 1974.

43. Ratshin RA, Karp RB, Kirklin JW, Kouchoukos NT, and Pacifico AD: Post-operative evaluation of aortic valve homografts using echocardiography (Abstr). Circulation (Suppl IV) *48*:206, 1973.

APPENDICES

The normal values presented here have been compiled from selected reports. Because such determinations depend on the techniques used in both recording and measuring cardiac structures, the source of each value is given. Thus the reader may make reference to the original reports in which the values are presented in the context of individual investigations.

Normal Echocardiographic Values in Adults

THE MITRAL VALVE

	RANGE	NUMBER OF SUBJECTS	REFERENCE
Mean EF Slope (mm/sec)			
103.0 ± 20.0	75.0–140.0	10	1
>80	—	—	2
—	70.0–150.0	50	3
85.0 ± 5.0	60.0–110.0	9	4
124.0 ± 29.0	—	15	5
Mean Opening Amplitude (mm)			
>20 mm	—	—	2
—	22.0–30.0	50	3
Mean Septal–Mitral Valve Distance (mm) at Onset of Ventricular Systole			
34.6	—	22	6
35.0	—	30	7
29.0	20.0–38.0	50	8
Mean Mitral Valve–Posterior Wall Distance (mm)			
9.8	—	—	6
Q_{ECG} Interval to Mitral Opening (Q-M) (sec)			
0.06 ± 0.003	—	14	9

THE AORTIC VALVE AND AORTIC ROOT

	RANGE	NUMBER OF SUBJECTS	REFERENCE
Aortic Root Dimension (cm)			
2.6 ± 0.3	—	23	13
—	2.7–3.5	20	31
3.27 ± 0.45	2.1–4.4	50	32
3.37 ± 0.4 (end-diastole)	—	42	33
3.50 ± 0.4 (end-systole)	—	44	33
Aortic Valve Leaflet Separation (cm)			
—	1.7–2.5	—	34
Aortic Valve Closure to A_2 (msec)			
12.0 ± 5.0	5.0–25.0	54	35
Aortic Root Systolic Amplitude of Motion (mm)			
10.4 ± 5.8	—	45	33
Aortic Root Wall Thickness (mm)			
5.7 ± 1.2	—	45	33

THE LEFT ATRIUM

	RANGE	NUMBER OF SUBJECTS	REFERENCE
Internal Dimension (cm)			
2.6 ± 0.6	—	23	13
3.23 ± 0.44	2.3–4.4	50	32
3.1 ± 0.5	1.8–4.0	21	42
2.9	1.9–4.0	72	11
Internal Dimension Index (cm/BSA^2)			
—	1.2–2.0	21	42
Ratio of Left Atrium to Aortic Root Dimension			
—	0.87–1.11	50	32

THE INTERVENTRICULAR SEPTUM

	RANGE	NUMBER OF SUBJECTS	REFERENCE
End-diastolic Thickness (cm)			
0.81 ± 0.04	—	16	14
0.99 ± 0.02	0.8–1.28	29	28
1.0	—	30	7
0.97 ± 0.06	0.8–0.10	16	16
1.0 ± 0.2	—	15	5
0.72 ± 0.07	—	25	29
End-systolic Thickness (cm)			
1.39 ± 0.06	—	16	14
1.42 ± 0.04	1.12–1.84	29	28
Percent Systolic Thickening			
75.9 ± 8.8	—	16	14
44.0 ± 2.1	30–64	29	28
Systolic Velocity (mm/sec)			
37.0 ± 2.3	—	16	14
Normalized Septal Velocity (sec^{-1})			
0.84 ± 0.06	—	16	14
0.61 ± 0.02	0.38–0.85	19	22
Amplitude of Left Septal Systolic Motion (mm)			
7.1 ± 0.3	5.0–10.0	29	28
5.0	3.0–8.0	10	26
4.2 ± 2.2	—	20	17
6.3 ± 1.7	3.0–8.0	17	27
Ratio of Septal to Posterior Wall Thickness			
1.03 ± 0.02	—	23	30
1.03 ± 0.07	0.9–1.1	16	16
1.17 ± 0.14	—	15	5

THE POSTERIOR WALL OF THE LEFT VENTRICLE

	RANGE	NUMBER OF SUBJECTS	REFERENCE
End-diastolic Thickness (cm)			
0.95 ± 0.2	—	23	13
0.78 ± 0.04	—	16	14
0.91 ± 0.13	—	25	15
0.9	—	30	7
0.94 ± 0.09	0.8 –0.11	16	16
0.92 ± 0.2	—	15	5
0.90 ± 0.14	0.65–1.10	20	17
1.1 ± 0.2	0.8 –1.3	17	18
End-systolic Thickness (cm)			
1.41 ± 0.06	—	16	14
1.50 ± 0.29	—	25	15
1.48 ± 0.30	0.95–2.15	20	17
Percent Systolic Thickening			
84.8 ± 6.3	—	16	14
Maximal Epicardial Systolic Velocity (cm/sec)			
2.5	1.9 –3.0	9	19
Mean Epicardial Systolic Velocity (cm/sec)			
2.2	0.5 –3.0	9	19
Mean Endocardial Systolic Velocity (mm/sec)			
42.3 ± 2.0	—	16	14
47 ± 11	26.0–64.0	15	20
27 ± 5.8	15.0–36.0	25	21
41 ± 7	30.0–58.0	30	25
44.4 ± 1.5	36.5–61.5	19	22
42.0	30.0–44.0	9	19
Normalized Endocardial Systolic Velocity (sec^{-1})			
0.97 ± 0.06	—	—	—
0.76 ± 0.03	—	25	23
0.95 ± 0.02	0.80–1.14	19	22
Maximal Endocardial Systolic Velocity (mm/sec)			
55 ± 10	36.0–70.0	15	20
37.0	20.0–46.0	11	24
41 ± 11	22.0–67.0	25	21
62 ± 14	43.0–100.0	30	25
51.0	37.0–56.0	9	19
Systolic Endocardial Amplitude (mm)			
11.5 ± 1.7	—	20	17
4.0	2.5 –6.6	11	24
7.2 ± 1.8	3.6 –10.4	25	21
14.0 ± 3.0	10.0–20.0	30	25
12.0	9.0 –14.0	10	26
12.9 ± 2.0	8.0 –16.0	17	27
Maximal Endocardial Diastolic Velocity (mm/sec)			
180 ± 30.0	130.0–240.0	30	25
Mean Endocardial Diastolic Velocity (mm/sec)			
94.0 ± 17.0	70.0–130.0	30	25

THE CHAMBER OF THE LEFT VENTRICLE

	RANGE	NUMBER OF SUBJECTS	REFERENCE
End-systolic Dimension (cm)			
2.7 ± 0.1	—	16	14
3.8 ± 0.36	—	10	43
2.86 ± 0.25	—	25	15
3.16 ± 0.13	—	10	44
3.4	—	30	7
End-diastolic Dimension (cm)			
4.5 ± 0.4	—	23	13
4.5 ± 0.2	—	16	14
5.0 ± 4.1	—	10	43
4.43 ± 0.29	3.8–5.0	25	15
4.81 ± 0.16	—	10	44
4.67 ± 0.10	3.9–5.4	19	22
—	3.0–5.3	—	2
5.0	—	30	7
4.6 ± 0.1	—	25	45
4.40 ± 0.28	—	20	17
4.5 ± 0.5	3.5–5.3	26	10
4.6	3.5–5.6	73	11
End-systolic Volume (ml)			
59.0 ± 17.0	—	10	43
40.1 ± 14.0	—	15	5
End-diastolic Volume (ml)			
92.6 ± 18.7	—	23	13
142.0 ± 24.0	—	10	43
125.4 ± 29.0	—	15	5
Ejection Fraction (%)			
62.2 ± 6.0	—	23	13
68.0 ± 8.0	—	15	20
59.0 ± 7.0	—	10	43
71.0 ± 2.0	—	10	44
74.3 ± 1.32	62.0–85.0	19	22
68.0 ± 6.0	—	15	5
Stroke Volume (ml)			
57.5 ± 12.9	—	23	13
83.0 ± 14.0	—	10	43
End-diastolic Dimension Index (cm/M^2)			
2.81 ± 0.29	2.2–3.31	17	27
Fractional Shortening (an index of V_{cf}) (%)			
33.5 ± 4.4	—	23	13
V_{cf} (circumferences/sec)			
1.24 ± 0.07	—	16	14
1.29 ± 0.23	0.84–1.83	15	20
0.92 ± 0.15	—	10	43
1.22 ± 0.05	0.91–1.89	25	23
1.10 ± 0.04	—	10	44
1.34 ± 0.16	1.03–1.62	15	46
1.26 ± 0.08	1.13–1.60	19	22
1.2 ± 0.02	—	25	45

THE RIGHT VENTRICLE

	RANGE	NUMBER OF SUBJECTS	REFERENCE
Internal Dimension (cm)			
1.5 ± 0.4	0.5–2.1	26	10
1.5	0.7–2.3	39	11
Internal Dimension Index (cm/M²)			
0.7	0.3–1.1	30	12

THE PULMONIC VALVE

	RANGE	NUMBER OF SUBJECTS	REFERENCE
"a" Wave Amplitude (mm)			
3.7 ± 1.2	2.0 –7.0	24	36
4.4 ± 0.46	3.0 –12.0	22	37
EF Slope (mm/sec)			
36.9 ± 25.4	6.0 –115.0	24	36
Amplitude of Opening (mm)			
13.9 ± 1.8	—	24	36
8.68 ± 0.92	—	22	37
RPEP/RVET			
0.24	0.16–0.30	45	38
Opening Slope (mm/sec)			
211.0 ± 12.7	100–300	22	37
Pulmonic Closure to P_2 Interval (msec)			
60.0 ± 13	30–75.0	14	35

THE TRICUSPID VALVE

	RANGE	NUMBER OF SUBJECTS	REFERENCE
Q_{ECG}-Tricuspid Opening (Q_{ECG}-T_1) (msec)			
90 ± 2	—	14	9
Mitral-Tricuspid Closure Interval (McTc) (msec)			
11.0 ± 8.0	0–30.0	11	39
20.0 ± 14.0	−5.0–50.0	40	40
EF Slope (mm/sec)			
—	60.0–125.0	31	41

Appendix B

Normal Echocardiographic Values in Neonates

THE MITRAL VALVE

	RANGE	NUMBER OF SUBJECTS	WEIGHT RANGE (kg)	REFERENCE
EF Slope (mm/sec)				
53.0	36.0–80.0	50	—	47
80 ± 1	60.0–130.0	200	—	49
Excursion (cm)				
1.0	0.6 –1.2	50	—	47
1.1	0.65–1.24	50	—	48
0.81 ± 0.01	0.6 –1.2	200	—	49
0.98 ± 0.13	0.85–1.11	46	2.27–2.70	50
1.02 ± 0.13	0.89–1.15	57	2.73–3.15	50
1.06 ± 0.13	0.93–1.19	50	3.18–3.61	50
1.10 ± 0.13	0.97–1.23	50	3.64–4.06	50
1.14 ± 0.13	1.01–1.27	37	4.09–4.51	50

THE AORTIC VALVE AND AORTIC ROOT

	RANGE	NUMBER OF SUBJECTS	WEIGHT RANGE (kg)	REFERENCE
Dimension (cm)				
1.02	0.80–1.10	48	—	48
1.00 ± 0.006	0.81–1.20	200	—	49
1.03 ± 0.10	0.93–1.13	46	2.27–2.70	50
1.07 ± 0.10	0.97–1.17	57	2.73–3.15	50
1.12 ± 0.10	1.02–1.22	50	3.18–3.61	50
1.17 ± 0.10	1.07–1.27	50	3.64–4.06	50
1.29 ± 0.10	1.11–1.31	37	4.09–4.51	50
Aortic Valve Leaflet Separation (mm)				
4.7 ± 0.7	4.0–5.4	46	2.27–2.70	50
5.0 ± 0.7	4.3–5.7	57	2.73–3.15	50
5.2 ± 0.7	4.5–5.9	50	3.18–3.61	50
5.5 ± 0.7	4.8–6.2	50	3.64–4.06	50
5.8 ± 0.7	5.1–6.5	37	4.09–4.51	50

THE LEFT ATRIUM

	RANGE	NUMBER OF SUBJECTS	WEIGHT RANGE (kg)	REFERENCE
Dimension (cm)				
0.9	0.6 –1.3	50	–	47
0.64	0.4 –1.05	50	1.9 –4.3	48
0.7 ± 0.01	0.5 –1.0	200	–	49
0.87 ± 0.18	0.68–1.05	46	2.27–2.70	50
0.93 ± 0.18	0.74–1.11	57	2.73–3.15	50
0.99 ± 0.18	0.80–1.17	50	3.18–3.61	50
1.05 ± 0.18	0.86–1.23	50	3.64–4.06	50
1.11 ± 0.18	0.92–1.29	37	4.09–4.51	50

THE INTERVENTRICULAR SEPTUM

	RANGE	NUMBER OF SUBJECTS	WEIGHT RANGE (kg)	REFERENCE
End-diastolic Thickness (mm)				
2.7 ± 0.04	1.8–4.0	200	–	49
2.7 ± 0.6	2.1–3.3	46	2.27–2.70	50
3.0 ± 0.6	2.4–3.6	57	2.73–3.15	50
3.2 ± 0.6	2.6–3.8	50	3.18–3.61	50
3.5 ± 0.6	2.9–4.1	50	3.64–4.06	50
3.7 ± 0.6	3.1–4.3	37	4.09–4.51	50

THE POSTERIOR WALL OF THE LEFT VENTRICLE

	RANGE	NUMBER OF SUBJECTS	WEIGHT RANGE (kg)	REFERENCE
End-systolic Thickness (mm)				
4.3 ± 0.1	2.5–6.0	200	–	49
End-diastolic Thickness (mm)				
2.6 ± 0.1	1.6–3.7	200	–	49
2.7 ± 0.7	2.0–3.4	46	2.27–2.70	50
3.0 ± 0.7	2.3–3.7	57	2.73–3.15	50
3.2 ± 0.7	2.5–3.9	50	3.18–3.61	50
3.5 ± 0.7	2.8–4.2	50	3.64–4.06	50
3.7 ± 0.7	3.0–4.4	37	4.09–4.51	50

THE CHAMBER OF THE LEFT VENTRICLE

	RANGE	NUMBER OF SUBJECTS	WEIGHT RANGE (kg)	REFERENCE
End-diastolic Dimension (cm)				
1.6	1.2 –2.0	50	—	47
1.6	1.2 –2.0	36	—	48
1.87 ± 0.03	1.2 –2.3	200	—	49
1.89 ± 0.28	1.61–2.17	46	2.27–2.70	50
1.93 ± 0.28	1.65–2.21	57	2.73–3.15	50
1.98 ± 0.28	1.70–2.26	50	3.18–3.61	50
2.03 ± 0.28	1.75–2.31	50	3.64–4.06	50
2.08 ± 0.28	1.80–2.36	37	4.09–4.51	50
End-systolic Dimension (cm)				
1.33 ± 0.03	0.8 –1.86	200	—	49
Outflow Tract (cm)				
1.0	0.7 –1.2	50	—	47
V_{CF} (circumferences/sec)				
1.51 ± 0.04	0.92–2.2	72	—	51

THE RIGHT VENTRICLE

	RANGE	NUMBER OF SUBJECTS	WEIGHT RANGE (kg)	REFERENCE
End-diastolic Internal Dimension (cm)				
1.3	1.0 –1.7	50	—	47
1.38	1.0 –1.75	50	—	48
1.25 ± 0.21	1.04–1.46	46	2.27–2.70	50
1.31 ± 0.21	1.10–1.52	57	2.73–3.15	50
1.37 ± 0.21	1.16–1.58	50	3.18–3.61	50
1.44 ± 0.21	1.23–1.65	50	3.64–4.06	50
1.50 ± 0.21	1.29–1.71	37	4.09–4.51	50

THE PULMONARY ARTERY

	RANGE	NUMBER OF SUBJECTS	REFERENCE
Dimension (cm)			
1.11	0.92–1.28	29	48
1.11 ± 0.02	0.94–1.30	200	49

THE TRICUSPID VALVE

	RANGE	NUMBER OF SUBJECTS	WEIGHT RANGE (kg)	REFERENCE
Diastolic Slope (mm/sec)				
43.0	34.0–56.0	50	—	47
93 ± 2	60.0–116.0	200	—	49
Excursion (cm)				
1.1	0.8 –1.4	50	—	47
1.1	0.8 –1.3	50	—	48
0.93 ± 0.02	0.7 –1.4	200	—	49
1.04 ± 0.16	0.88–1.20	46	2.27–2.70	50
1.08 ± 0.16	0.92–1.24	57	2.73–3.15	50
1.13 ± 0.16	0.97–1.29	50	3.18–3.61	50
1.17 ± 0.16	1.01–1.33	50	3.64–4.06	50
1.22 ± 0.16	1.06–1.38	37	3.09–4.51	50

Normal Echocardiographic Values in Children

AORTIC ROOT

BSA (M²)	MEAN (cm)	RANGE	NUMBER OF SUBJECTS	REFERENCE
0.5 or less	1.2	0.7–1.5	24	11
0.6–1.0	1.8	1.4–2.2	39	11
1.1–1.5	2.2	1.7–2.7	29	11
over 1.5	2.4	2.0–2.8	11	11

AORTIC VALVE OPENING

BSA (M²)	MEAN (cm)	RANGE	NUMBER OF SUBJECTS	REFERENCE
0.5 or less	0.8	0.5–1.0	24	11
0.6–1.0	1.3	0.9–1.6	39	11
1.1–1.5	1.6	1.3–1.9	29	11
over 1.5	1.8	1.5–2.0	11	11

LEFT VENTRICULAR INTERNAL DIMENSION

BSA (M²)	MEAN (cm)	RANGE	NUMBER OF SUBJECTS	REFERENCE
0.5 or less	2.4	1.3–3.2	24	11
0.6–1.0	3.4	2.4–4.2	39	11
1.1–1.5	4.0	3.3–4.7	29	11
over 1.5	4.7	4.2–5.2	11	11

LEFT VENTRICULAR AND INTERVENTRICULAR SEPTAL WALL THICKNESS

BSA (M²)	MEAN (cm)	RANGE	NUMBER OF SUBJECTS	REFERENCE
0.5 or less	0.5	0.4–0.6	24	11
0.6–1.0	0.6	0.5–0.7	39	11
1.1–1.5	0.7	0.6–0.8	29	11
over 1.5	0.8	0.7–0.8	11	11

LEFT ATRIAL DIMENSION

BSA (M²)	MEAN (cm)	RANGE	NUMBER OF SUBJECTS	REFERENCE
0.5 or less	1.7	0.7–2.4	24	11
0.6–1.0	2.1	1.8–2.8	39	11
1.1–1.5	2.4	2.0–3.0	29	11
over 1.5	2.8	2.1–3.7	11	11

THE RIGHT VENTRICLE

BSA (M²)	MEAN (cm)	RANGE	NUMBER OF SUBJECTS	REFERENCE
Internal Dimension				
0.5 or less	0.8	0.3–1.3	24	11
0.6–1.0	1.0	0.4–1.8	39	11
1.1–1.5	1.2	0.7–1.7	29	11
over 1.5	1.3	0.8–1.7	11	11
Internal Dimension Index (cm/M²)				
< 1.0	1.3	0.5–2.0	28	52
≥ 1.0	0.8	0.5–1.1		

Appendix References

1. DeMaria AN, Miller RR, Amsterdam EA, Markson W, and Mason DT: Mitral valve early diastolic closing velocity in the echocardiogram: Relation to sequential diastolic flow and ventricular compliance. Am J Cardiol, 37:693–700, 1976.
2. Goodman DJ, Harrison DC, and Popp RL: Echocardiographic features of primary pulmonary hypertension. Am J Cardiol, 33:438–443, 1974.
3. Segal BL, Likoff W, and Kingsley B: Echocardiography: Clinical application in mitral regurgitation. Am J Cardiol, 19:50–58, 1967.
4. Quinones MA, Gaasch WH, Waisser E, and Alexander JK: Reduction in the rate of diastolic descent of the mitral valve echogram in patients with altered left ventricular diastolic pressure-volume relations. Circulation, 49:246–254, 1974.
5. Abbasi AS, MacAlpin RN, Eber LM, and Pearce ML: Echocardiographic diagnosis of idiopathic hypertrophic cardiomyopathy without outflow obstruction. Circulation, 46:897–904, 1972.
6. Henry WL, Griffith JM, and Epstein SE: Mechanism of left ventricular outflow obstruction in patients with obstructive asymmetric septal hypertrophy (idiopathic hypertrophic subaortic stenosis). Am J Cardiol, 35:337–345, 1975.
7. Strunk BL, Guss SB, Hicks RE, and Kotler MN: Echocardiographic recognition of the mitral valve–posterior aortic wall relationship. Circulation, 51:594–598, 1975.
8. Joyner CR: Ultrasound in the Diagnosis of Cardiovascular-Pulmonary Disease. Chicago, Year Book Medical Publishers, 1974.
9. Waider W, and Craige E: First heart sound and ejection sounds. Am J Cardiol, 35:346–356, 1975.
10. Popp RL, Wolfe SB, Hirata T, and Feigenbaum H: Estimation of right and left ventricular size by ultrasound: A study of the echoes from the interventricular septum. Am J Cardiol, 24:523–530, 1969.
11. Feigenbaum H: Echocardiography. Philadelphia, Lea & Febiger, 1972.
12. Diamond MA, Dillon JC, Haine CL, Chang S, and Feigenbaum H: Echocardiographic features of atrial septal defect. Circulation, 43:129–135, 1971.
13. McDonald IG: Echocardiographic assessment of left ventricular function in aortic valve disease. Circulation, 53:860–864, 1976.
14. Cohen MV, Cooperman LB, and Rosenblum R: Regional myocardial function in idiopathic subaortic stenosis: An echocardiographic study. Circulation, 52:842–847, 1975.
15. McDonald IG, and Hobson ER: A comparison of the relative value of noninvasive techniques — echocardiography, systolic time intervals, and apexcardiography in the diagnosis of primary myocardial disease. Am Heart J, 88:454–462, 1974.
16. Henry WL, Clark CE, and Epstein SE: Asymmetric septal hypertrophy: Echocardiographic identification of the pathognomonic anatomic abnormality of IHSS. Circulation, 47:225–233, 1973.
17. McDonald IG, Feigenbaum H, and Chang S: Analysis of left ventricular wall motion by reflected ultrasound: Application to assessment of myocardial function. Circulation, 46:14–25, 1972.
18. Feigenbaum H, Popp RL, Chip JN, and Haine CL: Left ventricular wall thickness measured by ultrasound. Arch Intern Med, 121:391–395, 1968.
19. Ludbrook P, Karliner JS, London A, Peterson KL, Leopold GR, and O'Rourke RA: Posterior wall velocity: An unreliable index of total left ventricular performance in patients with coronary artery disease. Am J Cardiol, 33:475–482, 1974.
20. Cooper RH, O'Rourke RA, Karliner JS, Peterson KL, and Leopold GR: Comparison of ultrasound and cineangiographic measurements of the mean rate of circumferential fiber shortening. Circulation, 46:914–923, 1972.
21. Kraunz RF, and Kennedy JW: Ultrasonic determination of left ventricular wall motion in normal man: Studies at rest and after exercise. Am Heart J, 79:36–43, 1970.
22. Quinones MA, Gaasch WH, and Alexander JK: Echocardiographic assessment of left ventricular function: With special reference to normalized velocities. Circulation, 50:42–51, 1974.

23. Hirshleifer J, Crawford M, O'Rourke RA, and Karliner JS: Influence of acute alterations in heart rate and systemic arterial pressure on echocardiographic measures of left ventricular performance in normal human subjects. Circulation, 52:835–841, 1975.

24. Smithen CS, Wharton CFP, and Sowton E: Independent effects of heart rate and exercise on left ventricular wall movement measured by reflected ultrasound. Am J Cardiol, 30:43–47, 1972.

25. Fogelman AM, Abbasi AS, Pearce ML, and Kattus AA: Echocardiographic study of the abnormal motion of the posterior left ventricular wall during angina pectoris. Circulation, 46:905–913, 1972.

26. Jacobs JJ, Feigenbaum H, Corya BC, and Phillips JF: Detection of left ventricular asynergy by echocardiography. Circulation, 48:263–271, 1973.

27. Corya BC, Feigenbaum H, Rasmussen S, and Black MJ: Echocardiographic features of congestive cardiomyopathy compared with normal subjects and patients with coronary artery disease. Circulation, 49:1153–1159, 1974.

28. Rossen RM, Goodman DJ, Ingham RE, and Popp RL: Ventricular systolic septal thickening and excursion in idiopathic hypertrophic subaortic stenosis. N Engl J Med, 291:1317–1319, 1974.

29. Sawaya J, Longo MR, and Schlant RC: Echocardiographic interventricular septal wall motion and thickness: A study in health and disease. Am Heart J, 87:681–688, 1974.

30. Clark CE, Henry WL, and Epstein SE: Familial prevalence and genetic transmission of idiopathic hypertrophic subaortic stenosis. N Engl J Med, 289:709–714, 1973.

31. Hernberg J, Weiss B, and Keegan A: The ultrasonic recording of aortic valve motion. Radiology, 94:361–368, 1970.

32. Brown OR, Harrison DC, and Popp RL: An improved method for echographic detection of left atrial enlargement. Circulation, 50:58–64, 1974.

33. Gramiak R, and Shah PM: Echocardiography of the normal and diseased aortic valve. Radiology, 96:1–8, 1970.

34. Gramiak R, and Waag RC (Eds): Cardiac Ultrasound. St. Louis, The C. V. Mosby Co., 1975, p. 76.

35. Chandraratna PAN, Lopez JM, and Cohen LS: Echocardiographic observations on the mechanism of production of the second heart sound. Circulation, 51:292–296, 1975.

36. Weyman AE, Dillon JC, Feigenbaum H, and Chang S: Echocardiographic patterns of pulmonic valve motion with pulmonary hypertension. Circulation, 50:905–910, 1974.

37. Nanda NC, Gramiak R, Robinson TI, and Shah PM: Echocardiographic evaluation of pulmonary hypertension. Circulation, 50:575–581, 1974.

38. Hirschfeld S, Meyer R, Schwartz DC, Korfhagen J, and Kaplan S: The echocardiographic assessment of pulmonary artery pressure and pulmonary vascular resistance. Circulation, 52:642–650, 1975.

39. Farooki, ZQ, Henry JG, and Green EW: Echocardiographic spectrum of Ebstein's anomaly of the tricuspid valve. Circulation, 51:63–68, 1976.

40. Milner S, Meyer RA, Venables AW, Korfhagen J, and Kaplan S: Mitral and tricuspid valve closure in congenital heart disease. Circulation, 53:513–518, 1976.

41. Joyner CR, Hey EB, Johnson J, and Reid JM: Reflected ultrasound in the diagnosis of tricuspid stenosis. Am J Cardiol, 19:66–73, 1967.

42. Hirata T, Wolfe SB, Popp RL, Helmen CH, and Feigenbaum H: Estimation of left atrial size using ultrasound. Am Heart J, 78:43–52, 1969.

43. Fortuin NJ, Hood WP, Jr., and Craige E: Evaluation of left ventricular function by echocardiography. Circulation, 46:26–34, 1972.

44. Delgado CE, Fortuin NJ, and Ross RS: Acute effects of low doses of alcohol on left ventricular function by echocardiography. Circulation, 51:535–540, 1975.

45. Stack RS, Lee CC, Reddy BP, Taylor ML, and Weissler AM: Left ventricular performance in coronary artery disease evaluated with systolic time intervals and echocardiography. Am J Cardiol, 37:331–339, 1976.

46. Bennett DH, Evans DW, and Raj MVJ: Echocardiographic left ventricular dimensions in pressure and volume overload: Their use in assessing aortic stenosis. Br Heart J, 37:971–977, 1975.

47. Meyer RA, and Kaplan S: Echocardiography in the diagnosis of hypoplasia of the left or right ventricles in the neonate. Circulation, 46:55–64, 1972.

48. Godman MJ, Tham P, and Kidd BS: Echocardiography in the evaluation of the cyanotic newborn infant. Br Heart J, 36:154–166, 1974.

49. Hagan AD, Deely WJ, Sahn D, and Friedman WF: Echocardiographic criteria for normal newborn infants. Circulation, 48:1221–1226, 1973.

50. Solinger R, Elbl F, and Minhas K: Echocardiography in the normal neonate. Circulation, 47:108–118, 1973.

51. Sahn DJ, Deely WJ, Hagan AD, and Friedman WF: Echocardiographic assessment of left ventricular performance in normal newborns. Circulation, 49:232–236, 1974.

52. Tajik AJ, Gau GT, Ritter DG, and Schattenberg TT: Echocardiographic pattern of right ventricular diastolic volume overload in children. Circulation, 46:36–43, 1972.

Index